SETON HALL UNIVERSITY

S0-BIG-532

Public Health and Aging

An Introduction to Maximizing Function and Well-Being

Steven M. Albert, Ph.D., M.Sc., is Associate Professor of Clinical Sociomedical Science in the Department of Sociomedical Sciences (Mailman School of Public Health) and the Gertrude H. Sergievsky Center and Department of Neurology (College of Physicians and Surgeons), Columbia University. He is trained as an anthropologist and epidemiologist. His research centers on the assessment of health outcomes in aging and chronic disease (patient function, health service use, medical care costs, quality of life, clinical decision making).

Dr. Albert has recently received funding from the National Institutes of Health to investigate mental health and decision making in people living with ALS, and to investigate the cognitive and physical basis of independence in older people with disabilities. He has also been awarded funding from the Centers for Disease Control to examine attitudes toward health promotion in culturally insular New York City communities. He is the author (with Rebecca Logsdon) of the volume, *Assessing Quality of Life in Alzheimer's Disease* (New York: Springer Publishing Co., 2000).

Dr. Albert teaches courses on public health and aging, the epidemiology of aging, and measurement of quality of life in health care. He has consulted with hospitals, nursing homes, unions, foundations, and community organizations in efforts to improve the lives of staff and family caregivers to people with chronic disease.

Public Health and Aging

An Introduction to Maximizing Function and Well-Being

Steven M. Albert, PhD, MSc

SETON HALL UNIVERSITY
UNIVERSITY LIBRARIES
SO. ORANGE, NJ 07079-2671

 Springer Publishing Company

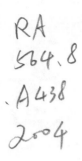

RA
564.8
.A438
2004

Copyright © 2004 Springer Publishing Company, Inc.

All rights reserved

No part of this publication may be reproduced, stored in a retrieval system, or transmitted in any form or by any means, electronic, mechanical, photocopying, recording, or otherwise, without the prior permission of Springer Publishing Company, Inc.

Springer Publishing Company, Inc.
536 Broadway
New York, NY 10012-3955

Acquisitions Editor: Sheri W. Sussman
Production Editor: Jeanne Libby
Cover design by Joanne Honigman

03 04 05 06 07 / 5 4 3 2 1

Library of Congress Cataloging-in-Publication Data

Albert, Steven M. (Steven Mark), 1956–
    Public health and aging : an introduction to maximizing function and well being / Steven M. Albert
        p. ; cm.
    Includes bibliographical references and index.
    ISBN 0-8261-2134-9
    1. Community health services for the aged.   2. Preventive health services for the aged.   3. Aged—Medical care.   4. Public health.   I Title.

    RA564.8.A438 2004
    362.198'97—dc22

                                                        2003057353

Printed in the United States of America by Integrated Book Technology.

Contents

9 Emerging Applications of the Aging and Public Health Paradigm **215**

List of Figures

List of Tables

Preface

My alumni magazine, which appears six times a year, recently reported 140 deaths. Sixty of the deaths were people who graduated from college in the 1920s. Thirty were graduates from the 1930s, 10 from the 1940s, 20 from the 1950s, and the remainder, 20, from between 1960 and 1990. In this very biased sample of deaths, the oldest group, people aged 90 to 100 in 2002, represented the largest proportion of deaths. The proportion of deaths sharply declined among more recent graduates, who, of course, were younger in 2002. There is the apparently exceptional case of graduates from the 1940s, who seem to have a lower death rate than expected. But this is entirely explained by the smaller pool of people in this college cohort, who attended college during a decade dominated by world war.

Thus, a look at a college alumni magazine (in this case, Cornell University) can reveal much about age, risk of death, and the influence of historical factors. The same issue reports on the oldest living graduate of the college, a man from the class of 1916, aged 108 in 2002. This long-time gardening columnist, though he does reside in an assisted living facility, apparently is not demented. Four generations of descendants attended his birthday party, which he remarked was "just a lot of fuss over me." This man's age puts him in a very select group, though the 2000 U.S. Census reports 1400 people over age 110 out of some 285,000,000.

If we turn to the back of the magazine to read what alumni of different ages report, we find further information relevant to aging and public health. The 1995 graduate (age 30 or so) exhorts his classmates in this way: "May all your weddings be perfect, babies brilliant, exams easy, jobs fun, and friends true." The 1945 graduate (age 77 or so) makes this report: "Nothing to do and not enough time to do it." The 1938 graduate (age 84 or so) reports, "I had angina in April, pacemaker in July, angioplasty in August. Otherwise fine." And the 1934 graduate reports: "My theme song now at 94 is 'Don't get around much any more!'"

These excerpts show that age is a dominating factor in health, as it is in so many social, psychological, and economic spheres. It is therefore a public health issue. The field of public health and aging, standing between clinical geriatrics and the demography and epidemiology of aging, asks how age matters for the experience of health and well-being, how care should be delivered to people who have lived long lives but who may still benefit from interventional medicine, what expectations for health and function are reasonable in the setting of physical and cognitive senescence, and finally, what about the first 50 years of life makes life better or worse when we enter the second 50 years.

Public health and aging is a developing field that has so far lacked a unified treatment or single framework. This book attempts to provide such a framework. Reasons for the lack of interest in aging by the public health community have been described elsewhere (Albert, Im, & Raveis 2002; CDC, 2003), but most likely have to do with a historical focus on infectious rather than chronic disease, and on maternal and child health rather than health in late life. Until recently there were also relatively few elderly, certainly not the 15–20% we can expect to see in most of the developed nations by 2050. But population pressures (such as declining fertility, greater life expectancy, and a convergence in age structure leading to similar proportions of people under age 15 and over age 65) now force the issue. How can we ensure a healthy old age? Why are some segments of society able to enter old age with greater physical and cognitive resources (setting aside obvious differences in economic status)? To what extent can physical and cognitive disability be prevented? To what extent can they be remediated once older people meet criteria for frailty or dementia? Does it make sense to speak of the prevention of frailty or other forms of primary prevention in late life?

This book examines these issues, provides tools for their investigation, and offers a first synthesis of a burgeoning literature in geriatrics, gerontology, occupational therapy, epidemiology, demography, neuropsychology, rehabilitation medicine, social work, and public policy. It is not encyclopedic or complete. Rather, it is a synthesis of what I see as the most productive measures, samples, studies, and clinical trials that address the question of age, health, and healthy old age.

No doubt readers will find something missing from this account, and certainly something in need of more extensive treatment. Given that this book is an introduction to a field, not everything can be covered, and certainly not at an equal level or depth. I have adopted the following strategy. In chapter 1, I identify key concepts and tools that define the field of public health and aging, such as primary prevention in late life, the life span view of health, the nature of age, "successful aging" and frailty, and cognitive and physical reserve. Chapter 2 introduces basic tools for this inquiry: cohort analysis, the life table, age-sex pyramids, risk stratification. Chapter 3 provides an overview of population processes related to age and historical changes in the structure of populations. Chapter 4 tackles age and mortality. Later chapters assess types of morbidity linked to underlying processes, such as declines in physical function and disability (chapter 5), changes in cognitive function and dementia (chapter 6), and the relationship between affective function and suffering, neglect, and isolation (chapter 7). A chapter on quality of life assessment tries to bring these approaches together in a unified model (chapter 8).

Chapter 9 is the most ambitious, as it tries to apply this emerging public health and aging paradigm to three central topics: preventing disability, promoting effective chronic disease management, and enhancing custodial care for the frailest, most vulnerable elders. In this chapter, I have made a point of reporting results from randomized clinical trials when possible, to show that rigorous clinical research is most likely to show what works and what does not, here as in other areas of research.

What is the basic goal of a public health approach to aging? It is to maximize function and well-being, as stated in the subtitle of this book. This is really the goal of all public health efforts, for all age groups; but it bears repeating in the case of older adults for a number of reasons. First, senescence is loss of function, and thus the focus on maximizing function implies working with a person's remaining strengths, using assistive technologies when possible, and making appropriate environmental modifications to reduce disability in the setting of senescent processes. Second, the goal of maximizing function and well-being implies concern for the person in an environment, rather than a focus on discrete physiological processes or clinical diagnoses. This approach is critical for older people. Geriatric syndromes cross-cut discrete disease entities, and good management of an older person's medical status requires attention to a variety of medical conditions and medications, as well as living situation, support networks, personal care preferences, and many other factors. Early on, Lawton (1969) suggested that care plans for older people be guided by function and behavior, rather than diagnoses. This advice continues to guide the best geriatric care (Gillick, 1994).

When describing his *Tractatus,* Wittgenstein spoke of two books: the one he had written, and the one he did not write while writing his book. The latter "virtual" book contained all the topics he did not include and many abandoned lines of reasoning and evidence that might help explain what did, in fact, appear in the book. Something like this is at work here too. Many important topics do not appear in the chapters that follow. For example, about 10% of people with HIV are over age 50. This proportion will likely increase as highly active antiretroviral therapy allows people with HIV to age. How will these people fare as they take potent medication regimens for 10 or 20 years? Will they face an increased risk of dementia or disability, since many are entering later life with HIV-related impairments? This topic was easy to leave out: very little data are available. For similar reasons we have not included extended discussion of alternative or complementary medicine in older people, anti-aging therapies, use of telemedicine in geriatric care, the status of older adults in developing countries, or innovative housing or behavioral interventions for frail elders.

Other omissions reflect relative emphasis. We do not include a chapter on minority aging in the United States. However, variation in the aging experience linked to minority status is covered in chapters devoted to demography, mortality, risk of disability, and cognitive assessment. The same is true for family caregiving, preferences for end of life care, long-term care options, and patterns of health care utilization. While the topics do not receive treatment as separate chapters, all are covered in the book within the framework outlined above.

Finally, some topics were simply too far afield for a book devoted to public health and aging, as we have tried to define it in chapter 1. We do not cover economic issues and public policy relevant to aging. Similarly, we have set aside the topics of work, retirement, and leisure, as well as family relationships and social supports. These topics are covered well in research in social gerontology and public policy. Instead, we have tried to emphasize age, health, and healthy old age and to marshal public health tools that allow us to promote this kind of aging.

This book's design, scope, insights (if any), and faults are all my own. I take full responsibility for the product. However, a number of people were kind enough to read chapters, suggest literature, and push me forward in this effort. These include Ursula Springer, Victoria Raveis, Ashley Im Love, Jane Bear-Lehman, and Mohamud Nizamuddin. Shiro Horiuchi kindly allowed me to reproduce unpublished figures from his work on three centuries of changing death rates and mean ages at death. I thank Sheri Sussman and Springer Publishing Company for bearing with my inability to meet deadlines. My colleagues at the Gertrude H. Sergievsky Center, Department of Sociomedical Sciences, Department of Neurology, and MPH Program in Aging and Public Health at Columbia University were helpful friends and critics, as always. Chapters of this book were written in New York and Israel.

Most of all, I thank Robin, Eli, and Charna for tolerating me while writing. They were the biggest help.

New York, 2002–2003

1

Between Clinical Geriatrics and the Epidemiology of Aging— Defining Public Health and Aging

C linical geriatrics is a medical specialty that centers on the health of the older person. It stresses medical management of chronic disease, rehabilitation in the face of disabilities related to these conditions, and increasingly "prehabilitation" (Gill, Baker, et al., 2002) to delay the onset of disability due to disease and frailty. The epidemiology of aging, by contrast, examines the health of older people as a population. It tracks the incidence of disease, factors that increase the risk of disease in defined subsets of older people, and outcomes following diagnosis. Increasingly, it is linked to health services research, so that hospitalization, program participation, and medical care costs have been included as outcomes.

The two fields are complementary in the sense that benefits in geriatric care should be visible in the health of the population of older persons. Also, epidemiologic research offers a chance to identify risk factors or adverse events due to treatment that might not be visible in clinical practice, especially in the case of uncommon diseases or therapies.

Somewhere between the two lies the field of public health and aging. Until now this field has not been well defined. It draws on geriatric medicine to promote health outside the clinic and beyond the clinician-patient encounter. It draws on epidemiology but often focuses on selected subgroups of the elderly, such as other adults with disabilities. It stands between the two fields and concentrates specifically on such intermediate areas as health promotion in late life, chronic disease self-management, behavioral interventions that complement clinical care, the social context of custodial care, and development of quality indicators for particular kinds of aging experience, such as dementia care, nursing home residence, physical frailty, home care, and independence through use of assistive technologies.

How does the field of public health and aging differ from gerontology? Public health and aging overlaps with clinical and behavioral gerontology to the extent that the latter focus on health. However, it differs from the two in its explicit focus on primary and secondary prevention of frailty, disease, and disability in late life. The field of public health and aging seeks to use the tools of public health, clinical geriatrics, and epidemiology to delay the onset of disease. Thus, a reasonable *primary prevention goal* for the field would be postponement of a disease with a long latency period, such as Alzheimer's disease, to a point later in the life span, so that people might avoid the extensive period of disability associated with the disease and die older from other, more benign conditions. A reasonable *secondary prevention goal* would be an increase in the so-far limited armamentarium of screening technologies used to identify people at risk for cognitive and physical frailty, falling, sensory deficits, and the diseases common to late life. A logical extension of this effort would be a series of randomized controlled trials to assess the benefit of such technologies and the treatments they might imply.

More generally, a central goal for public health and aging is to identify aspects of health in the first 50 years of life that predispose people to live a healthy second 50 years. This life span approach is underdeveloped, and yet a multitude of evidence suggests that people enter the second 50 years with great differences in the reserves and resources likely to predict healthy aging. These differences include level of completed education, occupational exposures, bone mineral densities, proportion of lean muscle mass, strength, VO_2 max, memory, health behavior profile, social support, wealth, and much else. We really know very little about the way these factors predispose an individual to poor or healthy aging. Take, for example, grip strength. Grip strength in midlife predicts disability and mortality risk up to 25 years later (Rantanen, Guralnik, Foley, & Masaki, 1999). But midlife grip strength is also related to grip strength at points much earlier in the life span (Kuh et al. 2002).

Perhaps the most productive approach to public health and aging would be identification of the factors in the first half of the life span that affect health in old age. This in turn would allow investigation of the extent to which modification of these factors might change the face of old age. However, this investigation would require prospective studies of birth cohorts through the life span into old age, a long and so-far incomplete task. Even such long-term cohorts as the British Medical Research Council 1946 birth cohort have only reached the mid-fifties as of this writing (Kuh et al., 2002).

PUBLIC HEALTH AND SUCCESSFUL AGING

It is salutary to try to explain the functions of public health and aging to the audience for our efforts, the people who have experienced old age and who confront the risk of frailty and chronic disease. One case will speak for many. Hannah is a 92–year-old woman I met in Israel. She has lived on a kibbutz, a collective settlement, for over 50 years, a hard but supportive environment for the elderly that has been shown to confer important health advantages (Ginzburg-Walter, et al., 2002). At age 92, she was quite frail and required 24–hour personal care assistance, which was provided by the kibbutz. She used a walker for indoor mobility, left her small home to go outside only rarely, and required help with dressing, toileting, and meal preparation. She had given up housework, shopping, and travel. On the other hand, she took medications and used the telephone independently, kept track of her affairs quite efficiently, and, despite pain from osteoporosis and some dyspnea from a heart condition appeared to be active within her home.

She asked what public health could do for her and whether she was an example of healthy aging. Put on the spot, I first asked her about her health. She explained that she suffered from many chronic conditions: heart disease, hypertension, osteoporosis, osteoarthritis, kyphoscoliosis, diabetes, and hearing and vision loss. She needed to take ten different medicines daily, from digoxin to diuretics. What could I do for her, she wanted to know, and what could she do to promote healthy aging? I then asked if she found her days more or less satisfying and interesting. "Oh yes," she said, "I am always reading, I hear from my daughter and grandchildren on the telephone every day, I make sure I check off medicines and meals on my chart throughout the day, and people come and visit all the time. I enjoy some of the shows on television and make sure I watch the news every day."

"You mean you find each day satisfying despite your poor health?"

"Of course."

"Well, then," I said, "I would say you are a very good example of healthy aging. Public health could learn from you. How is it that your days are so full and satisfying despite all the illness and pills?"

"My mind is clear, I have the help I need, and I still can appreciate books, friends and neighbors, and my children and grandchildren. But are you sure there is nothing else I should be doing?"

I demurred. Aside from checking for adverse effects from polypharmacy and perhaps some minor environmental modifications of the home, this 92–year-old serves as an excellent illustration of successful aging: engaged in daily projects, expert in self-care and disease management, maximally supported to promote independence in the face of frailty, well-connected to family and community, funny and feisty. And yet she clearly demonstrates the high risk of poor health and disability typical of very old age.

It is useful to compare this successful ager to traditional definitions of successful aging. Rowe and Kahn (1987) distinguished between "usual" and "successful" old age. Successful aging, in their view, consists of three elements: absence of disease and the risk factors for disease, maintenance of physical and cognitive abilities, and engagement in productive activities. They viewed the three elements as roughly hierarchical: absence of disease allows maintenance of physical and cognitive skill, and preservation of these skills in turn allows engagement in productive activity. Their key insight was recognition of variation in aging, which allows us to raise the bar for goals and expectations about health in old age. If successful aging is possible, then we can aim higher than "usual aging." As Rowe (2000) has stated, "There is more to aging than disease and disability, and there is more to successful aging than avoiding disease and disability. Successful aging includes avoiding disease and disability by taking a responsible approach toward usual aging. It also involves interventions that will enhance cognitive and physical function, and trying to develop a society that provides individuals opportunities of continuing engagement in life."

Rowe and Kahn (1987) did not specify what proportion of older people met this definition of successful aging, or, more critically, what proportion, given any particular age stratum, would be a reasonable goal for public health. Nor did they try to operationalize the three criteria. Attempts to use existing measures to partition the older population in this way (and relaxing criteria to stress minimal rather than absence of disease or disability) show that only 20–33% of community-resident older Americans meet criteria for successful aging (Strawbridge, Wallhagen, & Cohen, 2002).

An alternative approach stresses minimal interruption of usual activities and maintenance of social participation in the face of disease (Schmidt, 1994). By this criterion a majority of older adults, including the 92–year-old described earlier, could be considered successful agers. The mechanism for this preservation of activity and social participation has been described by Baltes as "selective optimization with compensation," that is, doing well with remaining strengths by recruiting preserved abilities to compensate, when possible, for areas of weakness (Freunde Baltes, 1998; Baltes, 1993).

A comparison of the Rowe and Kahn criteria with self-ratings of successful aging is instructive. Strawbridge and colleagues (2002) defined absence of disease, disability, and risk factors for disease fairly stringently: none of the eight most prevalent chronic diseases of late life (heart disease, stroke, bronchitis, diabetes, cancer, osteoporosis, emphysema, asthma); no limitation in the seven activities of daily living usually affected by disease (bathing, dressing, eating, using the toilet, moving from bed to chair, personal grooming, or indoor mobility); and absence of key risk factors for heart disease (cigarette smoking, obesity, hypertension). High physical function was defined as absence of difficulty walking a quarter of a mile, climbing stairs, or standing from a sitting position, and high cognitive function as absence of reports of difficulty with memory or word finding. Finally, active engagement was defined as contact with three or more close relatives or friends each month along with productive activity, such as working, volunteering, child care, or housecleaning. They applied these criteria to the Alameda County Study, a longitudinal cohort of older persons with a mean age of 75.

In the Alameda County sample, 18.8% met the three Rowe and Kahn criteria for successful aging. The proportion successfully aging varied by age (25% for people aged 65–69, 18.5% for people 70–79, and 11.6% for people 80–99), gender (women, 21.5%; men, 15.4%), and education (high of 21.7% for people with some college education, low of 10.8% for people who did not complete high school). Of people rating their health as excellent, only 43.2% met Rowe and Kahn criteria for successful aging.

In contrast to these results, half the Alameda County sample considered themselves to have aged successfully. Among respondents who met Rowe and Kahn criteria, fully a third (60/163) did not consider themselves successful agers. Likewise, less than a quarter of the people who considered themselves to have aged successfully met Rowe and Kahn criteria (103/436). In other words, the two hardly correspond. Self-perception and formal criteria for successful aging agreed in only about half the cases (474/867).

Which is the better measure of successful aging? One way to answer the question is to examine the extent to which the two definitions are associated with indicators of well-being, such as satisfaction with life, perceived control, and the relative balance of positive and negative affect. The set of well-being measures was related to both measures of successful aging. However, the difference in well-being scores was greater when the states of "successful" and "unsuccessful" aging were defined by self-ratings.

This result is not surprising: self-ratings of success in aging (or in anything else) are likely to be related to self-reports of well-being. On the other hand, it is surprising, at least at first glance, that older people define success in aging without giving priority to absence of disease and disability. Based on the Alameda County Study findings, it is possible to suffer chronic diseases and disability, or suffer physical and cognitive problems, or not be engaged in productive activity, and yet still consider one's aging to be successful, as did nearly three-quarters of those who considered their aging to be successful. How is this possible?

Unfortunately, Strawbridge and colleagues (2002) did not provide a breakdown of the number of subjects who failed to satisfy each Rowe and Kahn criterion, or the numbers who failed on two or three of the criteria. It is likely that older people failing to meet one of the criteria were more likely to consider their aging successful than people failing to meet two or three of the criteria. If this is so, then we might have evidence for the alternative definitions of successful aging described earlier. That is, older people who maintain activity despite health conditions, or who maintain high cognitive engagement despite physical limitation, or who manage productive contributions to households despite pain or weakness, all consider their aging to be successful. They have found ways to use remaining areas of strength to optimally participate in activity and maintain independence. This is successful aging, as already indicated by the 92–year-old kibbutz dweller mentioned above.

More complicated is the case of older adults who satisfied the Rowe and Kahn criteria and yet did not consider their aging to be successful. How can their self-rating be understood? Here we are on shakier ground. Again, further analyses would be useful. Two possibilities suggest themselves. First, we should ask if these people were younger than people who met criteria for successful aging and also considered themselves to have aged successfully. If so, this would suggest that this group is likely to have retained high expectations of health, function, and engagement in late life. This group could perhaps benefit from greater opportunity for engagement and productive involvement. Second, it may also be the case that this group has other comorbidities or functional limitations not adequately measured in the operationalization of the Rowe and Kahn criteria.

In any case, this study carries special importance for public health and aging. It teaches that health in late life must be considered along with successful adaptation to states of ill health. Both are reasonable goals for public health promotion, and the mix of emphasis on the two may change with age. That is, while health should be the goal of all medical care at all ages, with very old age the more critical goal may be promotion of successful compensation in the face of disease and disability. Our 92–year-old failed all three of the Kahn and Rowe criteria but had successfully optimized her remaining abilities to live satisfying days.

FOUR TYPES OF OLDER ADULT

Gillick (1994) has provided an excellent account of geriatric medical care. As a geriatrician with a primary care focus, one of the few who still makes home visits, her experience offers important guidance on what it is like to be old, ill, and in need of medical care. She begins her account with an overriding principle: "Only if we start with a deep understanding of what being sick is like can we hope to reach a consensus on what kind of health policy is appropriate for the elderly" (Gillick, 1994, p. 10).

In her account, she identifies four types of elder and has provided clinical vignettes of the particular medical challenges and opportunities specific to each type. These are worth reviewing here. Just as medical care goals will be different for each type of elder, so, too, will public health goals. Presentation of clinical vignettes for each type of elder allows a clear view of the different medical care and public health goals appropriate for each.

The Robust Elder

The robust elderly are "physically vigorous, mentally acute, a fount of wisdom and experience for their families, [and] busy accomplishing all the things they never previously had the time to undertake"(Gillick, 1994, p. 43). However, as Gillick reminds us, they typically have accumulated at least some chronic conditions in their 70 or 80 years of life, such as arthritis, hypertension, diabetes, hearing loss, glaucoma or macular degeneration, essential tremor, and other treatable but only minimally impairing conditions. Hence, "their date books are sprinkled with doctor's appointments; they carry a packet of their medicines in their pockets; their night tables are lined with containers for hearing-aids, glasses, and dentures"(p.43). A defining feature of this type of elder is lack of disability.

An example of a robust elder described by Gillick was Mrs. Landsman (a pseudonym), who at age 96 was quite active until she developed anemia, which led to detection of an advanced colorectal cancer. As a competent adult, she had to choose between surgery (and a risk of immediate death) and symptomatic treatment, where the progression of the cancer would ultimately lead to increasing morbidity and disability and later death. Gillick describes Mrs. Landsman's response in this way:

> Mrs. Landsman thought long and hard about the various options. She had no illusions about her own mortality, and in fact was quite ready to depart from this world. But there was one thing she was quite clear about: she did not wish to be a burden to others, nor did she wish to be dependent on others, which she regarded as equivalent. The prospect of repeated visits to the hospital for transfusions or treatment for chest pain or fractures was dismal. The prospect of fading away over an extended period of time, becoming increasingly dependent, was even more unappealing.
>   Mrs. Landsman opted for surgery. Ironically, an operation that would probably prove to be curative was performed because it provided the best palliation available. The simplest, most humane, and cheapest way to provide comfort for this very elderly woman was to perform major surgery. [1994, pp. 55–56]

This case history shows that maximally invasive treatment, surgery, may be appropriate and even be considered palliative, given advanced disease. We should not immediately exclude invasive treatment for the elderly, as some have counseled (Callahan, 1987). Apart from the fact that such treatments (open-heart surgery, transplantation, and hip replacement) can be associated with good outcomes in the elderly, the treatments may make sense even in a person who does not particularly want to live longer. Invasive treatments may actually be consistent with palliative care goals, as this case shows. Here the medical care goal of curing the cancer corresponded well with the public health goal of preventing frailty and disability.

The Frail Elder

Gillick describes frail older people as "hav[ing] no one overriding health problem. Instead they suffer from impairments in multiple domains . . . that collectively render them vulnerable to the slightest perturbation" (p.105).

She describes a Mr. Schaeffer, age 83, who suffered from diabetes, hypertension, congestive heart failure, psoriasis, and emphysema. Fatigue and weakness led him to live an increasingly less active life. He could not baby-sit for his grandchild on his own, did not go out unless he had a ride from someone, could not read the newspaper through without falling asleep, and used a homemaker to do grocery shopping, cooking, laundry, and cleaning. He then developed repeated bouts of pneumonia, which led to repeated hospitalizations. At the hospital he was diagnosed with aortic stenosis, which was treated with a valvuloplasty but he subsequently developed delirium, lost weight, acquired a nosocomial infection, and became increasingly less mobile. His family then recognized that he could not safely live independently and would not be able to return to his apartment. He became a candidate for the nursing home. He had a cardiac arrest, however, while still in the hospital, which led to the last of his three intubations. However, this time he could not be revived and died.

These are the prosaic but important details of medical care for the frail elder. They are not glamorous. As Gillick writes, "Autobiographical and fictional accounts of aging focus on the drama, but seldom on the prosaic details that make all the difference to the frail older person. I have yet to read a story in which the elderly protagonist describes his intense embarrassment upon suddenly developing incontinence, only to be rescued by a geriatric consultant who determines that his problem has been caused by the new blood pressure medicine he has been taking" (p. 106).

Medical care goals for the frail elder are complex. The upper bound is the maximum medically tolerable intervention, the lower bound beneficence, not doing harm, and potentially withholding treatment if it is in the best interest of the patient. The public health goal for this type of elder is to maximize function. This typically takes two forms: environmental modification to reduce task demand (as Mr. Schaeffer did by using a homemaker and choosing which activities he preferred to do, given his fatigue), and rehabilitation to increase capacity and adapt spared abilities (which was evidently not available to Mr. Schaeffer). We take up these issues in chapter 5.

The Demented Elder

Dementing disease is one of the central challenges of geriatric care. While many diseases cause the global, progressive, irreversible impairment in cognitive function we call "dementia," the most prevalent sources are vascular disease (stroke) and Alzheimer's disease. These are diseases of later life, for the most part, and pose extreme challenges to caregiving families and medical providers. As Gillick remarks,

> The dilemma of when to stop treating, or when to provide less than maximally intensive care, is never more poignant than with the elderly person who has Alzheimer's disease or one of several types of dementia. Dementia, the gradual loss of multiple facets of the mind such as memory,

language, and judgment, robs people of their ability to understand what is happening to them when they get sick. Illness becomes as incomprehensible to these patients as its treatment. Moreover, the future they are vouchsafed if they are successfully cured of pneumonia or appendicitis is one of relentless decline. If they live long enough, they will likely pass from a state of mild forgetfulness to apathy and incontinence, and ultimately to a bed-bound existence. [p. 7]

We examine cognitive function and dementia in chapter 6. The medical care goals of the demented elder are maximization of function, reduction of treatable and hence excess morbidity, and, ultimately, palliation. The public health goals for this type of elder include excellent custodial care and, when possible, physical and cognitive remediation.

The Dying Elder

"Late life," as the term implies, is the period of life closest to death. While it is not always clear when the dying process starts (and, as a result, when medical care goals should shift further toward palliation), care of the dying elder is clearly a key component of geriatric care and an important consideration in public health and aging.

One first problem for medical care and public health goals for this population is the lack of realistic appraisal of the risk of dying by patients and their families, which is in some cases unfortunately encouraged by clinicians. These unrealistic appraisals may lead to poor choices in medical care, such as recourse to invasive procedures with little or no chance of success. Clinicians may be as uncomfortable with end of life choices as patients are. But with proper communication of risk, this situation may change. As Gillick writes, "If instead of being told that they had a 10% or 20% chance of survival with ICU care, patients were told they had an 80% to 90% chance of dying with ICU treatment, and a 99% chance of dying without it . . . how many in fact would choose the ICU?" (p. 80). This is an interesting question worth a study in itself.

A second challenge for medical care goals for this type of elder is the issue of control and autonomy at the end of life, which may be further complicated by mental health issues. We take up these issues in chapter 7. Gillick describes a Mrs. Renan, dying of cancer. She sought physician-assisted suicide and would not accept reasonable medical management of her condition, which included blood transfusions, or easily available palliative treatments. Says Gillick, "She accused me of abandoning her because I said I would not and could not give her a lethal injection." Gillick distinguishes reasonable medical care goals, such as strategies to reduce disability and relieve symptoms, and inappropriate goals, such as elimination of existential suffering.

Was I a failure as a doctor if I could not cure . . . her overwhelming sadness and rage over aging? My role was supportive. I could try to make Claire as functional as possible during her final months or years. This entailed such things as blood transfusions to improve her strength and prescribing a wheelchair to help her maintain some degree of mobility. I could try to make her as comfortable as possible by treating her arthritic pain with medication and trying to regulate her bowels with a judiciously selected combination of stool softeners and cathartics. I could provide relief by simply being there, by acknowledging her misery and promising not to abandon her. But [I do not] think that physicians must at all costs obliterate suffering, if necessary by causing death. [p. 90]

This type of patient, who, we should add, refused adequate treatment for her depression, may be the most challenging. Medical care goals here are clear: "upstreamed" palliative care, that is palliative care delivered from the beginning of the dying process, so far as we can discern it. Public health goals include reduction of isolation for this type of patient and maximization of information and choice about end of life care. Ensuring opportunity for a "good death" should be a goal, but some patients and families may not be able to avail themselves of this opportunity, as illustrated by the difficult case of Mrs. Renan.

Table 1.1 summarizes medical care and public health goals for the four types of elder. We take up these issues mostly in chapters 5, 6, and 7.

TABLE 1.1 Types of Aging Experience and Goals of Medical Care and Public Health

Type of Elder	Goal of Medical Care	Goal of Public Health
Robust	Life prolongation, cure	Prevention of frailty and disability
Demented	Maximization of function, palliation	Prevention of excess morbidity; excellent custodial care
Dying	Palliation ("upstreamed")	Reduction of isolation, maximization of choice
Frail	*Upper bound*: maximum medically tolerable intervention *Lower bound*: medical care based on best interest of patient	Environmental modification to reduce task demand; rehabilitation to increase capacity by developing spared abilities

HOW THE FIRST 50 YEARS MATTER FOR HEALTH RISKS IN THE SECOND 50 YEARS

As mentioned earlier, despite decades of gerontological research, we still do not have a single prospective cohort study that has followed people from birth to old age. Thus, it is difficult to study the ways in which health and risk behaviors in the first half of life may affect health in the second. Gerontological research cohorts usually begin at age 65, or perhaps 55. We do not have direct evidence of health at earlier ages. As a result, we are forced to use proxy measures to summarize health and risk experience in the first half of life. These proxies typically include such factors as:

- Occupation, to assess environmental exposures during work years
- Education and literacy, to assess cognitive engagement over the life span
- Parent occupation and education, to assess perinatal and childhood conditions
- Household income, to assess access to health services over the life span
- Birthplace, to assess environment and access to health care in migrating populations
- Stature, to assess nutritional status in early life
- Race and ethnicity, to assess the effects of culture and potentially restricted access to health services.

Recent progress in molecular genetics, environmental health, and imaging technologies now allow derivation of biological indicators, in some cases, for these lifelong factors. For example, some genes are more common in particular racial or ethnic groups, such as *APOE*. If a sociocultural group is more at risk of a disease associated with this gene, such as a cardiovascular condition or Alzheimer's disease, we can now begin to separate sociocultural and genetic factors. Similarly, long-term environmental exposures leave a DNA signature, just as long-term cognitive engagement, evident in educational attainment and literacy, may be visible in functional MRI images. Still, we await the definitive cohort study that will allow precise measurement of risk factors in early life and relate them to outcomes in late life. In the absence of such a study, we must rely on these proxies and their expression in biology.

We turn now to two cases that illustrate well the different legacies from the first 50 years that affect the health resources older adults have when they enter later life. These examples also show some of the difficulties involved in public health research, where biologic and clinical factors are often confounded with socioeconomic status.

Entry into Late Life with Lower Cognitive Reserve

African Americans face a higher risk of Alzheimer's disease (AD) than white Americans. This difference remains when we stratify samples by *APOE* e4 status, a well-validated risk factor for Alzheimer's disease. Figure 1–1 compares the incidence of AD in whites, African-Americans, and Hispanic Americans living in northern Manhattan, New York City. Only people with the e3/e3 variant of *APOE* (the so-called wild type) are included, thus removing the effect of this genetic risk factor. The cumulative incidence curves in the figure plot the risk of the disease by age in the three race-ethnicity groups. As in all incidence studies, people included in the analysis were free of the disease initially, and all were followed at regular intervals with a common cognitive assessment battery to identify the age at which people first met criteria for AD.

As the figure shows, minorities were significantly more likely to meet criteria for AD. By age 75, 2% of the whites and 9% of the minorities developed the disease. By age 80, about 9% of the whites and 21% of the minorities met AD criteria. These large differences in incidence persisted even with statistical control for differences between the race-ethnicity groups in a great variety of risk factors for AD, such as years of school, family history of AD, number of comorbid chronic disease conditions, and behaviors such as smoking and head injury. Tang and

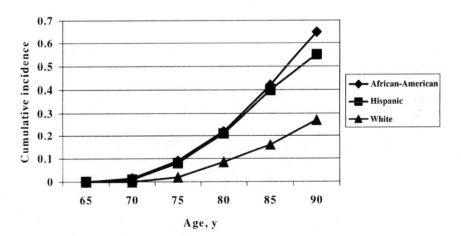

FIGURE 1.1 Cumulative Risk of AD, by Race-Ethnicity, Limited to *APOE*.

From Table 1, Tang et al., 1998. Reprinted with permission, American Medical Association.

colleagues (1998) also recalculated incidence using a stricter definition of dementia to identify only clear and obvious cases of AD. This strategy eliminated more mild forms of AD as "cases" and, as a result, should also help eliminate subtle diagnostic biases, either from clinicians interpreting cognitive tests or from the tests themselves, and in this way reduce any differential misclassification. Even with this conservative approach to diagnosis, differences between the race-ethnicity groups persisted.

These differences in the risk of AD raise important questions. Do we overdiagnose minorities (and if so, why?), or do we underdiagnose whites (and again, if so, why?). Graphically, is the cumulative incidence curve for minorities too high, or is the cumulative incidence curve for whites too low? Why should minorities be at greater risk of developing AD? Is it because they enter later life already with poorer abilities, so that they start follow-up closer to the threshold of low cognitive ability used to define AD? Or do they enter late life with abilities similar to whites, but decline at a faster rate in old age? The first factor suggests an effect in the first 50 years of life, the second an effect in the second.

We investigated this issue in a related sample of 871 older adults drawn from the same community and assessed with the same clinical battery and diagnostic paradigm (Albert & Stern, 2001). We selected people who had at least three cognitive assessments, where the AD diagnosis, if made for a respondent, was made at the last of the series of assessments. Of the 871 people, 138 met criteria for AD at their last assessment, whereas the remainder never met criteria for AD.

To assess whether the race-ethnicity groups entered old age with different cognitive resources, we examined scores on the Selective Reminding Test, a test of memory, at baseline, that is, when no one had yet met criteria for dementia. The test asks respondents to repeat a list of 12 words over 6 trials, for a maximum score of 72 and minimum of 0. Mean scores at baseline were significantly lower among minorities. If we divide the distribution into tertiles (upper third, middle third, lower third), the lower third included scores with a range from 8-34. 16.3% of whites scored in the lowest tertile, but 32.4% of African Americans and 44.4% of Hispanics scored in this range. This difference strongly supports the claim of early-life events as a predictor of a key late-life outcome. Minority elders enter later life with poorer memory scores and hence less cognitive reserve.

By contrast, the slope of memory score change over the serial assessments, that is, the mean rate of decline, was not significantly different across the three race-ethnicity groups. Age, education, and initial memory score were all independently associated with rate of decline in memory performance, but in a regression model that included these factors race-ethnicity was not significantly associated with rate of decline. Thus, cognitive performance in minorities did not decline at a faster rate. Baseline differences, differences that predate old age, appear to be responsible for the higher risk of AD among minorities. Of course, poorer memory performance at baseline very likely reflects an early stage of disease progression, prodromal AD. But this too is consistent with early-life experience as the source of greater risk of AD in late life.

Entry into Late Life with Different Health Risk Profiles

Rantanen, Guralnik, and colleagues (1999) examined a cohort of men aged 45 to 68 and found that grip strength at this age was a strong predictor of disability 25 years later. These men, all from the Honolulu Heart Program—Asia Aging Study, were first assessed from 1965 to 68 and were reassessed between 1991 and 1993, when participants were 71-93 years old. Grip strength is correlated with strength in other muscle groups and for this reason is considered a good indicator of overall strength. Grip strength performance was assessed with a hand-held dynamometer, and hand strength at mid-life was categorized into low (< 37 kg), middle (37-42 kg), and high (> 42 kg) performance tertiles.

Men with low performance in mid-life were significantly more likely to report disability in late life. These men reported nearly twice as much disability as men in the upper tertile in doing heavy household work (25% vs. 14%), walking (26% vs. 15%), bathing (8% vs. 3%), and a variety of other indicators of disability and functional limitation (i.e., walking speed, ability to rise from a chair). Men in the middle tertile fell between these two groups in risk of disability in late life. The increased risk of disability in old age associated with low grip strength in mid-life persisted in regression models that controlled for age, height, weight, education, occupation, smoking, physical activity, and chronic conditions at the exam in which disability status was established.

This finding is extremely important. "Muscle strength is found to track over the life span: those who had higher grip strength during midlife remained stronger than others in old age" (Rantanen et al., 1999). For this reason, these men entered late life with a greater reserve in strength, and this reserve helped forestall onset of disability. Rantanen and colleagues mention a number of alternative hypotheses for this finding, which are also of note: (1) grip strength may be a marker of physical activity, which may itself prevent disability; (2) low grip strength may reflect early disease processes that later progress and cause disability; and (3) grip strength may be related to motivation to stay fit and through this mechanism lower the risk of disability in late life. Each of these hypotheses merits investigation, but all suggest the critical role of health factors in midlife as predictors of late life outcomes.

It turns out as well that grip strength in midlife is related to birth weight. In the UK Medical Research Council National Survey of Health and Development, 2,815 men and 2,547 women born in 1946 have been followed through 1999, when they were 53 years old (Kuh et al., 2002). Men and women in the highest fifth of the distribution of birth weight had 10% greater grip strength at age 53, compared to people in the lowest birth weight group. A 1 kg increase in birth weight was associated with a 1.9 kg increase in grip strength for men and a 1.2 kg increase for women 53 years later. This relationship persisted even with control for weight and height and "suggest[s] the importance of prenatal influences on muscle development that have persisting consequences through to later adulthood," (Kuh et al., 2002, p. 632).

Thus, grip strength in middle age is at least partly related to prenatal environment, and grip strength in mid-life is related to disability in late life. These investigations represent a rare case in which a single important risk factor or health indicator has been investigated across the whole life span and related to outcomes at different points in the life span. They suggest the unity of the lifespan, where a risk factor acquired at the earliest ages is expressed in different ways across the life span. More research of this type will be required if we are to understand health outcomes in late life.

THE STATE OF HEALTH PROMOTION AND DISEASE PREVENTION FOR OLDER ADULTS AT THE START OF THE 21ST CENTURY

As these remarks suggest, public health and aging is a young field. The idea of primary prevention in late life still strikes some people as strange. We have been unable to identify any comprehensive treatment of the subject. Even the field of preventive or interventional geriatrics, which is further along, is still relatively new. In fact, efforts toward this end are underway in a number of fields, from neuroscience to occupational therapy, and continued progress toward primary prevention in late life is reported nearly weekly. Still, no comprehensive account is available. In this section, we bring together some of this research in the form of a brief overview. We return to many of these areas in later chapters.

Current recommendations from the U.S. Preventative Services Task Force Guide to Clinical Preventive Services, 1996, 2002; **http://**

www.ahcpr.gov/clinic/uspstf/uspstables.htm) for standard geriatric care for older adults, by modality and strength of evidence for efficacy, can be summarized in a single table (Table 1.2). These geriatric care recommendations fall into three types: recommendations based on findings from medical history, physical exam, and

TABLE 1.2 Current Recommendations (USPSTF)

Condition	Intervention	Grade
Identification by History		
Malnutrition	dietary counseling	I
Deconditioning	exercise counseling	I
Substance abuse	counseling on lifestyle	I
TIA	chemoprophylaxis	I
Functional decline	assessment/environment	I
Identification by Physical Exam		
Hypertension	sphygmomanometry	I
Obesity	weight counseling	I
Skin cancer	exam	IIIH
Hearing deficit	audiology	I
Impaired vision	vision test	I
Dentition	dental screening	I
Oral cancer	visual inspection	IIIH
Carotid artery disease	auscultation	IIIH
Breast cancer	palpation	I
Valvular heart disease	cardiac auscultation	II
Aortic aneurysm	palpation	II
Ovarian cancer	pelvic untrasound	III
Peripheral artery disease	palpation	IIIR
Dementia	MMSE	IIIR
Depression	GDS	IIIR
Abuse/neglect	general exam	IIIR
Falls	gait assessment	I
Identification by Screening Procedure		
Colorectal cancer	stool hemoccult, colonoscopy	IIIH
Breast cancer	mammography	I (to age 75?)
Cervical cancer	Pap smear	IIIH
Tuberculosis	PPD	IIIH
Thyroid disease	TSH (women)	I
Hypercolesterolemia	Blood cholesterol	I
Diabetes	Fasting plasma glucose	IIIH
Coronary heart disease	Electrocardiogram	IIIH

I, recommended for person aged 65+; II, insufficient evidence to recommend for or against; III, not recommended for general population aged 65+; IIIR, not recommended but be alert for; IIIH, recommended for high-risk groups only.

screening procedures. The first set involves evidence of malnutrition, physical deconditioning, substance abuse, transient ischemic stroke (TIA), and functional decline. These are risk factors for health decline and disability, or disease conditions that, if unchecked, put people at risk for further health decline. Interventions in these cases include dietary counseling, exercise counseling, lifestyle modification, aspirin or heparin chemoprophylaxis to prevent stroke, and modification of home environments to reduce task demands or promote safety. These recommendations are backed with evidence of the highest quality.

The second set of risk factors or diseases is identified on physical exam. Thus, a person with evidence of falls should have a gait assessment. Someone reporting trouble chewing should have a dental exam. An elder reporting vision difficulty should have an opthalmological exam, and a person reporting trouble with memory or attention should be screened for dementia. These recommendations are commonly followed, though evidence for their efficacy is mixed, and some are reserved for high-risk populations only. Thus, an exam for oral cancer might be undertaken only in an elder with mouth lesions.

Finally, screening procedures currently adopted for geriatric medicine include the fecal occult blood test (FOBT) and colonoscopy for colorectal cancer, mammography for breast cancer, Pap smear for cervical cancer, PPD test for tuberculosis, TSH test in women for thyroid disease, blood cholesterol for hypercholesteremia, fasting plasma glucose levels for diabetes, and electrocardiogram for coronary heart disease. Again, some of these procedures, as indicated in Table 1.1 are reserved for patients with a high index of clinical suspicion, and some are recommended only up to certain ages (as in the case of mammography).

Goldberg and Chavin (1997) have extended this approach with an evaluation of preventive medicine and screening in older adults. They include a variety of vaccinations and newer supplementary therapies proposed, for example, for prevention of osteoporosis. Their recommendations are summarized in Table 1.3.

An enhanced vision of prevention in old age divided into primary, secondary, and tertiary prevention and based on a wider review of literature, is shown in Table 1.4. For primary prevention, we seek *to arrest disease processes by reducing or eliminating risk factors for disease.* For this effort we rely on vaccination (immunoprophylaxis for flu and pneumonia), drug therapies (statins, anti-inflammatory agents, chemoprophylaxis for heart disease and possibly dementia), counseling (exercise, psychological support, occupational therapy strategies), and prostheses (hip protectors, grab bars and other environmental modifications to prevent falls, for example).

Secondary prevention involves *early detection and treatment of disease to minimize morbidity and risk of disability.* These efforts

TABLE 1.3 Preventive Medicine and Screening in Older Adults

Screening	Rating
Blood pressure	I
Cholesterol	I
Clinical breast exam	I
Mammogram	I
Pelvic exam/Pap smear	I
FOBT, colonoscopy	II
Audiology	III
Auscultation, palpation (mouth, nodes, testes, skin, heart, lung)	III
Glucose	III
TSH	III
Electrocardiogram	III
Vision/glaucoma screening	III
Mental/functional status	III
Osteoporosis (bone mineral density)	III
Prostate exam (PSA)	III
Chest x-ray	III
Prophylaxis/Counseling	
Exercise	I/II
Influenza vaccine	I/II
Pneumococcal vaccine	I/II
Tetanus-diphtheria vaccine	I/II
Calcium supplementation	II
Estrogen, SERM, bisphosphonate	II
Aspirin	I/II

I, Evidence from randomized trials; II, evidence from non-randomized or retrospective studies; III, expert opinion or other considerations.

Adapted from Goldberg & Chavin, 1997; http://members.aol.com/Tgoldberg/prevrecs.htm, 2002/

involve screening to detect disease at an early, asymptomatic stage. Examples include checks for bone mineral density for osteoporsis, glucose metabolism for diabetes, cognitive assessment for dementia, and hypertension screening.

Finally, we stress tertiary prevention, which seeks *appropriate disease management to reduce disability.* Examples of tertiary prevention include education to support patient self-care, telemedicine to monitor clinical chemistries, "lifeline" devices that allow elders to report medical emergencies, podiatry in diabetics, inhalers for pulmonary disease, and perhaps most critically a single medical provider to coordinate care.

The position of the three types of prevention over the life course and their effect on quality of life is shown schematically in Figure 1.2.

TABLE 1.4 Enhanced Prevention

Primary: arrest disease process by *reducing or eliminating risk factors*
- Vaccination—immunoprophylaxis—prevention of flu, pneumonia
- Drug therapy (e.g., statins, anti-inflammatory agents)—chemoprophylaxis—prevention of heart disease, dementia
- Counseling—exercise, OT, psychological support—prevention of disuse syndromes
- Prostheses—hip protectors, grab bars—prevention of falls

Secondary: *early detection and treatment of disease* to minimize morbidity
- Screening to detect disease in asymptomatic stages: bone mineral density for osteoporosis, glucose metabolism for diabetes, cognitive assessment for dementia, hypertension screening

Tertiary: *appropriate disease management* to reduce disability
- Education to support patient self-care
- Telemedicine for monitoring of clinical chemistries
- "Lifeline" devices for falls
- Podiatry in diabetes
- Inhalers for asthma and COPD
- Single medical provider to coordinate care

The y-axis represents a composite measure of health-related quality of life or some indicator of wellness (see chapter 8). The ABC pathway represents an individual's trajectory in the absence of prevention efforts of the sort summarized above. At age 70 (A), frailty or preclinical disability begins and initiates a steady decline in well-being, such that at

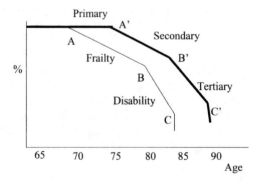

FIGURE 1.2 Leverage Points for Prevention.

TABLE 1.5 Types of Elder and Prevention Goals

		Prevention Goals				
		Frailty	Disease	Disability	Iatrogenesis	Injury
Prevention Types	Primary	H	H			
	Secondary		H	F, D	F, D	F, D
	Tertiary			Dy	Dy	

Cells indicate most important and common prevention strategy for elder type.

H, robust elderly (60–75% of older people), little or no chronic disease, no disability

F, frail-disabled elderly (20–35% of older people), several non-curable diseases, several prescription medicines, some disability, hospitalized for disease exacerbation

D, demented elderly (5–10% of older people), many severe chronic conditions, disabled, frequently hospitalized, may be institutionalized

Dy, dying elderly (5% of older people), primarily hospice, nursing home, and hospital population

age 78 (B) frank disability sets in. The trajectory of declining well-being accelerates between ages 78 and 84 (C), when this hypothetical individual dies.

Now imagine a different trajectory for this individual, indicated by the A'B'C' trajectory, which represents the effects of successful prevention. Because of primary prevention efforts at age 70, this person does not reach the frailty endpoint until age 75 (A'). Then, because of effective secondary prevention, the trajectory of decline to the point of frank disability is more gradual, such that the disability endpoint is not reached until age 84 (B'). Tertiary care is not very different in this hypothetical figure, but the gains from primary and secondary prevention have allowed this individual to die at a much older age, 89 (C'), and to experience greater wellness or health-related quality of life in both the states of frailty and disability. The area between the two curves represents the additional quality of life adjusted years, or well years, added to this person's life through prevention efforts.

Finally, we can link these thoughts about prevention to the public health goals mentioned earlier in our thoughts about the different types of aging experience. Major public health goals that are broadly applicable for all elderly include prevention of frailty, disease, disability, iatrogenesis (morbidity caused by medical or hospital treatment), and injury. Table 1.5 is a grid that cross-classifies these goals with types of prevention. The cells of the table show which type of elder can be expected to benefit most from the particular prevention strategy for the different public health goals.

SUMMARY

Definition of Public Health and Aging

The field of public health and aging stands between clinical geriatrics and the epidemiology of aging. It examines health promotion in late life, chronic disease self-management, behavioral interventions that complement clinical care, the social context of custodial care, and development of quality indicators for particular kinds of aging experience, such as dementia care, nursing home residence, physical frailty, home care, and independence through use of assistive technologies. In addition to promoting primary and secondary prevention in old age, a central goal for public health and aging is to identify aspects of health and behavior in the first 50 years of life that predispose people to live a healthy second 50 years.

"Successful Aging"

Rowe and Kahn (1987) distinguished "usual" from "successful aging." Their key insight was recognition of variation in aging, which allows us to raise the bar for goals and expectations about health in old age. If successful aging is possible, then we can aim higher than "usual aging." They did not specify what proportion of older people meet this definition of successful aging, or, more critically, what proportion of "successful aging," given any particular age stratum, would be a reasonable goal for public health. Nor did they operationalize the three criteria. Attempts to use existing measures to partition the older population in this way show that only 20-33% of community-resident older Americans meet these criteria for successful aging.

In one recent study, only 18.8% met the three Rowe and Kahn criteria for successful aging. However, half considered themselves to have aged successfully. In this study, self-ratings of successful aging and Kahn and Rowe criteria hardly corresponded. Self-perception and formal criteria for successful aging agreed in only about half the cases. One way to interpret this disparity is to recognize that successful adaptation to states of ill health can also be considered "successful aging." Both maintenance of health and compensation in the face of declining health are reasonable goals for public health in late life.

Four Types of Older Adult

It is useful to identify different types of "old age." Four prominent types in geriatric care include the robust, frail, demented, and dying elder.

Just as medical care goals will be different for each type of elder, so too will public health goals.

In the case of the robust elder, the medical care goal of cure corresponds well with the public health goal of preventing frailty and disability. Medical care goals for the frail elder are complex. The upper bound is the maximum medically tolerable intervention, the lower bound beneficence: not doing harm and potentially withholding treatment if it is in the best interest of the patient. The public health goal for this type of elder is to maximize function. This typically takes two forms: environmental modification to reduce task demand, and rehabilitation to increase capacity and adapt spared abilities.

The medical care goals of the demented elder are maximization of function, reduction of treatable and hence excess morbidity, and ultimately palliation. The public health goals for this type of elder include excellent custodial care and, when possible, physical and cognitive remediation.

Medical care goals for the dying elder include "upstreamed" palliative care, that is, palliative care delivered from the beginning of the dying process, so far as we can discern it. Public health goals include reduction of isolation for this type of patient and maximization of information and choice about end-of-life care.

How the First 50 Years Matter for Health in the Second 50 Years

Despite decades of gerontological research, we still do not have a single prospective cohort study that has followed people from birth to old age. Thus, it is difficult to study the ways in which health and risk behaviors in the first half of life may affect health in the second 50 years.

Grip strength illustrates well the unity of the life span with respect to risk factors and later health outcomes. This is a measure of general muscle strength, easily obtained with a hand dynamometer. Grip strength in mid-life is related to prenatal environment, and grip strength in mid-life is related to disability in late life. These investigations represent a rare case in which a single important risk factor or health indicator has been investigated across the whole life span and related to outcomes at different points in the life span.

Prevention in Late Life

For primary prevention in old age, we seek to arrest disease processes by reducing or eliminating risk factors for disease. For this effort, we rely on vaccination, drug therapies, counseling, and prostheses.

Secondary prevention involves early detection and treatment of disease to minimize morbidity and risk of disability. These efforts involve screening to detect disease at an early, asymptomatic stage. Examples include checks for bone mineral density in the case of osteoporosis, glucose metabolism for diabetes, cognitive assessment for dementia, and hypertension screening.

Finally, tertiary prevention seeks appropriate disease management to reduce disability. Examples of tertiary prevention include education to support patient self-care, telemedicine to monitor clinical chemistries, "lifeline" devices that allow elders to report medical emergencies, and perhaps most critically a single medical provider to coordinate care.

2

A Public Health Framework for Thinking About Aging

Aging is the maturation and senescence of biological systems. "Maturation" and "senescence" imply time-dependent changes. With time, our minds and bodies change in a variety of ways; these changes are what we mean by "aging." With each additional decade of life, adults will see slowing in reaction time, psychomotor speed, and verbal memory; declines in strength and walking speed; a decreased rate of urine flow; loss of skeletal muscle; and greater mortality, among many other changes. On the whole, they will also see declines in addictive behaviors and crime, reduction in severe psychiatric disorders, and stability in psychological well-being; continuing increases in vocabulary; greater selectivity in friendship and increased contact with close family; less need for novel stimuli; and increases in wealth, leisure time, and altruistic behaviors, also among many other changes. The popular understanding of aging mostly stresses the first set, the negative changes, but a more complete and accurate understanding would more profitably stress both kinds of change because both are relevant to a public health perspective on aging.

These changes, positive and negative, occur with the longer life or greater age of the organism. But it is useful to distinguish between two meanings of "aging." The first is simply the number of years an organism has survived. The second is the ticking of some kind of clock mechanism that governs the "maturation and senescence" of biological systems.

The changes described above, such as a decline in urine flow or loss of skeletal muscle, are more prevalent among older adults than in younger people. These changes may be more prevalent because they are, in fact, expressions of senescence and maturation, suggesting that the changes reflect movement of a biological clock mechanism. Or they may be more prevalent simply because of the greater length of time older people have lived, and hence the greater opportunity they have had to experience the risks or exposures that produce these effects.

This is a key distinction. More than likely, some combination of true senescence and greater exposure to risk factors is likely to be responsible for the changes we consider "aging." For example, the highest audible pitch people can hear declines with greater age, suggesting that this change is a senescent feature of the auditory system. But it is likely also that long years of occupational exposure to noise, untreated ear infections during childhood, neurologic conditions, or an accumulation of minor injuries might also contribute to loss of hearing in old age. Senescent changes, long periods of exposure to disease risk factors, and the interaction between the two are confounded in the lay understanding of aging but a successful public health approach to aging must distinguish between them.

AGING AND SENESCENCE

Senescence is the progressive, cumulative deterioration in function or loss of physiological capacity associated with greater chronological age. Current thinking suggests it is a biological feature of many physiological systems and that it is best measured as decreased reserve and reduced resistance to stressors. It is evident in a "diminished availability of redundant systems necessary for physical and social well-being" (Crews, 1990. p.12). For example, research suggests that loss of skeletal muscle and lean body mass, sarcopenia, is a universal, involuntary change that is distinct from pathological wasting syndromes (such as those common in cancer) and cachexia (seen in patients with rheumatoid arthritis, congestive heart failure, or end-stage renal disease). Nonetheless, these senescent changes put older people at risk for pathologic changes and in this sense can be considered "the backdrop against which the drama of disease is played out" (Roubenoff & Castaneda, 2001. p. 1230). A senescent change, such as sarcopenia, puts the body at risk for disease and also poor recovery from disease; for example, "a body already depleted of protein because of aging is less able to withstand the protein catabolism that comes with acute illness or inadequate protein intake" (Roubenoff & Castaneda, 2001).

Hence senescence and disease are related but distinct. We only see senescence in organisms that have lived a long time, but a longer time alive also means a greater opportunity to develop disease or suffer health insults that are actually distinct from these senescent changes.

To take another example, think of cancer. It is often said to be a disease of aging. This presumption is likely based on the higher death rate from malignant neoplasms evident among older adults. Indeed, the mortality rate from cancer among adults aged 65+ in 1999 was 1,129.3 per 100,000, much higher than the rate of 25.1 for people aged 25-44 and 229.3 among people aged 45-64 (Kochanek, Smith, & Anderson, 2001, Table 7). Of the 546,552 deaths due to cancer in the U.S. in 1999, 390,070, or 71.4%, involved older adults. But the larger number of cancer deaths in older adults does not mean that cancer is a feature of aging. In fact, cause-specific mortality from cancer is actually higher in the 45-64 age group; 135,748 of the 391,994 deaths in this age group, or 34.6%, were due to cancer, compared to 21.7% of the deaths in the older age group (390,070 cancer deaths of 1,797,451 deaths total). Cancer incidence is also lower in the seventh and eighth decade of life, compared to the fifth and sixth decades (Hadley, 1992). Here again we see confounding between old age as a time for longer exposure to disease agents that may lead to cancer, and old age as an expression of senescent changes that may lead to cancer directly (i.e., dysregulation of cellular processes, such as apoptosis), or that put one at risk for cancer (such as slower bowel motility, development of polyps, and onset of colorectal cancer).

We can also think of senescence as the changes typical of an organism that is approaching the maximum life span of a species. With larger numbers of people now living long enough to become centenarians, we can now characterize the state of our minds and bodies when people approach this maximum. Marie Calment, who died at age 122 and has the distinction of being the oldest person ever identified (as documented by reliable birth records), died blind and unable to walk, but without dementia (Robine & Allard, 1998). Novelists have gone a step further to imagine senescent changes unchecked by death. Jonathan Swift gives a chilling picture of a people damned to age endlessly without death (much like the character Tithonus, of Greek myth):

> At ninety they lose their teeth and hair, they have at that age no distinction of taste, but eat and drink whatever they can, without relish or appetite. The diseases they were subject to continue without increasing or diminishing. In talking they forget the common appellation of things, and the names of persons, even of those who are their nearest friends and relations. For the same reason, they can never amuse themselves with reading because their memory will not serve to carry them from the beginning of a sentence to the end. [Swift on the *struldbrugs*, *Gulliver's Travels*]

Another way to distinguish between the senescent changes of aging and the increase in disease risk associated with greater age is to try to separate *age-related* changes from *age-determined* changes. Only the latter can be considered true senescent changes. The greater prevalence of cancer and cancer mortality seen at older ages is likely to be a mixture of the two: a longer exposure time to etiologic agents that increase susceptibility to disease (age-related factor), along with genetically determined intrinsic factors, such as changes at the cellular level, that predispose to disease (age-determined change).

This combination of age-related and age-determined factors complicates public health efforts for older adults. In the setting of late-life declines in physiologic reserve, what is normal aging and what is disease? Age-related phenomena that have a particular pathology or follow a predictable course, such as the greater incidence of cancer in later life, can be called "disease." But Evans (2002) reminds us that it is wrong to then conclude that aging without disease is "normal" or "successful." Age-determined changes that are not usually considered "disease" also should be considered targets for intervention efforts if they lead to loss of reserve and put one at risk for disease.

Figure 2.1, which presents findings from the Berlin Aging Study, shows how easy it is to draw false conclusions about aging and disease (Linderbenger & Baltes, 1997), in this case in the setting of cross-sectional research. The upper panel shows a simple scatterplot of the relationship between age and a composite measure of intelligence. The correlation is negative,-0.57, showing a strong and significant decrease in intelligence with greater age. One would be tempted to conclude from this figure that normal aging includes declines in intelligence.

The lower panel, however, shows the same relationship, only this time adjusted for performance on measures of balance, gait, and sensory ability. The correlation is now-0.06, hardly any relationship at all. Clearly, the decline in intelligence shown in the top panel is an artifact. With greater age, older people are likely to develop deficits in balance, gait, and sensory ability; decline in these abilities leads to lower performance on tests of intelligence. Thus, declines in intelligence with age are not normal aging but instead reflect declines in balance and sensory ability. If declines in intelligence are not part of normal aging, should declines in balance and sensory ability, then, be considered part of normal aging? They may be part of the senescent processes associated with aging, or they may be consequences of pathologic changes in other physiologic systems. How much of the decline associated with age should be considered part of "normal aging"?

A useful, if rough, model of the relationship between senescence, disease, and the public health outcome most important in aging, disability, is shown in Figure 2-2.

Senescence, defined here as "physiologic changes of aging, not disease-based," is itself associated with frailty (i.e., weakness, poor

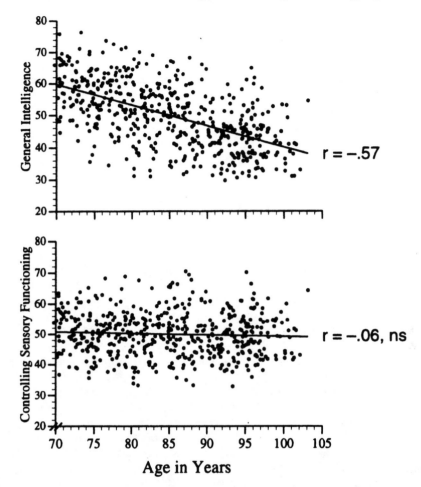

FIGURE 2.1 The Age Relation of Individual Differences in General Intelligence Before and After Controlling For Main Effects of Balance—Gait, Hearing, and Vision.

Source: Lindenberger & Baltes, 1997. Reprinted with permission, American Psychological Association.

endurance, slowness [Fried et al., 2001]), even in the absence of any identifiable disease process. Frailty, in turn, puts older people at risk for disability, defined as difficulty with basic household and personal self-maintenance activities severe enough to threaten independent living. Senescent changes can be accelerated in the presence of disease and can also predispose older people to develop frank disease; hence the double arrow connecting senescent change and disease. Disease can

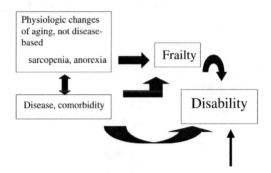

FIGURE 2.2 Sources of Frailty and Disability.
Source: Albert, Im, & Raveis, 2002. Reprinted with permission, American Public Health Association.

also cause disability directly (think of an older person with Alzheimer's dementia or a young person with an isolated medical condition). Thus, senescence is important for its independent association with frailty as well as its association with disease. From a public health standpoint, aging as a risk factor for poor health outcomes is best understood both as senescent changes, such as sarcopenia and hypometabolism, and the interaction of these changes with disease. Note, however, that senescence and disease do not exhaust the causes of disability. The third arrow, in the right hand corner of the figure, illustrates that there are other causes of disability as well, which are also important in a public health approach to aging. These include environmental factors (the degree to which daily living conditions serve to underchallenge or overwhelm people [Lawton 1980]), inadequate access to assistive and prosthetic technologies, and weak social and psychological resources.

Wallace (1997) describes some of the different ways disease and age-determined changes may be related, and which further complicate public health efforts. First, the pathogenesis of some diseases is likely to be altered with age. Declines in immune response, for example, a feature of aging, may turn a viral infection into pneumonia rather than a less complicated respiratory infection. Second, an age-determined change in one physiologic system (which may not cause overt disease in that system) may increase susceptibility to disease in another system. An example mentioned by Wallace is an increase in stroke related to age-determined hypotension. Third, age-determined changes can make older people more susceptible to disease when exposed to environmental challenges. Older adults develop reductions in glucose tolerance, for example, which may lead to frank diabetes under certain conditions. Wallace also points out, however, that some age-determined changes may actually retard development of disease. Lactose intolerance, an age-determined change to the extent that it increases with age, may lead to less fat intake and reduced risk of atherogenesis.

If we make this distinction between senescent change and disease, we avoid some confusion in thinking about health and aging. For example, consider this definition of aging: "the accumulation of deleterious changes in physiology and their external manifestations, which occur from the time of conception until death" (cited in Crews, 1990). This definition does not distinguish between disease and aging, between age-related and age-determined changes, and between changes that are deleterious and changes that are neutral or even positive.

BIOMARKERS OF AGING

Wallace (1997) reminds us that "no one has yet discovered a single biological process that is called 'aging'." He goes on to say, "there is no single chemical or metabolic activity or genetic timer that proceeds inexorably and irreversibly, dictating how long we will live."

What are usually called "biomarkers of aging" are not genetic timing mechanisms of this sort, but rather physiologic changes that are correlated with chronological age. One recent study identified over 100 physiologic changes that have been shown, at least in cross-sectional studies, to be correlated with age (Sehl & Yates, 2001). These correlations are mostly in the low to moderate range. Averaging across indicators within particular physiologic domains, Sehl & Yates conclude that beginning at age 18, each additional year of life is associated with a 1-3% decline in these parameters. This applies to indicators of respiratory and cardiac function, working memory, visual reaction time, gait speed, sensory discrimination, and other more typical indicators of age. But it must be stressed that these findings are based on cross-sectional studies, so that different cohorts of people are assessed rather than a single cohort followed over time, and that the highest correlation between any of the parameters and age was no more than 0.50 (Bortz, 1989), so that no more than 25% of the variance in hearing (highest audible pitch), for example, could be explained by age differences.

None of the proposed biomarkers of age truly represent an underlying mechanism of senescence. In any sample of older people we will find a wide range of performance on every one of the parameters. But this is simply another way of saying that any random sample of older people of any given age will include both highly functional, robust elders and impaired, frail people with disabilities severe enough to require nursing-home levels of care.

PHENOTYPES OF "FRAILTY" AND "SUCCESSFUL AGING"

Given this heterogeneity of aging and health, it would be useful to identify phenotypes of poor, normal, and successful aging. What combination of features best characterizes these health states? Reasonable definitions would be useful for guiding genetic studies, in which we might seek to determine the degree to which high function in late life, for example, is heritable. That is, if a person reaches age 80 or 85 without any difficulty or need for help in the activities of daily living (ADL), is it likely that his or her sibling will also reach this age without ADL disability? Longevity clearly has a heritable component (Perls et al. 2002), and many of the diseases of late life, including Alzheimer's disease (Green et al., 2002), also fall into this category: first-degree relatives of probands with the condition face a higher risk of having the condition than first-degree relatives of unaffected probands. Twin studies also suggest strong genetic components to many features of aging, such as cognitive ability and even some behaviors.

Apart from the utility of such definitions for genetic studies, it is worth dwelling on these phenotypes because they force us to define what we mean by frailty or successful aging. Successful aging certainly would have to include independence in the activities of daily living and absence of dementia. Should we also include other criteria, such as absence of heart disease, bone mineral densities greater than some minimum, and high scores in visual reaction time and gait speed? And why stop here? Why not include measures of psychological and social health, such as engagement in leisure activities, absence of depression, satisfying social networks, and high scores on measures of self-efficacy? We are driven to consider these many features because health in late life is not a matter of discrete physiologic systems. Impairments in vision, hearing, lower extremity strength, and affect increase the risk of falls, incontinence, and ADL dependency (Tinetti et al., 1995). These relationships were already indicated in Figure 1.2, which shows that disease interacts with senescent processes to increase the risk of frailty and disability.

If successful aging is hard to define, perhaps it is easier to define what successful aging is not, that is, "frailty." One proposed frailty phenotype, already mentioned earlier, consists of the following components: shrinking (unintentional loss of 10 lbs or more), weakness (scores in the lowest 20% of the distribution of grip strength values), poor endurance (reports of exhaustion when performing daily activities), slowness (scores in the lowest 20% of the distribution of timed gait speeds), and low activity (scores in the lowest 20% of activity profiles, as determined by estimated expenditure of calories). Older adults with three or more of these characteristics were considered to be frail (Fried et al., 2001).

This is a useful definition, though one could easily imagine other components that could be added. It is largely limited to physical elements. Going back to Figure 2.2, we can ask how well this definition of frailty "works": Is it a precursor to self-reported disability? Is it highly correlated with the presence of comorbid medical conditions? We know already from the figure that the correspondence will not be perfect because disability has other sources. Also, in the absence of a time element and longitudinal sample, we cannot truly examine causal chains.

Still, Fried and colleagues (2001) provide important data on the strengths and limitations of this frailty phenotype. Of 363 older adults with self-reported disability in ADL, only 28% also met these criteria for frailty. This is an important finding. If the features of frailty identified in this approach truly represent senescent changes that are relatively free from disease processes, then the majority of self-reported disability is due to disease and not to the inevitable slowing, weakening, and shrinking typical of aging. These data are only a first start in what will surely become an important stream of research, but they suggest that most of the disability seen in older populations is attributable to disease, rather than aging per se. If so, optimal disease management and primary prevention of disease will likely continue to reduce disability to even lower levels.

In this sample of 363 older adults with ADL disability, note too that 54%, not the remaining 72%, had identifiable comorbid medical conditions without meeting criteria for frailty. Thus, disease without frailty accounted for the largest proportion of people reporting disability but still did not exhaust the sources of disability. Of these disabled elders, 18% did not meet criteria for frailty and did not have comorbid disease, either. Their disability was the result of unmeasured frailty or disease, or more likely resulted from the complex of environmental, psychological, and social factors indicated in the third, independent pathway to disability shown in Figure 2.1.

If we assume that this breakdown of the sources of disability in late life is correct, we can see that prevention of disability involves public health efforts—primary, secondary, and tertiary—targeted to frailty, disease, and behavioral-environmental factors. Roughly speaking, these data suggest that perhaps half of the old-age disability we see is due to disease, a quarter to direct senescent processes relatively independent of disease, and another quarter to behavioral-environmental factors. All are modifiable.

AGING AND DISABILITY: REASSESSMENT OF THE WHO MODEL

Figure 2.3 presents the WHO model (1981) of the relationship between survival, disability, and frailty. (Note that "frailty," "impairment," and "morbidity" have all been used interchangeably to identify changes that precede frank disability and presumably represent preclinical states of disability.) The shape of the disability and frailty curves is hypothetical, but these presumably follow the shape of the survival curve, which reflects the increasing and accelerating risk of mortality with greater age.

Survival curves are generated by applying prevailing death rates at each age to a hypothetic cohort (radix) born at a given time. Conventionally, we begin with 100,000 births. The death rate for each age group removes people from the population. The survivors then experience the death rate prevailing for the next age group. We assume no changes in death rates and no other sources of entry or exit from the cohort. By age 100 or 110 we assume that the cohort is extinct, though some individuals will pass this age milestone.

As shown in the survival plot in Figure 2.3, mortality is extremely low until people reach age 40 or so (hence the flat curve until this age, with nearly 100% survival; life tables for the U.S. population in the 1990s, for example, suggest that only 4% of people die before age 40 [Erickson, Wilson, & Shannon 1995]). The doubling of mortality every 7 or so years (after its nadir between ages 5 and 15) is evident in the steep slope beginning in mid-life.

In this model, the proportion of older people in a birth cohort is shown on the ordinate and age on the abscissa. In the figure, 50% of

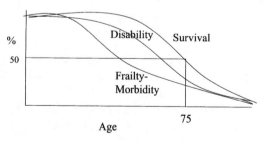

FIGURE 2.3 Partitioning Survival by Functional Status: WHO Model (slightly modified).
Source: WHO, 1981.

elders are still alive at age 75. The area under the survival curve indicates the total person-years lived by the cohort. Thus, if everyone in the cohort died at the same age, say 85, the survival curve would appear rectangular, and the total person-years lived by the cohort would simply be 100,000 x 85, 850,000, with an obvious life-expectancy at birth of 85 (850,000 /100,000). We return to this model in more detail in chapter 3. For now we need simply note that survival in this model can be partitioned according to functional status. We assume that the risk of disability and frailty follows the pattern established for survival: an increasing, accelerating risk with age. We assume too that they are nested: frailty precedes disability, so that people reach frailty before disability, and that everyone with disability has passed through a period of frailty. Similarly, states of disability, of varying duration, precede mortality. Our prior discussion, of course, suggests that this is too simple a model, but it is important nonetheless to understand the model because it is well established and offers an important tool for thinking about aging and public health.

Returning again to the figure and people aged 75, we see that 50% have died, and that of the 50% still alive, roughly 20% are disabled and frail, perhaps another 5% frail without disability, and the remaining 20% neither frail or disabled. In this simple approach, then, about half the surviving elders at age 75 might be considered to have aged successfully, with the other half frail or disabled.

Looking at the aging of the cohort as a whole, we can calculate person-years of disability, frailty without disability, and optimal function over the complete experience of the cohort. Person-years lived with disability are represented by the area between the survival and disability curves. Similarly, person-years of frailty or preclinical disability are indicated by the area between the disability and frailty curves. Remember, however, that the frailty and disability curves shown here are completely hypothetical. Evidence is available for the nesting of frailty within disability only for particular, narrowly-defined domains. For example, older adults lose the ability to climb stairs with risers that are 16 inches high before they lose the ability to climb stairs that are 10 inches high. If risers on stairways are typically 10 inches, then loss of the ability to manage a 10–inch riser is disability; upon reaching this point, elders lose the ability to climb stairs. Many elders who cannot climb stairs with 16–inch risers, however, can still climb stairs with 10–inch risers; and people who have lost the ability to climb stairs with 16–inch risers are likely to be at risk for later inability to climb stairs with 10–inch risers. Hence they are frail without being disabled, and the nesting of frailty within disability shown in the figure is reasonable for such fairly narrowly defined tasks that depend on a common set of physiologic or biomechanical properties.

The model is especially valuable for tracking differences in population health. Across populations, we can compare survival and disability-free survival. Within populations we can examine changes over time to determine if gains in life expectancy are associated with a gain or loss of disability-free survival. Robine (1992) has shown that arguments regarding the compression of morbidity and rectangularization of aging can be sharpened (and tested empirically) using this model. Increases in life expectancy mean that the survival curve in Figure 2.3 is shifting upward and to the right. The key question is whether the disability curve is shifting in the same direction at the same pace. If it does not change at all, then all additional years gained from the increase in life expectancy are years lived with disability, clearly an unwelcome outcome. If the disability curve is shifting in the same direction but at a slower pace than increases in life expectancy, then the net effect of gains in life expectancy will also be an increase in the proportion of years lived with disability, still an unwelcome outcome. If the disability and survival curves are moving outward in tandem, then the proportion of years lived with disability remains unchanged, still not the best outcome from a public health perspective. Only if the disability curve moves outward at a rate faster than the survival curve will the volume of disability across the life span be reduced. In fact, evidence is mounting that this has happened in the U.S. over the past 20 years (see chapter 5).

AGING AND "SOCIAL AGE"

When people think of old age, they usually think of years or some other indicator of the passage of time (for example, in societies where people do not use year-based calendars, these indicators might include number of harvests completed, number of ritual cycles conducted, or number of relocations of dwellings). But even in contemporary American culture, "old age" is not simply a matter of chronologic age or the biologic expression of senescence. Fry (1980) used a technique drawn from cognitive anthropology to show that cultural dimensions, such as productivity, vulnerability, and reproductive potential, underlie judgments of "young," "middle-aged," and "old." In her pile sort study, respondents were asked to group hypothetic age-linked social statuses according to similarity. Multidimensional scaling analyses revealed a clear chronologic age dimension, but also second-and third-order dimensions, showing, for example, that respondents also grouped old people and children together as opposed to people of middle age. This finding is consistent with research on the "infantilization" of older people (Ryan, Bourhis, & Knops, 1991; Albert & Brody, 1996). "Baby talk" and terms typically reserved for children are often applied to older people with cognitive impairment or other disabilities. For example, older people are often spoken of as "cute" and elicit the same protective urge seen with infants, such as a desire to hug or comfort.

The reverse is also true. Younger adults who are not active, not interested in new experiences or travel, not willing to switch careers, or who are slow, deliberate, or narrow-minded, are often called "old before their time." These negative features of aging—negative, at any rate, when applied to younger people—are meant to criticize or embarrass young people. This use of language also suggests a social component in our understanding of aging. People are old not just because of their age but also because of their behavior, their health, their attitudes, their choices, and even their politics.

More generally, evidence from cross-cultural studies suggests that the defining characteristics of old age include chronologic age but also many other criteria, such as achieved social status, having grandchildren, holding political office, oratorical skill, and physical changes associated with age. In societies with high mortality and short life expectancy, having children reach adulthood is associated with change in status to "elder" and associated honorific terms (Albert & Cattell, 1994). Again, the other side to social age needs to be mentioned. In American society, adults can refuse to "grow up," and people can insist on "not acting their age." This can take a variety of forms: not leaving a parent's home, not marrying at a so-called appropriate age, refusing to establish clear career goals, marrying someone much younger than you are, even buying consumer products associated with a different age stratum.

Thus, old age has a social dimension. For public health efforts, this social component is most relevant in its bearing on expectations for health and function in later life. Even this brief discussion of the use of age criteria to label behaviors suggests that attitudes toward aging and old age are mostly negative. Old age is seen as a time of decline, withdrawal, and vulnerability. In this view, aging is not welcome, and little should be expected for older people, except perhaps to ease decline, provide care, and protect them from exploitation or danger related to their increased vulnerability. These are the elements of "ageism" (Butler, 1969; Palmore, 1999): assumptions of disability, lack of ability, or vulnerability (and hence need for protection) based on age, rather than actual competencies.

The pervasiveness of ageism should not be underestimated. The older person who misses a word because of a hearing problem is considered too old for conversation and patronized with simplified language. Words may be put in his mouth and his opinion ignored. Older people who forget a name are called "senile," dissatisfaction with illness-related activity restrictions is called "crankiness," and expressions of sexual interest make one a "dirty old man or woman." Even medical personnel are not above recourse to ageist stereotypes.

This sort of ageist thinking has consequences for public health. If missing a word is considered a feature of "getting old," families (and older people themselves) may not take advantage of tertiary treatments available to manage hearing loss, such as hearing aids. Losing track of names may indicate mild cognitive impairment, not just aging; people with mild cognitive impairment may benefit from cognitive prostheses, environmental modification, anti-dementia drugs, or increased supervision by family members. "Crankiness" may be depression, genuine dissatisfaction with unpalatable symptoms, a complaint against undesirable housing, or simply a bad mood, any of which would otherwise be understood as features of daily life for people of any age. From a public health perspective, these expressions of ageism are doubly damaging. They falsely label potentially treatable medical conditions (such as memory or hearing loss) as "aging," and also turn everyday complaints, dissatisfactions, interests, and behaviors into pseudo-medical aging syndromes ("crankiness," "childishness," "the dirty old man").

Ageist thinking is revealed for what it is when one compares preconceptions about older people to the facts at hand. For example, younger people mostly imagine old age as a time of sickness, disability, and loss of autonomy. In fact, nearly 80% of people aged 65+ have no disability of any sort and less than 5% reside in nursing homes. For all our fears of cognitive decline and Alzheimer's disease as invariant features of aging, it is mainly a disease of the very old. Most surveys find an Alzheimer's disease prevalence of 6% for people aged 75–84 and 20% for people aged 85+ (Brookmeyer, Gray & Kawas, 1998). Recent evidence also suggests that the prevalence and incidence of both physical and cognitive disability may be declining (Manton & Gu, 2001; Freedman, Hakan & Martin, 2001). Clinical depression is also not more common in older people (see chapter 7); it is often a comorbid feature of physical illness and bereavement, and for this reason seems more common among older people.

Many of these ageist attitudes have been elicited using questionnaires, such as "What is Your Aging IQ?" (Special Committee on Aging, United States Senate, 1991). The questions present typical preconceptions about aging and in this way highlight ageist thinking. One version of the questions is shown here, with suggested correct answers:

TRUE OR FALSE?

1. Everyone becomes "senile" sooner or later, if he or she lives long enough. *False.*

2. American families have by and large abandoned their older members. *False.*
3. Depression is a serious problem for older people. *True.*
4. The numbers of older people are growing. *True.*
5. The vast majority of older people are self-sufficient. *True.*
6. Mental confusion is an inevitable, incurable consequence of old age. *False.*
7. Intelligence declines with age. *False.*
8. Sexual urges and activity normally cease around age 55–60. *False.*
9. If a person has been smoking for 30 or 40 years, it does no good to quit. *False.*
10. Older people should stop exercising and rest. *False.*
11. As you grow older, you need more vitamins and minerals to stay healthy. *False.*
12. Only children need to be concerned about calcium for strong bones and teeth. *False.*
13. Extremes of heat and cold can be particularly dangerous to old people. *True.*
14. Many older people are hurt in accidents that could have been prevented. *True.*
15. More men than women survive to old age. *False.*
16. Deaths from stroke and heart disease are declining. *True.*
17. Older people on the average take more medications than younger people. *True.*
18. Snake oil salesmen are as common today as they were on the frontier. *True.*
19. Personality changes with age, just like hair color and skin texture. *False.*
20. Sight declines with age. *False.*

A second version includes these questions:

1. Baby boomers are the fastest growing segment of the population. *False.*
2. Families don't bother with their older relatives. *False.*
3. Everyone becomes confused or forgetful if they live long enough. *False.*
4. You can be too old to exercise. *False.*
5. Heart disease is a much bigger problem for older men than for older women. *False.*
6. The older you get, the less you sleep. *False.*
7. People should watch their weight as they age. *True.*
8. Most older people are depressed. Why shouldn't they be? *False.*
9. There's no point in screening older people for cancer because they can't be treated. *False.*

10. Older people take more medications than younger people. *True.*
11. People begin to lose interest in sex around age 55. *False.*
12. If your parents had Alzheimer's disease, you will inevitably get it. *False.*
13. Diet and exercise reduce the risk of osteoporosis. *True.*
14. As your body changes with age, so does your personality. *False.*
15. Older people might as well accept urinary accidents as a fact of life. *False.*
16. Suicide is mainly a problem for teenagers. *False.*
17. Falls and injuries "just happen" to older people. *False.*
18. Everybody gets cataracts. *False.*
19. Extremes of heat and cold can be especially dangerous for older people. *True.*
20. You can't teach an old dog new tricks. *False.*

The questions elicit ageist stereotypes well. They reflect unrealistic fatalism and therapeutic nihilism ("everybody gets cataracts," "falls and injuries just happen to older people," "there's no reason to treat older persons with cancer," "most older people are depressed"), false assumptions about the aging process ("you can't teach an old dog new tricks," "people begin to lose interest in sex after age 55," "the older you get, the less you sleep") and overestimates of the heritability of late-life disease ("if your parents had Alzheimer's disease, you will inevitably get it"), sociological naïveté ("American families have by and large abandoned their older members"), and under-recognition of true negative aspects of aging, such as the increased risk of suicide among older white men and greater use of prescribed medicines. Sometimes the difficulty is a misplaced recognition of a problem, such as the claim of less sleep with greater age. It is true that older people sleep for shorter durations; this is related to poorer quality of sleep. However, older people also nap more during the day, resulting, in fact, in greater amounts of sleep overall than younger people.

Together, these prejudices suggest that aging is mostly misunderstood. Overall, negative features are exaggerated and positive features ignored. This social or cultural component of aging should be recognized as a potential obstacle to successful public health interventions for older people.

WHEN DOES OLD AGE BEGIN?

So far, we have examined aging and older persons without specifying when someone is old. From what we have said already, we see that the question is unreasonable. There is no single age at which we can say that people cross the threshold into old age. People age at different rates; hence, for any given age, there will be great variation in all proposed biomarkers of aging. Old age does not have a biological definition, only a social one. For example, in the United States, establishment of the Social Security system linked old age to the age of 65. This definition of old age was more a product of social perceptions and economic necessity than anything else.

But people do have an idea of when people become old. A number of surveys have asked at what age someone is old. The start of old age can be assigned to a wide chronologic range. This assigned age may reflect attitudes toward aging and older persons. For example, dating the start of old age to increasingly older ages means that many aspects of aging, once considered hallmarks of old age, now fall short of making someone old. It also stands to reason that many features of respondents, such as age and social status, are likely to be related to judgments of the start of old age. One might imagine that minority groups with a shorter life expectancy might date the onset of old age earlier than other more advantaged groups.

Someone who reports that old age begins at age 55 clearly has a different attitude toward aging than someone who asserts that it begins at age 75. In the one case, a larger portion of the life span is considered the period of old age, with the physical and psychological changes of the fifth and sixth decade already considered signs of senescence. In the other, only changes typical of the seventh decade and beyond qualify as old age, and senescence is pushed ahead to a point closer to death and the maximum biologic life span. Respondent choices of an age for old age tell us the decade when people are expected to slow down, retire, and focus on self-maintenance rather than on new careers or goals.

Figure 2.4 shows the age at which respondents consider women to be old. These data are drawn from the National Council on Aging's Myths and Realities of Aging survey, conducted in 2000 in a national probability sample of the United States. The data are weighted to reflect the sampling scheme and over-representation of older people and minorities. The figure plots the mean age "the average woman" is said to be old by respondents' age and sex.

Note the strong relationship between a respondent's age and his or her report of when women are old. Clearly, young people consider the start of old age to be much earlier than older people do. For people around age 20, women are old are at age 50. By the time, people reach the sixth and seventh decades, old age is pushed back to the late 60s and early 70s. Note too that women date the start of old age later than men do, whatever the respondent's age. Women consider old age

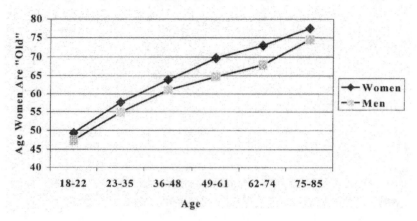

FIGURE 2.4 Age Women Are "Old," by Respondent Age and Sex, U.S.
Source: National Council on Aging, 2000 (weighted data).

to begin 2-4 years later than men. They push old age further back than men not just for themselves, but also in their reports of the start of old age for men (Albert, O'Neil, Muller, & Butler, 2002). Moreover, the age at which old age is said to begin appears now to be far more correlated with one's own age than it was in earlier surveys.

SUMMARY

This chapter has shown that "old age" is not obvious. It is hard to define biologically, prone to social judgment and bias, and evolving with changing life expectancies and health trajectories in later life. From the perspective of public health it is important to remember that we are really talking about aging, not old age; lifespan health, not gerontological health. What happens in the first 50 years of life affects health in the second 50 years, and it makes little sense to divide the lifespan into young and old periods according to some age criterion. This chapter has established the following points:

Aging and Senescence. Senescence is the progressive, cumulative deterioration in function or loss of physiological capacity associated with greater chronological age. It is related to disease but distinct. We only see senescence in organisms that have lived a long time, but a longer time alive also means a greater opportunity to develop disease or suffer health insults that are actually distinct from these senescent changes.

Biomarkers of Aging. What are usually called "biomarkers of aging" are not genetic timing mechanisms, but rather physiologic changes that are correlated with chronological age. They do not truly capture an underlying mechanism of senescence. In any sample of older people we will find a wide range of performance on every one of the proposed parameters. This is simply another way of saying that any random sample of older people of any given age will include both highly functional, robust elders, as well as impaired, frail people.

Phenotypes of "Frailty" and "Successful Aging." Successful aging certainly would have to include independence in the activities of daily living and absence of dementia, major threats to independence in late life. There is no shortage of other elements to consider in defining successful aging: absence of heart disease, youthful bone mineral densities, and high scores in visual reaction time and gait speed. And why not include measures of psychological and social health? Frailty may be easier to define. One proposed frailty phenotype includes "shrinking," weakness, poor endurance, slowness, and reduced activity. Yet in one sample of older adults with self-reported disability in ADL, only about a quarter also met these criteria for frailty. This is an important finding. If suggests that the majority of self-reported disability is due to disease and not to the inevitable slowing, weakening, and shrinking typical of aging.

Aging and Disability: Reassessment of the WHO Model. In the WHO model of the relationship between survival, disability, and frailty, the onset of frailty and disability is presumed to follow the shape of a population's survival curve, so that all three processes reflect an increasing and accelerating risk of reaching the endpoints with greater age. Yet, evidence suggests that frailty precedes disability only for particular, narrowly-defined domains that share common biomechanical or physiologic properties. More typical of health in late life are geriatric syndromes that combine features of frailty and disability. For example, impairments in vision, hearing, lower extremity strength, and affect together increase the risk of falls, incontinence, and ADL dependency.

The WHO model requires refinement but still allows us to assess improvements in population health and functional status. In this model, we see that the volume of disability across the life span will be reduced only if the disability curve moves outward at a rate faster than the survival curve. Evidence, examined later, suggests that this has happened in the U.S. over the past 20 years, a welcome finding.

Aging and "Social Age." When people think of old age, they first think of years or some other indicator of the passage of time. But a more careful look suggests that people are considered "old" not just because of their age but also because of their behavior, their health, their attitudes, their choices, and even their politics. The use of age criteria to label behaviors suggests that attitudes toward aging and old age are mostly negative. Old age is seen as a time of decline, withdrawal, and vulnerability. Such expressions of ageism are damaging for public health efforts. They falsely label potentially treatable medical conditions as "aging" and also turn everyday complaints, dissatisfactions, interests, and behaviors into pseudo-medical aging syndromes.

When Does Old Age Begin? We have seen that there is no single age at which we can say that people cross the threshold into "old age." For Americans, the strongest predictor of judgments about the start of old age is one's own age, suggesting considerable social variability in our thinking about age.

Clearly, with age come changes in function, health, and psychology. The popular understanding of aging mostly stresses negative changes, but a more complete and accurate understanding would more profitably stress both positive and negative changes. This approach alerts us to the strengths older people retain and the need to work with these strengths to compensate for deficits, a key element in a public health approach to aging.

3

Public Health and the Demography of Aging

In 2000, there were 35 million people aged 65 or older in the United States, 12.4% of the U.S. population. Over 4 million Americans were aged 85+, 1.5% of the total population (U.S. Census, 2000, Preliminary Results). The number of older Americans is ten times higher now than it was at the turn of the twentieth century, when there were only 3 million people aged 65+. At that time, older people accounted for only 4% of the total population (Federal Interagency Forum, 2000). By 2030, the number of older people will double to 70 million, and by that date the proportion of people in the U.S. aged 65+ will approach 20% of the total population. This increase in the proportion of older people represents the continuation of a longstanding trend. In 2000, there were over 50,000 centenarians in the United States, about 1 in every 5600 Americans. There were nearly 1400 people aged 110+ (U.S. Census, 2000, Preliminary Results).

The age-sex pyramid for the United States population in 2000 is shown in Figure 3.1. This is perhaps less a pyramid than an emerging rectangle or pillar, a typical shape for countries that have already undergone the demographic transition in which an equilibrium of high mortality and fertility is replaced by one of low mortality and fertility (see below). The figure shows that ages 35 to 54, representing a bulge in the center of the figure, are the most populous ages. These age strata contain the aging baby-boomers, people born between 1946 and 1965. Lower fertility after this period, which continued over the next three decades, has led to fewer people at younger ages and hence absence of a wide base for the pyramid. The median age in the U.S. in 2000 was 35, again showing absence of a wide base for the pyramid.

The age-sex pyramid (or rectangle) in 2000 shows the strong preponderance of women over men in later life. Among people aged 65+,

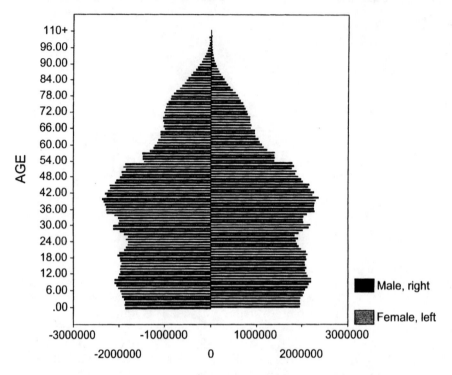

FIGURE 3.1 U.S. Age-Sex Pyramid, 2000.
Source: United States Census 2000 Summary Files 1 (SF1) 100-Percent Data.

the sex ratio (number of women for each man) is 1.4; for people aged 85+ it is 2.5, and for people 100+ it is 4.0. This asymmetry affects living arrangements and marital status in important ways, leaving older women more likely to live alone, depend on children when frail, and enter nursing homes at higher rates than men.

Aggregating across the strata of the pyramid also shows the size of the young (0–17) and older population (65+) relative to people aged 18–64. In 2000, people under age 18 made up 25.7% of the population, and people aged 65+ 12.4%. Together, these so-called dependent sectors made up 38.1% of the U.S. population. There are thus some 1.6 people aged 18–64 for each person in the dependent sectors, a grim picture if these sectors were truly dependent. Comparing people aged 18–64 to people aged 65+ yields the so-called support ratio, which was 5:1 in 2000. In fact, only a minority of people aged 65+, about 20%, can be considered dependent, at least according to need for help in one or more of the personal self-maintenance activities, or activities of daily living (ADL: bathing, dressing, grooming, feeding, using toilet) (Manton, 1992). This proportion has declined between 1983 and 1999 (Manton & Gu, 2001). Increasingly, people aged 65+ are not retiring, continue to provide increasingly large intergenerational transfers of resources to their children in the 18–64 age group, and contribute to child-rearing support for grandchildren. The dependency and support ratios of people aged 18–64 to people on either side of this age band no longer measures anything very useful, at least in the United States (and probably elsewhere as well), a testament to the changing social and health profile of older people.

EPIDEMIOLOGIC TRANSITION I: DECLINING DEATH RATES ACROSS THE LIFE SPAN

The epidemiologic or demographic transition describes a sweeping change in the age structure of populations. Agrarian, nonindustrialized societies have high birth and death rates. Historically, these societies averaged 35–45 deaths and births per 1000 people. Industrialized, urban societies have far lower fertility and mortality, about 10–15/1000 (Mausner & Kramer, 1985). Each of the two conditions is characterized by a rough parity, so that there is little or no absolute increase in population under each regime. However, historically, death rates have fallen before birth rates in this transition, leading to huge increases in population, as, for example, in Europe, between 1790 and 1900.

The mortality side of this transition is clearly seen for death rates in Sweden over three centuries, summarized by Horiuchi (2003). Data for this comparison are not easily available, because the comparison requires nearly 300 years of continuous, complete mortality data on a national scale. Sweden is one of the few countries with vital registration systems that have collected such data. Figure 3.2 shows death rates for three cohorts of Swedish women, the first born between 1751 and 1755, the second between 1876 and 1880, and the third between 1951 and 1955. The figure (which graphs mortality on a logarithmic scale) shows little difference in mortality risk for the first two cohorts. Mortality is well over 10% per person-year in the first 1–2 years of life, reaches its nadir (< 1%) at about age 10, hovers around 1–3% until age 35 or so, and then climbs exponentially (i.e., doubling every 7 years or so).

The mortality risk is completely different for the third birth cohort (1951–1955), born 100 years later. Mortality in the perinatal period for this cohort is <1%, the mortality nadir is again around age 10 (as it is in all human populations) but is well under 1/1000, and mortality

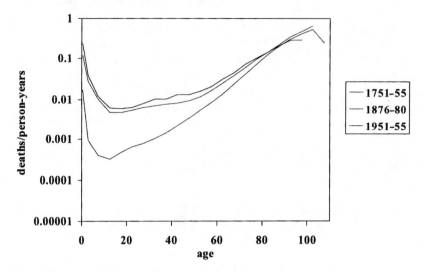

FIGURE 3.2 Death Rates by Age for Swedish Females, Selected Periods.

Source: Prepared by Shiro Horiuchi, using Human Mortality Database, http://www.mortality.org (Horiuchi, S. Age patterns of mortality. In P. Demeny & G. McNicoll (Eds.), *Encyclopedia of Human Population,* Farmington Hills, MI: MacMillan Reference, 2003).

risk does not reach 1% until age 60 or so. At every age, except perhaps when people reach their 80s, mortality for the most recent birth cohort is vastly lower than it is in the prior cohorts.

It is useful as well to plot the distribution of deaths by age for the three cohorts. Figure 3.3 is a plot of their ages at death. It shows what proportion of deaths occurred at each age across the lifespan. For the eighteenth and nineteenth century birth cohorts, a relatively high risk of death prevails at all ages. Certainly, there are modes at both very young and very old ages, but high numbers of people are also dying at all ages across the life span. With the more recent twentieth century birth cohort, the age distribution of deaths is quite different. Here deaths are concentrated at the oldest ages, as shown in a large shift to the right in the distribution of deaths. The vast majority of deaths now occur in people over age 60. Aside from perinatal mortality, mortality linked to trauma, and a low level of chronic and infectious disease at young and middle age, almost all deaths are concentrated in the 60–100 year-old group, presumably reflecting the effect of long-term chronic diseases.

If we add an even more recent birth cohort and plot its age distribution at death, as Figure 3.4 does, we see that this trend continues into

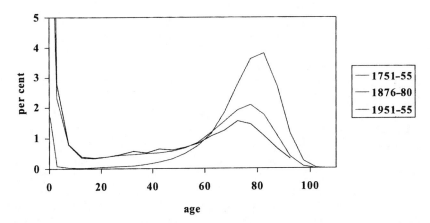

FIGURE 3.3 Age Distribution of Deaths for Swedish Females, Selected Periods.

Source: Prepared by Shiro Horiuchi, using Human Mortality Database, http://www.mortality.org (Horiuchi, S. Age patterns of mortality. In P. Demeny & G. McNicoll (Eds.), *Encyclopedia of Human Population,* Farmington Hills, MI: MacMillan Reference, 2003).

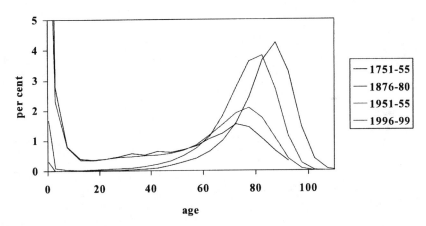

FIGURE 3.4 Age Distribution of Deaths for Swedish Females, Selected Periods.

Source: Prepared by Shiro Horiuchi, using Human Mortality Database, http://www.mortality.org (Horiuchi, S. Age patterns of mortality. In P. Demeny & G. McNicoll (Eds.), *Encyclopedia of Human Population,* Farmington Hills, MI: MacMillan Reference, 2003).

our own era. The age distribution of death for Swedish women born from 1996 to 1999 is pushed even further to the right and is even more clearly unimodal. Almost all deaths are concentrated in later life, with a mode above age 80. These data suggest we have not yet reached a limit to the increasingly greater concentration of deaths at later and later ages.

Wilmoth and Horiuchi (1999) present these data in an alternative form that captures this transition in mortality risk extremely well. Again, using data available from Sweden over the past 250 years, they calculated the interquartile range for age at death. The interquartile range specifies the age range for the middle 50% of people dying in a given year. To establish this range, we begin with the complete distribution of ages at death and establish the ages at which the youngest and oldest 25% of deaths occur. The middle 25%–75% of ages at death, then, represents the upper and lower age at death for the interquartile range, which is expressed as the difference in these ages. Wilmoth and Horiuchi tracked changes in this interquartile range over two and a half centuries for Swedish men and women, as shown in Figure 3.5.

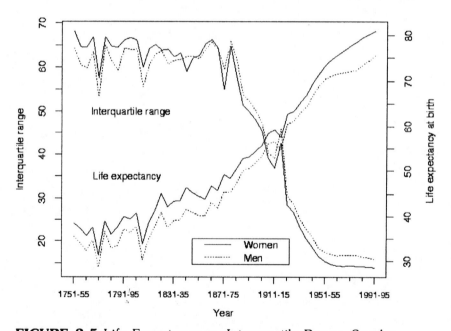

FIGURE 3.5 Life Expectancy vs. Interquartile Range, Sweden.

Source: J. R. Wilmoth and S. Horiuchi (1999). Rectangularization revisited: Variability of age at death within human populations. *Demography* 36:475–495, 1999. Reprinted, with permission, Population Association of America.

In Figure 3.5, the interquartile range for age at death is shown on the left axis and life expectancy at birth on the right. Until 1871–1875, the interquartile range for age at death extended across almost the entire lifespan, both for men and women. It remained steady at about 65 years, showing that 50% of people died within an age range as wide as 5–70 years of age, say, or 2–67. Starting in 1871, this range began to narrow, dropping from 65 to only 15 years in less than 100 years. Thus, in 1951 the middle 50% of deaths occurred in people in a much narrower age band, from 65–80 or perhaps 60–75. One consequence of the epidemiologic transition, then, is for the age at death to become increasingly compressed and pushed out to older ages. While some people have always died at late ages, the likelihood now is for most people to die at later and later ages. As Wilmoth and Horiuchi (1999) summarize, "Death has always been certain, but certainty regarding the timing of death has varied widely in historical perspective" (p. 494).

EPIDEMIOLOGIC TRANSITION II: INCREASING LIFE EXPECTANCY

This later age at death is shown by the axis on the right in Figure 3.5: life expectancy at birth. Over the same time period, life expectancy increased from 35 to greater than 75 years. Indeed, Swedish females born between 1991 and 1995 have life expectancies at birth of 80+ years, a pattern typical of countries that have completed the epidemiologic transition, such as Japan, the United States, Israel, and nations of western Europe.

Increases in life expectancy over time are visible in the shifting position of survival curves. These curves display the proportion of people surviving until progressively greater ages. That is, of 100% alive at birth, we track the proportion still alive at every age, for example at ages 1, 10, 50, and beyond, until all members of the birth cohort have died. In low-mortality, low-fertility societies that have completed the demographic transition, its characteristic form is flat (after a small decline in the perinatal period), with nearly 100% survival until age 40 or so. After this age, the curve declines steeply. This pattern reflects the increased mortality risk associated with greater age (Kirkwood, 1985). With increasing life expectancy, these curves shift upward and to the right, as shown in Figure 3.6, and assume an increasingly rectangular form.

One way to mark this shift is to examine the age at which half a population has already died. The survival curve for people born in

52   *Public Health and Aging*

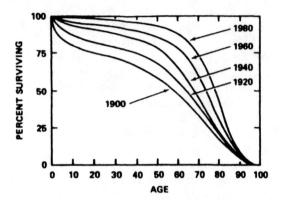

FIGURE 3.6 Changes in Survivorship Curves in the United States in the Twentieth Century.

Reprinted with permission from J. F. Fries and L. M. Crapo, *Vitality and Aging* (San Francisco: W. H. Freeman, 1981).

1900 in the U.S., the lowest curve in the figure, shows that half of Americans (as indicated by the 50% mark on the ordinate) were dead by age 56 or so. For later birth cohorts, this age steadily increased, indicating that a greater and greater number of people survived to older ages. In 1920, the 50% mark was reached at age 64; in 1940, at age 68; in 1960, at age 72; and in 1980, at about age 78.

As suggested earlier, with each successive birth cohort, survival curves appear increasingly rectangular, suggesting that survival may be approaching some kind of maximum, biologically-driven life span (Fries, 1983), though this remains controversial. Deaths are pushed to increasingly later ages, allowing successive birth cohorts to live more years in the aggregate, or otherwise said, to accumulate an increasing number of person-years over the life span. The total person-years lived by the cohort is simply the sum of the number of years lived by each person in the cohort. As mentioned in chapter 2, by convention, standard life table models begin with the birth of 100,000 people. The total person-year measure is obtained by summing across ages at death until the oldest survivor dies. The survival curve indicates this total person-year aggregate. It is the area under the curve. Thus, the area between adjacent curves in Figure 3.6 represents the additional person-years lived by each successive cohort.

While we cannot give a full description of lifetable functions here (see Pollard, Yosuf & Pollard. 1974 for an excellent account), life expectancy is such a function and cannot be understood without at least a basic familiarity with the lifetable. Essentially, the stationary lifetable model applies the mortality risk prevailing at a given time to a birth cohort, say, the 100,000 people born at this time. Mortality rates for each age are then applied to the cohort. An abridged lifetable for the United States in 1988 is shown in Table 3.1.

The function $_nq_x$ is simply the mortality rate for each age group in that year. Plotting $_nq_x$ on the ordinate and age on the x-axis reveals the bathtub or j-shaped curve typical of mortality for human populations: a small but sharp upturn in the perinatal period, a decline that reaches its nadir at ages 5–15, and a slow but steady increase after this age.

The function l_x is the number of people entering each age interval; by convention the starting number, or radix, is usually 100,000. The number of people entering each age interval reflects the number of deaths in the prior interval.

The function $_nd_x$ is the number of people dying in each age interval. If we multiply the mortality rate $(_nq_x)$ by the number of people entering each age interval (l_x), we obtain the number of deaths. The number of people dying in each age interval is subtracted from the total and yields the number of people surviving to enter the next interval.

The function $_nL_x$ is the number of person-years lived by the cohort in each age interval. The total number of person-years is the product of l_x and the number of years that define the age interval (1 year in a standard lifetable; 5 years in the abridged lifetable shown in Table 3.1, with the exception of the first year of life). In calculating $_nL_x$ we need to make an assumption about the timing of death. Did people die at the beginning or end of the age interval? This assumption clearly affects the total person-years contributed by the cohort in the age interval. By convention, we assume that people die in the middle of the age interval, except for the 0–1 age interval, which demands more sophisticated treatment because most deaths are concentrated near the time of birth.

The function T_x is the sum of $_nL_x$. It is the total number of person-years lived by the birth cohort in the given age interval and in all subsequent ones. Thus, the T_x entry in the first row of the lifetable is the sum down the column of all $_nL_x$ entries and gives the total number of person-years lived by the birth cohort, 7,494,642 years. The second row T_x value shows that cohort members who survived the first year of life lived a total of 7,395,495 years. People who survived to age 85 lived a total of 179,948 person-years in this and subsequent years until the last person died.

If we divide T_x by l_x in any given age interval, we obtain e^x, life expectancy at a given age. Thus, life expectancy at birth for the U.S. population in 1980 was 7,494,642/100,000, or 74.9 years. Life expectancy at age 50 was 28.6 years; people who survived to age 50 had a life expectancy of 78.6 years. Similarly, life expectancy at age 80 was 8.1 years; people who survived to age 80 had a life expectancy of 88.1 years.

TABLE 3.1 Abridged Life Tables by *Race* and *Sex*: United States, 1988

Age Interval	Proportion Dying	Of 100,000 Born Alive		Stationary Population		Average Remaining Lifetime
Period of Life between two exact ages stated in years, race, and sex	Proportion of persons alive at beginning of age interval dying during interval	Number living at beginning of age Interval	Number dying during age	In the age interval	In this and all subsequent age intervals	Average number of years of life remaining at beginning of age interval
(1) x to $x + n$	(2) $_nq_x$	(3) l_x	(4) $_nd_x$	(5) $_nL_x$	(6) T_x	(7) e_x
ALL RACES						
0–1	.0100	100,000	999	99,147	7,494,642	74.9
1–5	.0020	99,001	198	395,540	7,395,495	74.7
5–10	.0012	98,803	120	493,688	6,999,955	70.8
10–15	.0014	98,683	134	493,155	6,506,267	65.9
15–20	.0044	98,649	431	491,767	6,013,112	61.0
20–25	.0058	98,118	565	489,206	5,521,345	56.3
25–30	.0061	97,553	696	486,274	5,032,139	51.6
30–35	.0074	96,957	717	483,035	4,545,865	46.9
35–40	.0096	96,240	924	479,021	4,062,830	42.2
40–45	.0126	95,316	1,204	473,785	3,583,809	37.6
45–50	.0189	94,112	1,777	466,443	3,110,024	33.0
50–55	.0300	92,335	2,766	455,194	2,643,581	28.6
55–60	.0473	89,569	4,298	437,869	2,188,387	24.4
60–65	.0728	85,831	6,208	411,976	1,750,628	20.5
65–70	.1055	79,123	8,344	375,656	1,338,552	16.9
70–75	.1568	70,779	11,096	327,120	962,896	13.6
75–80	.2288	59,683	13,654	265,113	636,776	10.7
80–85	.3445	46,029	15,858	190,715	370,663	8.1
85 and over ..	1.0000	30.171	30,171	179.948	179,948	6.0

TABLE 3.1 (continued).

MALE

Age						
0–1	.0100	100,000	999	99,147	7,494,642	74.9
0–1	.0110	100,000	1,104	99	7,150,218	71.5
1–5	.0022	98,896	220	395,074	7,051,163	71.3
5–10	.0014	98,676	138	403,003	6,666,089	67.5
10–15	.0017	98,598	165	492,389	6,163,086	62.5
15–20	.0062	98,373	615	490,489	5,670,697	57.6
20–25	.0087	97,758	854	486,701	5,180,208	53.0
25–30	.0089	96,904	865	482,334	4,693,507	48.4
30–35	.0107	96,030	1,024	477,665	4,211,173	43.8
35–40	.0134	96,015	1,275	472,046	3,733,508	39.3
40–45	.0170	93,739	1,592	464,990	3,261,462	34.8
45–50	.0246	92,147	2281	456,603	2,796,472	30.3
50–55	.0385	89,886	3,457	441,337	2,340,989	26.0
55–60	.0610	86,429	6,273	419,704	1,899,632	22.0
60–65	.0941	81,156	7,839	387,689	1,479,928	18.2
65–70	.1360	73,517	9,996	343,533	1,092,259	14.9
70–75	.2022	63,521	12.842	286,233	748,726	11.8
75–80	.2931	50,679	14.852	216,396	462,493	9.1
80–85	.4239	35,827	15,189	140,288	246,097	6.9
86 and over	1.0000	20,638	20,638	105,809	105,809	5.1

FEMALE

Age						
0–1	.0089	100,000	890	99,243	7,831,495	78.3
1–6	.0018	99,110	175	396,021	7,732,252	78.0
5–10	.0010	98,936	101	494,400	7,336,231	74.2
10–15	.0010	98,834	100	493,954	6,841,831	69.2
15–20	.0024	90,734	240	493,108	6,347,877	64.3
20–25	.0028	98,494	272	491,802	5,854,769	59.4
25–30	.0033	98,222	321	490,324	5,362,967	54.6
30–35	.0041	97,901	405	488,539	4,872,643	49.8

TABLE 3.1 (continued).

Age Interval	Proportion Dying	Of 100,000 Born Alive		Stationary Population		Average Remaining Lifetime
Period of Life between two exact ages stated in years, race, and sex	Proportion of persons alive at beginning of age interval dying during interval	Number living at beginning of age Interval	Number dying during age	In the age interval	In this and all subsequent age intervals	Average number of years of life remaining at beginning of age interval
(1) x to $x+n$	(2) $_nq_x$	(3) l_x	(4) $_nd_x$	(5) $_nL_x$	(6) T_x	(7) e_x
FEMALE						
35–40	.0058	97,496	687	486,163	4,384,104	45.0
40–45	.0084	96,929	817	482,754	3,897,941	40.2
45–50	.0135	96,112	1,293	477,562	3,415,187	35.5
50–55	.0219	94,819	2,077	469,225	2,937,626	31.0
55–60	.0347	92,742	3,217	456,141	2,468,400	26.6
60–65	.0637	89,525	4,810	436,300	2,012,259	22.5
65–70	.0793	84,715	6,716	407,664	1,575,959	18.6
70–75	.1210	77,999	9,435	367,619	1,168,295	15.0
75–80	.1843	68,564	12,640	312,711	800,676	11.7
80–85	.2981	55,924	16,671	239,106	487,965	8.7
85 and over	1.0000	39,253	39,253	248,859	248,859	6.3

Source: National Center for Health Statistics.

56

Life expectancy, then, is simply the total number of person-years lived by a birth cohort divided by the number of people in the cohort. It is the average number of years a person can expect to live, given his current age—with, we must hasten to add, all the assumptions that go into the stationary-population lifetable model. The major assumption in these models is a fixed mortality rate; the models assume that prevailing mortality rates do not change over the life span of the cohort. They also assume a fixed birth cohort, with no loss or gain to immigration. As Table 3.1 shows, life expectancy at birth does not mean that everyone dies by this age, or that everyone can expect to live to this age. It is simply the aggregate number of person-years lived by the birth cohort divided by the number of people who make up this cohort.

Increased life expectancy is the product first of reductions in perinatal mortality, second of improvements in health and living conditions in the first half of the lifespan, and only most recently of improvements in medical care for older people. For example, in the nineteenth century control over infectious disease in childhood (leading to reduction in perinatal and child mortality) and a shift away from manual labor (resulting in major improvements in health and living conditions in midlife) already led to an increase in life expectancy and reduction in disability in later life (Costa, 2000). The life-extending technologies of modern medicine and the more effective adult and geriatric medicine available today have had a more modest impact on life expectancy. Olshansky, Carnes and Cassel (1990), for example, have shown through simulations that even complete elimination of cancer, cardiovascular disease, and diabetes (an unlikely prospect) would raise life expectancy no higher than age 86.4 for men and 94.1 for women.

As the lifetable in Table 3.1 shows, life expectancy calculations depend heavily on perinatal and childhood mortality. Deaths at the earliest ages lower a cohort's life expectancy severely. These early deaths remove people from the cohort before they can contribute any person-years to the cohort's survival experience. Thus, with high infant mortality, as is typical of the high-mortality, high-fertility countries that have not yet undergone the demographic transition, life expectancy will be low and never rise above the fourth or fifth decade. However, in these societies people who survive childhood can still expect to live to old and even very old ages. In South Asian countries, for example, life expectancy is much lower than that of North America and European societies. Yet India still had about 47 million people aged 65+ and 6 million aged 80+ in 2000, despite a life expectancy (62.5 years) nearly 20 years lower than the 80.0 years typical of these societies. Life expectancy in Zimbabwe in 2000 was 42.6 years; yet even here over 400,000 people lived to age 65+. Thus, a society with low life expectancy may still suffer an epidemic of the chronic diseases of late life.

EPIDEMIOLOGIC TRANSITION III:
POPULATION AGING

One last consequence of the reduction of fertility and mortality characteristic of the demographic transition is population aging: a narrowing of the base of the age-sex pyramid and an increase in the number of people at older ages. Demographic indicators of population aging include an increase in the median age of a population, a greater proportion of people aged 65+, and a more equal distribution of the population across age strata. Hence the transformation of the age-sex pyramid into an age-sex rectangle or pillar.

In 2000, Japan and the European societies were the oldest populations. In Italy, 18.2% of the population was aged 65+, making it the oldest population in the world. Sweden (17.2%), Greece (17.2%), Belgium (17.1%), and Japan (17.0%) were close behind (U.S. Census Bureau, International Data Base, 2002). With 12.4% of its population aged 65+, the United States was not in this league. However, with current demographic trends, most of the developed nations will have increasingly older populations. In the more developed countries, the proportion of the population aged 65+ will approach 20% (Manton, Suzman & Willis, 1992).

The same trend is at work in the less developed countries. Figure 3.7 shows the transformation in age structure underway in Pakistan. In the 25 years separating the first two panels of Figure 3.7, the proportion of the population aged 65+ will rise from 4.1% to 5.6%, 5.8 to 12.0 million people. In this period, life expectancy will also rise from 61.1 to 69.8 years. The major engine of this demographic transformation is declining fertility. In the same period, the number of births per 1000 women will decline from 32 to 6, and completed fertility will drop from 4.6 children per woman to 2.3 (U.S. Census Bureau, International Data Base, 2002). With fewer children born, the base of the age-sex pyramid shrinks and the mean (or median) age of the population must rise, since people already alive continue to age. If this trend continues, as is expected, all of the world's populations will eventually have the same pillar-like shape.

AGING AND RISK OF DEATH

Earlier, we noted that most of the rise in life expectancy is due not to medical advances, but rather to improvements in public health and living conditions. For example, between 1820 and 1920 mortality in

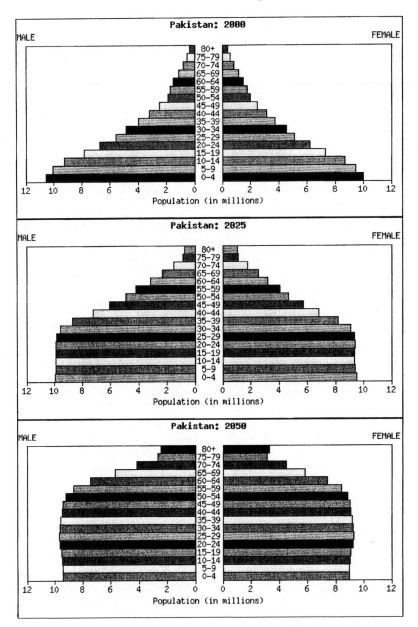

FIGURE 3.7 Age-Sex Pyramids, Pakistan, 2000, 2025, 2050.

Source: U.S. Census Bureau, International Data Base, 2000. http://www.census.gov/cgi-bin/ipc/idbpyrs.pl?cty=pk&out=s&ymax=250

Table 3.2 Rates of Mortality Due to Tuberculosis, Males, Massachusetts

Age	Year of Observation				
	1900	1910	1920	1930	1940
40–49	253	253	175	118	86
50–59	267	252	171	127	92
60–69	304	246	172	95	109
70+	343	163	127	95	79

Source: Pollard, Yusef, & Pollard, 1974.

New York City dropped from 30 to 10 per 1000 (Mausner & Kramer, 1985). Improvements in sanitation reduced deaths from cholera, typhus, and diphtheria, all when medicine was still rather primitive. Death rates in this early period also declined among older people, as shown in Table 3.2 and plotted in Figure 3.8.

In the time-specific lifetable, table entries are the age-specific death rates for a series of successive birth cohorts. Row entries indicate age and columns year of observation. The experience of each birth cohort is summarized in the diagonals of the table. Thus, people who were 40–49 in 1900 were 50–59 in 1910, 60–69 in 1920, and 70–79 in

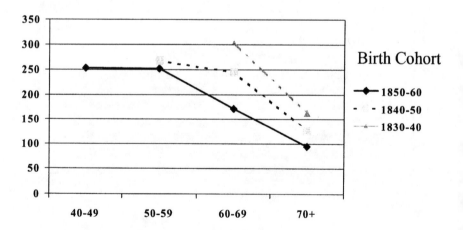

FIGURE 3.8 Plot of Cohort Mortality from Tuberculosis: Age-Specific Mortality, Tuberculosis (males, Massachusetts).
Source: Pollard, Yusuf, & Pollard, 1974.

1930. They were born between 1850 and 1860. The prior cohort was 50–59 in 1900, 60–69 in 1910, 70–79 in 1920, and accordingly born between 1840–1850. If we plot these mortality rates by birth cohort, an important finding emerges that would not be evident from plots of the row or column entries alone. Mortality from tuberculosis in Massachusetts men in the first part of the century declined with each successive birth cohort, even at the oldest ages. The risk of dying from tuberculosis was lower at every age.

These data should be kept in mind when examining the declining death rate in late life in the last half century. Earlier, we saw that mortality rises with age, such that the risk of death approaches 35% and even 50% per year for people aged 80+. Yet between 1950 and 2000 the rate of death has declined for people aged 80+. This decline is shown in Figure 3.9 for England and Wales, France, Sweden, and Japan. Between 1950 and 1990 death rates declined from 170 to 90 per 1000 (Vaupel, 1997). Stratifying by age and plotting death rates by year shows that death rates fell even for people aged 90 and 95.

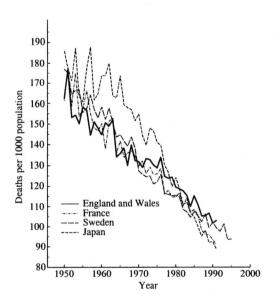

FIGURE 3.9 Improvements in Mortality from 1911–1991 in England & Wales for Females Ages 85, 90, and 95.

Source: compiled by author from data in the Kannisto-Thatcher oldest-old database, Odense University, Odense, Denmark. Reprinted with permission, The Royal Society, Vaupel, 1997.

Why should death rates in the oldest-old be declining? Some of the decline is likely due to medical advances applied specifically to the diseases of the very old. Most of it is likely due to improvements in health and living conditions over the whole lifespan. The latter changes appear to have allowed a subset of people with some kind of long-life genetic endowment—"longevity genes"—to reach old age. While this genotype must have always been present in a subset of the human population, only in the twentieth century have health and living conditions improved to the point where accidental mortality (such as death from trauma or infection) has been controlled well enough for substantial numbers to reach later life.

Recent empirical investigation of aging and mortality has confirmed this heterogeneity in populations. Carey, Liedo, Muller, Wang, and Vaupel (1998) and colleagues followed 1.2 million medflies born at the same time (whose median survival is about 15 days) in a controlled environment. They carefully recorded deaths each day and established death rates at every age (i.e., day). Figures 3.10a and b present results from this study.

Figure 3.10a shows a single mode for deaths at around the 15–day mark, and the vast majority of medflies were dead by age 45. However,

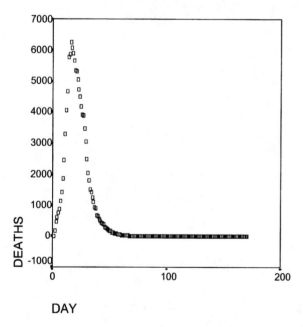

FIGURE 3–10a. Medfly Survival: Number Dying by Follow-Up Day.
Source: Carey, Liedo, Orzco, & Vaupel, 1992.

Log of Mortality Rate by Day

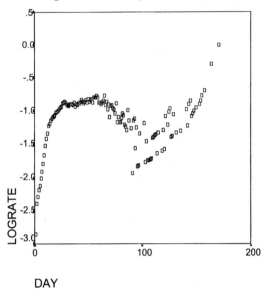

DAY

FIGURE 3–10b. Mortality Rate by Age, Medflies: Log of Mortality Rate by Day.
Source: Carey, Liedo, Orzco, & Vaupel, 1992.

a small number lived much longer; in fact, the last member of this birth cohort died at 151 days. Such unexpected longevity suggests heterogeneity in genetic endowment. A second finding was unexpectedly strange behavior in the relation between age and mortality risk in this small set of long-lived survivors. As shown in Figure 3.10b, which plots the log of the mortality rate against age, this rate increased with age in exponential fashion only up to a certain age; after that it leveled off, declined, and even behaved quite chaotically. Medflies who survived to extreme old ages actually faced a declining mortality risk.

A DEMOGRAPHIC PORTRAIT OF THE OLDEST OLD IN AMERICA

We conclude this chapter with a brief demographic portrait of the "oldest old" in the United States. The oldest old are typically defined as people aged 85+ (Hadley, 1992). These are some of the characteristics of this group:

- They are high consumers of custodial care, with 25% residing in nursing homes and another 25% receiving paid, or formal, home care. Yet even in this age group 50% live in the community and report no need for help in daily personal care activities.
- They are the fastest growing segment of the older population in the U.S.; in fact, the U.S. will have the largest number of oldest old of any country in the next 50 years. This is a paradox because the U.S. will not have the most elderly (age 65+).
- They are largely female: the sex ratio (number of men per 100 women) is expected to decline from 75.4 (1930) to 59.9 (2050). Men are more likely to live in a family setting (59%) than women (37%).
- They are largely white (2.8/3.0 million in 1990), but note that people aged 65+ are becoming increasingly more racially diverse.
- They are less likely now than in the past to have family caregivers. Familial-aged dependency ratios (persons 85+/persons 65–69) are increasing (12 in 1950 to 88 in 2050).
- They are largely widowed: 82% of 85+ women in 1980 were widowed compared to 33% among women aged 65–69. Half of men age 85+ are widowed.
- In the 1990s they were largely a low income group, especially if female and living alone (73% of this group were living below the poverty index).
- They are increasing well educated. Educational attainment in this group has increased dramatically: 29.1% completed high school in 1985, and 63% of this age group is expected to have completed high school in 2015.
- Fewer women in this age group will be childless, compared to the young-old, though few will also have 5+ offspring. This may affect the availability of family caregivers. (Hadley, 1992)

SUMMARY

Aging Populations and Alteration of Shape of Age-Sex Pyramid. In most societies, the age-sex "pyramid" is now less a pyramid than an emerging rectangle or pillar, the typical shape for countries that have completed the demographic transition, in which an equilibrium of high mortality and fertility is replaced by one of low mortality and fertility.

"Support" and "Dependency Ratios." Comparing people aged 18–64 to people aged 65+ yields the so-called "support ratio," which was 5:1 in the United States in 2000. In fact, only a minority of people aged 65+, about 20%, can be considered dependent, at least according to need for help in one or more of the personal self-maintenance activities or activities of daily living, and this proportion has declined between 1983 and 1999. Increasingly, people aged 65+ are not retiring in the traditional sense, continue to provide increasingly large intergenerational transfers of resources to their children aged 18–64, and contribute to child-rearing support for grandchildren.

Historical Changes in the Age Distribution of Deaths. Over the past 250 years, deaths have become increasingly concentrated at the oldest ages. In societies that have completed the demographic transition, the vast majority of deaths now occur in people over age 60. This change is evident in the increasingly rectangular shape of survival curves.

Increases in Life expectancy. Life expectancy is the total number of person-years lived by a birth cohort divided by the number of people in the cohort. It is the average number of years a person can expect to live, given his current age, assuming a fixed birth cohort and no change in mortality rates over the life span of the cohort. Life expectancy at birth does not mean that everyone dies by this age, or that everyone can expect to live to this age. Life expectancy calculations depend heavily on infant mortality. Thus, even in societies with low life expectancies, a large number of people who survive the perinatal and childhood periods can expect to reach old age.

Older Populations. In 2000, Japan and the European societies were the oldest populations. In Italy, 18.2% of the population was aged 65+, making it the oldest population in the world; Sweden (17.2%), Greece (17.2%), Belgium (17.1%), and Japan (17.0%) were close behind. In the more developed countries, the proportion of the population aged 65+ will approach 20% by 2050 (Manton, Suzman, & Willis, 1992). The same trend is at work in the less developed countries.

Declining Risk of Death Over Successive Birth Cohorts. In the time-specific lifetable, table entries are the age-specific deaths rates for a series of successive birth cohorts. Row entries indicate age and columns year of observation, and the experience of each birth cohort is summarized in the diagonals of the table. Plots of mortality by birth cohort reveal declining aggregate and cause-specific death rates even among older people beginning with the 19th century, before the availability of modern medicine. The trend continues in the latter half of the 20th century, with declining death rates among people aged 80+.

Sources of the Declining Risk of Dying. Why should death rates in the oldest-old be declining? Some of the decline is likely due to medical advances applied specifically to the diseases of the very old. Most of the decline is likely due to improvements in health and living conditions over the whole lifespan. The latter changes appear to have allowed a subset of people with some kind of long-life genetic endowment to reach old age. This genotype must have always been present in a subset of the human population, but only in the 20th century have health and living conditions improved to the point where accidental mortality (such as death from trauma or infection) has been controlled well enough for this genetic potential to be expressed, with substantial numbers now reaching increasingly older ages. For example, in the United States the 2000 Census identified some 50,000 centenarians and 1500 people over the age of 110. The limits of this trend and the true biological maximum life span remain unclear.

4

Mortality

Mortality has already has been discussed in prior chapters, first as the end product of senescence and disease, and second as a key determinant of the age structure of populations. We also examined historical change in the age distribution of deaths, variation in life expectancy across populations, and what these differences may imply about the genetics of aging and likely limits to extension of the human life span. Still, mortality requires more detailed treatment. It is clearly a central outcome in aging and public health, but it is also more complex than usually recognized. Dying in late life almost always includes frailty, multiple diseases, and additional intervening medical events. Once we move beyond simple counts of total or cause-specific mortality to measurement of mortality as a sequence of events over a potentially long period, we are forced to recognize that it is often difficult to state when dying begins and what someone actually died of.

Alzheimer's disease is a case in point. It has a long latency period, perhaps even 20-40 years, over which brain lesions develop. These are the characteristic neuritic plaques and neurofibrillary tangles that obstruct amyloid clearance and that are evident in neuropathologic studies (autopsy confirmation of the disease). At some point in disease progression, these neuropathologic changes begin to affect cognition and motor function. The characteristic cognitive changes include deficits in short-term memory and language; typical motor findings include extrapyramidal signs (slowness, rigidity, tremor) (Stern et al., 1997). When these symptoms become severe enough to interfere with the performance of ordinary daily tasks, such as work, household maintenance, or shopping, the patient has reached a new milestone in disease progression. We say he has made the transition from subclinical to clinical disease; indeed, it is only at this point that a patient typically presents to the internist or neurologist and is diagnosed, perhaps after neuropsychological testing and brain imaging to rule out other causes of dementia. He then goes home to live another 7–8 years, on average, before dying, along the way crossing additional milestones of progressively more severe disability (Stern, et al., 1994). He finally dies during a hospitalization, let's say, after being transferred from a nursing home. He may have been transferred to the hospital because of a pneumonia that did not respond to oral antibiotics, but by this point he likely had already developed a wasting syndrome, severe weakness in the lower extremities, poor skin integrity, and exacerbation of intercurrent heart disease.

Did this man die of pneumonia or wasting, Alzheimer's or heart disease, or some broader complex of aging-related disease? The answer is not obvious.

CAUSES OF DEATH

People die of something, and this "something" is listed on death certificates. Death certificates distinguish between "underlying" or "primary" causes of death and "contributory" causes. "Underlying causes" indicate proximal or immediate conditions that led to the death, while "contributory causes," indicate more distal or remote causes, that is, longstanding chronic conditions that may have played a role in the death. Accordingly, public health surveillance of mortality makes use of underlying cause, contributory cause, or both (total cause) for attributing deaths to disease and tracking changes in cause-specific mortality.

The death certificate also includes information on age, race (as well as Hispanic origin), sex, and residence. Age is rarely missing; well under 1% of death certificates lack information on age at death (Pickle, Mungiole, Jones, & White, 1996). Every death in the United States is recorded on these certificates, which are sent to local departments of health and then to the National Center for Health Statistics. For example, the average number of deaths recorded in the United States over the period 1988-92 was 2,131,977 per year. Heart disease was responsible for 33.9% of the deaths, cancer 23.3%, and stroke 6.7%. The three conditions are the biggest killers of Americans and together account for nearly two-thirds of deaths in any given year. These causes, all chronic diseases that predominantly affect the elderly, should be contrasted with external causes of death, such as injuries (including motor vehicle accidents), suicide, and homicide. Together, these account for just 6.7% of deaths in a year (4.2%, 1.4%, and 1.1%, respectively; Pickle, et al., 1996).

The quality of cause-of-death information on death certificates appears to be good, though some problems have been identified. Currently, a computerized algorithm is used to apply World Health Organization coding for all medical conditions reported. Indicators of quality of cause-of-death information suggest that the system works reasonably well. Exercises in which experts code medical information show high agreement with algorithm assignments. Also, the proportion of certificates with unclassifiable causes of death (residual or nonspecific category of the International Classification of Disease [*ICD-9* categories 780-799]) has declined considerably, while the number of medical conditions reported on death certificates has increased, suggesting increased specificity.

Still, while underlying cause information in death certificates agrees well with hospital records, validity of cause-of-death information is less sure for deaths outside of medical settings (Pickle, Mungiole, Jones, White, 1996), some 40% of all deaths. More generally, when the person completing cause-of-death information does not have a detailed understanding of a person's medical condition, "underlying" and "contributing" causes of death may be confused. Pickle and colleagues illustrate this problem in the case of long-term diabetics. Diabetics are at high risk of death from stroke and heart disease, which are likely to appear on their death certificates. Diabetes, however, is underreported on the death certificate for people who died of stroke or heart disease. The result is an underestimate of the mortality burden of diabetes.

Hadley (1992) has pointed out the difficulty of maintaining the distinction between "underlying" and "contributing" causes of death for the older population. It may not be possible to identify what is "underlying" and what is "contributory" in older people, where multiple pathologies are common and chronic conditions interact in complex ways. What should be listed as the underlying or contributory cause of death in a person who died from a fall or pneumonia but also had longstanding diabetes, osteoporosis and a recent stroke? The more important question is to determine how this set of chronic conditions may have led to the fall or pneumonia, or how these conditions may have made this fall or pneumonia lethal.

More generally, we can ask why longstanding chronic conditions ultimately kill older people. Is the death simply the result of continued progression of the disease? Or is the death the result of greater vulnerability to pathology of a given severity because of frailty or some other chronic condition? Or, finally, is the death actually the result of some new pathology that has emerged because of the person's chronic disease status? It may be difficult to separate these factors in death certificates, which have traditionally not listed chronic conditions as contributory causes of death, or in autopsy series, which are not representative of the universe of deaths.

UNITED STATES DEATH RATE PER 100,000
POPULATION BY AGE, CAUSE, RACE, AND SEX

The *Atlas of United States Mortality* (Pickle et al, 1996) and the yearly compendium on *Deaths, United States, 2000* (CDC, 2002) are key documents for understanding mortality in a society that has already undergone the demographic transition (see chapter 3). Figure 4.1 presents death rates by age, race, and sex for 15 disease conditions, key results from the *Atlas*. The figure plots the rate of death (on a logarithmic scale) against age for each disease condition. Each line in the graph summarizes the experience of four race-by-sex groups (white males, black males, white females, black females).

The graph in the bottom right-hand corner shows all-cause mortality and presents the j-shaped curve mentioned in prior chapters. The death rate is high in the perinatal period and first year of life, reaches its nadir at about age 10, and then increases steadily. Across the four groups, the death rate per 100,000 is about 50 at age 10 and increases to 100 at age 20, 500 at age 40, 1,000 at age 60, and over 10,000 at age 80. A closer look reveals considerable variation across the four groups, with white women showing the lowest rates and black men the highest, but the relationship between age and mortality risk is consistent across the groups.

This j-shaped pattern is sharply defined for many of the cause-specific mortality plots. Heart disease, many of the cancers (for example, lung, prostate, and breast), stroke, pneumonia/influenza, and perhaps liver and chronic obstructive pulmonary disease (COPD) all follow this pattern. Death from these diseases (and also incidence) is strongly related to age and increases across the entire life span. Thus, the risk of stroke mortality begins at about 1 per 100,000 for people aged 20 and increases to 10 at age 40, 100 at age 60, and nearly 1,000 at age 80.

A variant of this pattern is evident for mortality from some of the cancers and liver disease. Mortality from these causes appears to plateau in the sixth decade and perhaps even decline at older ages.

Finally, note the very different pattern for external, accidental causes of death and the special case of suicide. Mortality from unintentional injuries, motor vehicle accidents, homicide, and suicide is highest for young people and reaches its peak at about age 20. Mortality from these causes may continue to increase over the lifespan (unintentional injuries), remain more or less flat (motor vehicle accidents, suicide, firearm suicide), or decline (homicide, firearm homicide).

These broad patterns once again confirm the centrality of age for chronic disease incidence and mortality. The postponement of death to later ages means an increasing mortality burden for chronic disease.

DEATH RATES BY AGE AND SEX: CHANGES OVER THE LAST 50 YEARS

Figure 4.2 shows trends in the crude and age-adjusted death rates over the past half-century or so. The trend in the crude death rate, while declining, vastly underestimates the reduction in mortality in the United States in the twentieth century. Because the U.S. population grew increasingly older over the century (and because age is a risk factor for mortality), it is necessary to standardize the population in each year to ensure that populations of similar age structure are being compared. The age-adjusted death rate includes this correction factor and shows that annual mortality has declined by half over the century, from about 1,100 to less than 500 per 100,000 people.

Disaggregating this trend by age shows that mortality has declined for just about every age group. These trends are shown in Figure 4.3. All three of the oldest age groups show declines in mortality over the past 50 years. In 1950, for example, the death rate per 100,000 was 5,000 for men aged 65-74, 10,000 for men aged 75-84, and 20,000 for men aged 85+. By 1998, these rates were 4,000, 7,500, and about 19,000, respectively. While the largest declines are evident in childhood mortality (especially the under 1–year group), the reduction in late life is also impressive. By all accounts, the downward trend continues. Between 1997 and 1998, for example, mortality in people aged 85+ declined by 4% among white men, 3.4% among black men, 0.4% among white women (who already experienced the lowest mortality in this age group), and 0.9% among black women (CDC, 2000).

An alternative way of measuring this mortality reduction is to look at declines in the years of life lost to disease, given declines in cause-specific mortality. With declines in cause-specific mortality, the number of years of life lost to disease should also decline. We capture this effect of mortality reduction as a decline in "years of potential life lost before age 75." This is the number of years of life these people would have lived, per 100,000 people, if they had not died before age 75 from disease. The total years of life lost to disease was 10,448 in 1980, 9,086 in 1990, and 8,322 in 1996. It has continued to fall about 200-300 person-years per 100,000 people every year, at least through 1998 (National Center for Health Statistics, 2001).

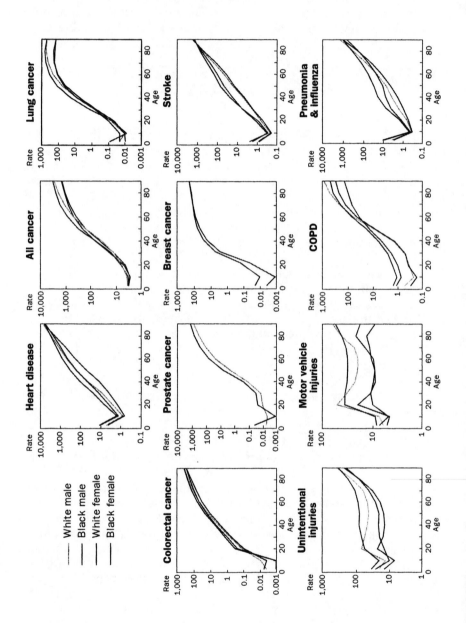

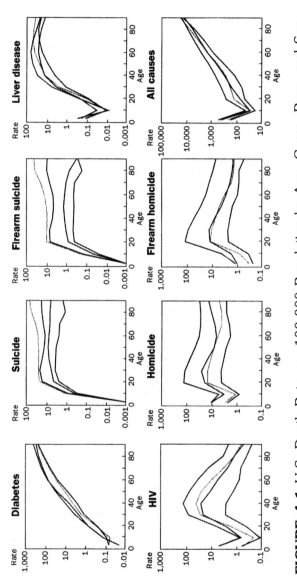

FIGURE 4.1 U.S. Death Rate per 100,000 Population by Age, Cause, Race, and Sex.

Note: For plotting purposes, rates equal to 0 are shown as 0.001 per 100,000 population.

Source: From *Atlas of United States Mortality* by L. W. Pickle, M. Mungiole, G. K. Jones & A. A. White, 1996. Hyattsville, MD: National Center for Health Statistics, p. 15.

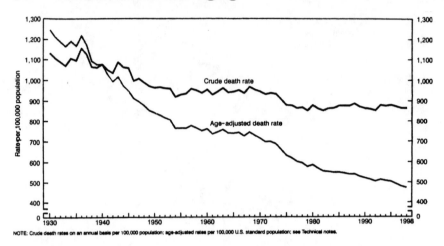

FIGURE 4.2 Crude and Age-Adjusted Death Rates: United States, 1930–1998.

Source: CDC, *Deaths, United States, 2000.* National Vital Statistics Report, Vol. 48, No. 11, P. 4. July 24, 2000. Hyattsville, MD: National Center for Health Statistics.

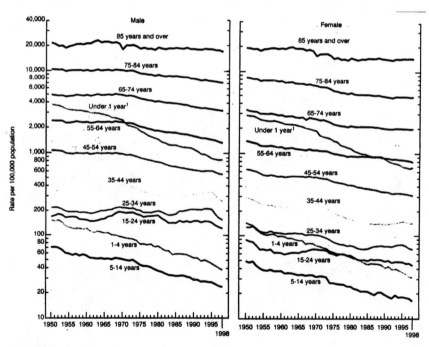

FIGURE 4.3 Death Rates by Age and Sex: United States, 1950–1998.

Source: CDC, *Deaths, United States, 2000.* National Vital Statistics Report, Vol. 48, No. 11, P. 4. July 24, 2000. Hyattsville, MD: National Center for Health Statistics.

This decline in years of potential life lost before age 75 is consistent across diseases and extends to unintentional injuries, suicide, and homicide. Evidently, improvements in health and environment across the life span have pushed the risk of death from disease out to later and later ages, resulting in lower death rates and fewer years of life lost to disease. Also, changes in safety standards (seatbelts, traffic patterns, law enforcement, occupational health efforts) may have helped reduce years of life lost to unintentional injuries. Finally, it may be that the decline in the mortality burden of suicide (392 to 363 years of life lost per 100,000 between 1980 and 1998) may be due at least in part to improved mental health services and broader changes in help-seeking patterns.

CHANGES IN RANK ORDER OF CAUSES OF DEATH AT OLDER AGES

In 1980, 1,341,848 people aged 65+ died. The ten most prevalent causes of death were heart disease, cancer, stroke, pneumonia and influenza, chronic obstructive pulmonary disease, atherosclerosis, diabetes, unintentional injuries, kidney disease, and liver disease. Heart disease, cancer, and stroke together accounted for 74.5% of these deaths.

In 1999, 1,797,451 people aged 65+ died (remember that there were many more people aged 65+ in 1999 compared to 1980, so that this absolute increase actually represents a smaller proportion of people aged 65+). The ten leading causes of death were much the same, with heart disease, cancer, and stroke again accounting for the preponderance of deaths (now 63.8%). However, atherosclerosis and liver disease no longer appeared as leading causes of death in 1999. They were replaced by Alzheimer's disease (seventh place) and septicemia (tenth place).

It is hard to know what to make of these changes. Surely people had, and died from, Alzheimer's disease in 1980. Part of the change can be attributed to revision in coding conventions (the shift from *ICD-9* to *ICD-10* coding between 1980 and 1999), and part to public recognition of Alzheimer's disease as a cause of death in its own right. These nonmedical factors must be considered when interpreting vital statistics.

SOCIOECONOMIC STATUS AND MORTALITY RISK

Educational attainment, typically measured by how many years of school someone has completed early in life, as well as other indicators of socioeconomic status (SES) (income, wealth, race, ethnicity, occupation),

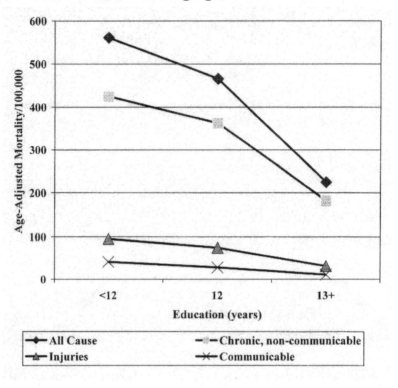

FIGURE 4.4 Education and Cause-Specific Mortality, 1998: Ages 25–64.

Source: Based on data from: CDC, *Deaths, United States 2000.* National Vital Statistics Reports, Vol. 48, No. 11. July 24, 2000. Hyattsville, MD: National Center for Health Statistics.

are strong predictors of disparities in late-life disability, health status, and mortality risk. What is true for education applies to all socioeconomic indicators.

Figure 4.4 shows the effect of early educational attainment on mortality for people aged 25-64; the yearly compendium of U.S. mortality does not provide this breakdown for people aged 65+. Mortality per 100,000 people is shown for all-cause mortality and for non-communicable chronic disease, communicable disease, and injury. Mean mortality risk is shown for people who did not complete high school (<12 years), for people who completed high school (12 years), and for people who had schooling beyond high school (13+ years).

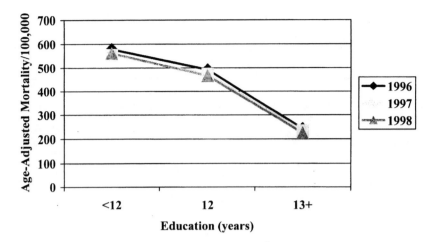

FIGURE 4.5 Education and All-Cause Mortality, 1996–1998, Ages 25–64.

Source: Based on data from: CDC, *Deaths, United States 2000.* National Vital Statistics Reports, Vol. 48, No. 11. July 24, 2000. Hyattsville, MD: National Center for Health Statistics.

Mortality in this age group is strongly related to educational attainment. People who have completed one or more years of post-high school education face about half the risk of dying evident in people who did not complete high school. The same difference in risk appears for all three of the cause-specific mortality measures. This similar risk difference, evident across such very different sources of mortality, suggests that education lowers mortality in some general way. It is associated with reductions in risk behaviors (i.e., smoking, multiple sex partners, driving while intoxicated) linked to all three sources of mortality, with more effective health-seeking behaviors once disease becomes apparent, and with greater wealth and hence access to medical care.

This difference in mortality risk by educational attainment persists despite a more general decline in U.S. mortality, as shown in Figure 4.5. Figure 4.5 plots all-cause mortality by education group for three years; 1996-1998. Mortality has declined for all three of the education groups, but the gap between the groups has not narrowed.

Elo and Preston (1996) have shown that this relationship holds in late life as well, though it is slightly attenuated. They examined death rates per 1000 in the period 1979–85, breaking out mortality risk by age (25–64, 65–89) and gender. They treated education more carefully than most studies. The plots for the older age group are shown as Figure 4-6, which show age-standardized adjusted risk.

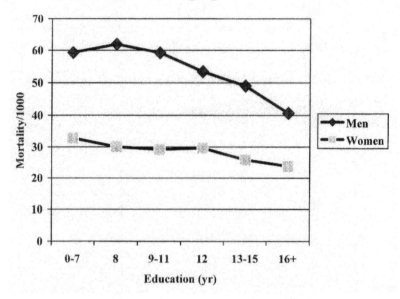

FIGURE 4.6 Mortality Risk, U.S., Aged 65–89, 1979–1985.
After Elo & Preston, 1996.

These results clearly show the protective effect of early education on late-life mortality. Women have an advantage at every educational level, but men and women each face lower mortality risk with increasing education. An education gradient applies across the entire range of education but becomes most pronounced with completion of high school and more advanced schooling.

Not shown is the comparable figure for people aged 25-64. At younger ages, however, the education effect is even stronger, as might be expected because education has greater scope to affect death rates (which, on the whole, are much lower). Relative to men with high school education, men in the younger age group with 16+ years of school face a mortality risk of 0.67 and men in the older age group a mortality risk of 0.76. For women, the comparable risk ratios are 0.84 and 0.80, respectively. These data show that the protective effect of education is indeed attenuated in late life.

Still, given the great significance of education for mortality risk and the increasingly educated older population, it is interesting to imagine postponement of mortality from this factor alone, apart from improvements in medical care. Figure 4.7 shows the increasing proportion of women by birth cohort, who have completed high school. As the figure shows, over 30 years (comparing women born between 1916 and

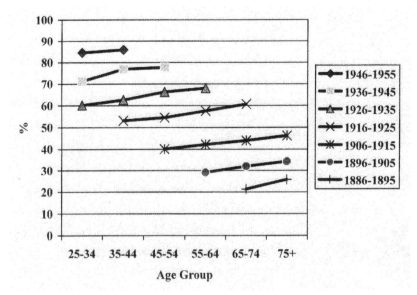

FIGURE 4.7 Proportion Completing High School, by Birth Cohort, U.S. Women.
Source: Based on data from: Daphne Spain and Suzanne M. Bianchi, *Balancing Act.* Table 3.1. 1996. New York: Russell Sage Foundation.

1925 and 1946 and 1955), the proportion completing high school increased from 55% to 85%. We can expect an increasingly educated older population to have a very different experience of health and dying in coming decades.

CHANGES IN DISEASE-SPECIFIC MORTALITY AMONG BIRTH COHORTS

The cohort analysis model described in chapter 2 allows further insight on declining mortality at older ages. Manton (1992) has analyzed birth certificate information from successive birth cohorts to show that mortality from specific diseases, whether indexed by underlying cause or total-mention data, has been declining in some cases even at very late ages. Mortality rates for six white male cohorts, all born between 1884 and 1888 and 1909 and 1913, were plotted against age group. In this way, he examined differences in mortality in people of the same age who were born at different times. Declines in mortality at late age in these birth cohorts may indicate changes in exposure to risk factors earlier in life. Manton (1992) suggests that these changes may also indicate changes in the basic disease process, for example, slower progression.

Figure 4.8a reproduces Manton's cohort plot for total mention occurrences of cerebrovascular disease, and Figure 4.8b for underlying cause occurrences. The plots show lower mortality from cerebrovascular disease at each age across the successive birth cohorts. For example, people born from 1899 to 1903 and 1904 to 1908 reached ages 75-79 in 1974-1978 and 1979-1983, respectively. Mortality from cerebrovascular disease was much lower in the more recent cohort, as the figures show. This trend is true for other adjacent birth cohorts who reached comparable ages.

These results suggest that cause-specific mortality is truly declining for some (but, of course, not all) of the major diseases of late life. The results imply that deaths from these conditions are being postponed to later ages, either because people contract the disease at later ages or because they are living longer with it. Or it may be that people are dying of other causes, but again these deaths also appear to be postponed to later ages, since most of the major diseases show similar reductions in mortality across adjacent birth cohorts. Of course, postponement of disease to later ages is preferable to living longer with disease. Both outcomes are consistent with reduction in mortality in

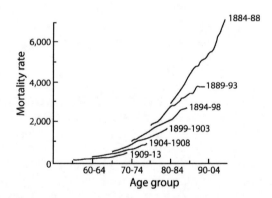

FIGURE 4.8a Cohort Plot of Six White Male Cohorts Born 1884–1888 to 1909–1913 for Total Mention Occurrences of Cerebrovascular Disease.

Source: Manton, K. G., "Mortality and life expectancy changes among the oldest old," in R. Suzman, K. G. Manton, D. P. Willis (Eds.), The oldest old (p. 173), 1992. New York: Oxford University Press. Reprinted with permission, Oxford University Press.

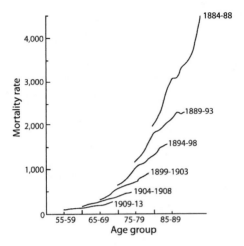

FIGURE 4.8b Cohort Plot of Six White Male Cohorts Born 1884–1888 to 1909–1913 for Underlying Cause Occurrences of Cerebrovascular Disease.

Source: Manton, K. G., "Mortality and life expectancy changes among the oldest old," in R. Suzman, K. G. Manton, D. P. Willis (Eds.), *The oldest old* (p. 173), 1992. New York: Oxford University Press. Reprinted with permission, Oxford University Press.

late life and longer life expectancy. Investigation of this issue requires a careful look at disability and active life expectancy, covered in chapter 5.

TRAJECTORIES OF DYING

Lynn (2001) distinguishes three trajectories of dying: a relatively compressed period of disability followed by death from cancer; a longer period of declines, recoveries, and relapses in function that ends with death from organ failure; and a much longer period of slow dwindling and decline typical of increasing physical and cognitive frailty (i.e., dementia).

Lunney, Lynn, and Hogan, (2002) have proposed an alternative typology based on Medicare claims for decedents. They identified four trajectories based on three criteria: medical expenditures, length of illness, and diagnostic category. They identified one trajectory characterized by a short but expensive death; this kind of dying is typical of death from cancer, accounts for about a quarter of American deaths, and entails a mean cost of $31,000 in the last year of life. A second trajectory summarizes dying with dementia and physical frailty; this trajectory of dying accounts for about half the deaths of older people and carries a mean cost of $25,000 in the last year of life. The third trajectory is typical of deaths due to organ failure; about 20% of deaths follow this pattern, which carries a cost of $37,000 in the last year of life. Finally, a fourth trajectory summarizes the experience of people who die suddenly and with little medical care contact in the last year of life. This trajectory accounts for the smallest proportion of deaths, some 7%, and is the least expensive; Medicare costs for this kind of dying run about $2,000 in the last year of life.

The four trajectories show great variation in the experience of dying at old ages, both in clinical features and associated health care costs. These differences become apparent after death, when we can look back at the last year of life; it is, of course, harder to know in advance that someone has entered the last year of life. Yet, as we have seen, time until death, rather than age, is likely to be the better indicator of health status and biologic age (Evans, 2002). It is also a better predictor of medical care costs. Miller (2001) has shown that Medicare costs are strongly associated with time until death and only weakly with age. For example, for people aged 75 who were five years from death, annual Medicare costs were $3,000. These costs rise to $13,500 for people of the same age in the last year of life. This pattern holds for all age groups and hence "the correlation between age and Medicare costs appears to be explained largely by time until death. Therefore age is a poor measure of health status and cannot reliably be used as a basis for forecasting" (Miller, 2001; p. 217).

Miller also shows that medical care costs decline with older age, especially in the last year of life. Medicare costs in the last year of life were $13,500 per enrollee for people aged 75, $10,700 for people aged 85, and $7,000 for people aged 95. In fact, medical care costs in the oldest age groups were lower even 3-4 years before death. For example, 3 years before death, annual medical care costs per enrollee were $4,200 for people aged 75, $4,000 for people aged 85, and $3,200 for people aged 95. This decline is most likely a result of implicit rationing, such as decisions to limit surgery or diagnostic procedures for the very old, but may also reflect greater frailty at older ages. Frailty means that people approach death with less reserve. As a result, their dying is likely to be quicker and hence allows less time or opportunity for expensive interventions.

From these trends, Miller (2001) suggests that increasing longevity may actually result in a decrease in Medicare expenditures. Increasing longevity, if accompanied by delays in late-life morbidity and disability, should postpone the period of high health-care costs associated with the end of life. In pushing death to later and later ages, we also push the last year of life to later ages, when frailty and implicit rationing make dying less expensive. Evidence for increasing longevity is indisputable, and evidence for decreasing morbidity and disability is accumulating (see chapter 5). It is therefore possible and perhaps even likely that progress in keeping people alive to older ages will lower medical care costs in the last year of life, the major source of expense to Medicare. These costs have remained constant at about 30% of Medicare's budget (Hogan, Lunney, Gabel & Lynn, 2001; Lubitz & Riley, 1993), despite major changes in the use and cost of medical technologies over the past three decades. This consistency may reflect the trend toward less expensive deaths associated with increasing longevity.

MAPPING TRAJECTORIES OF DYING

The dying process can be mapped or measured in a number of ways. One approach is to mark the location and flow of older persons through the health care system as they move from community residence to hospital or nursing home care and finally to death. Figure 4–9 maps this process and gives an indication of the magnitude of each pathway to death.

Of the 1,966,000 deaths of non-institutionalized older people tracked in 1990 (6.7% of the total non-institutionalized population), about 60% died in hospitals, another 22% after nursing home placements, and the

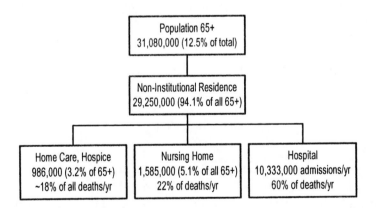

FIGURE 4.9 Location and Flow of Older People Approaching Death.
Source: After Ford, A. B., "An overview of community-based long-term care." In E. Calkins, C. Boult, E. H. Wagner, J. T. Pacala (Eds.), *New ways to care for older people: Building systems based on evidence* (p. 137). 1999. New York: Springer Publishing Co.

remainder in home settings, with or without hospice care. The figure simplifies the flow of older people as they approach death in a number of ways. First, nursing home deaths follow two routes. One route involves admission to nursing homes from the community followed by death, with or without hospitalization. In 1990, 697,000 older people (2.4%) entered nursing homes directly from the community, while another 1,334,000 (4.6%) entered nursing homes from hospitals. The two streams together yield 2,031,000 people entering nursing homes in the year. However, about a quarter of these admissions is temporary, with elders returning to community-based care or independence after short-stay respite or rehabilitation.

A second simplification involves hospital admissions. The non-institutionalized population had about 10,333,000 admissions in the year, which followed a total of some 159,490,000 visits to physicians. Thus, about 6.5% of physician visits, or 1 in 20, were followed by hospitalization. From these admissions, 1,180,000 died in the hospital, so that about 1 in every 10 admissions was followed by death in the hospital. The number is obviously higher if we add deaths among patients transferred to hospitals from nursing homes.

Pulling these data together is no easy task; some 10 different data sources were consulted in constructing the composite figure! However, there is no other way to get a sense of the complex flow of people and settings as death approaches.

Finally, it is reassuring to examine the complement of the figures described above. Over 93% of non-institutionalized elders did not die in the year. A similar proportion avoided spending any days in nursing homes. The vast majority of physician visits were not followed by hospitalization, and the vast majority of hospitalizations were followed by discharges back into the community.

A second way to map trajectories to death is to examine changes in quality of life among people who are dying. These changes are most easily captured in studies of the last year of life. A key case-control study compared the last year of life in a group of dying elders to an ordinary year of life among surviving elders (Lawton, Moss, & Glicksman, 1993). The study was retrospective and identified dying elders from obituary notices. Next of kin, identified by death certificate, were contacted and interviewed about the dying person's experience 12 months, 3 months, and 1 month before death. Surviving elders were identified in the same neighborhood and matched by age, gender, and source of information. Lawton and colleagues found that virtually all quality of life indicators declined over the 12 months compared to trends in the survivor group, with the exception of visits from family and friends, which increased. Still, they noted that across the many different indicators of quality, most of these dying elders had good scores on a majority of the measures, suggesting that most experienced relatively good quality of life at the end of life.

Results from the National Mortality Followback Survey suggest that the quality of life among people who are dying may also be improving (Liao, McGee, Cao, & Cooper, 2000). In the Followback Survey a random sample of deaths is drawn from death certificates, with next of kin contacted and interviewed about the last year of life of the decedent. A comparison of results from the 1986 and 1993 surveys shows important gains in quality of life at the end of life. For example, among decedents aged 65-84, the proportion avoiding a hospital admission increased from 21.6% to 25.1% among men and 19.6% to 24.9% among women. Gains were even greater among decedents aged 85+. In this group, the proportion avoiding hospitalization increased from 22.3% to 29.1% among men, and 30.7% to 40.6% among women. The proportion without a nursing home admission also increased in all groups except the younger men. These are welcome findings because they suggest that more people were able to live the last year of life in their own homes, a result consistent with large increase in hospice use in the same period (see below).

This comparison also revealed better physical and cognitive status in decedents over the decade, a trend especially pronounced among the oldest old. The proportion in the most severely disabled categories declined for all groups. Similarly, a composite measure of quality of life based on time in hospital or nursing homes, restriction in daily activities, and cognitive status showed improvement for the oldest old. Because the burden of disability in the last year of life declined between 1986 and 1993, the authors conclude that the related decline in hospital and nursing home use was at least partly due to better health even in the last year of life.

THE HIGH COSTS OF DYING

Medical care in old age is more expensive than medical care for younger age groups because of the greater burden of chronic disease borne by older people. However, as shown earlier, medical management of the chronic diseases of old age is less a burden to Medicare than medical management of dying. About 30% of all Medicare expenditures occur in the year in which people die, that is, the last year of life (Lubitz & Riley; Miller, 2001). The constancy of this proportion of Medicare spending over a number of decades is impressive, given the huge increases in overall Medicare spending. Between 1976 and 1988, costs in the last year of life increased from $3,488 to $13,316, on average, per decedent. Costs per year for non-decedents rose from $492 to $1,924 in the same period. Thus, both groups saw nearly a four-fold increase over this decade and a half, and accordingly end-of-life care as a proportion of the total Medicare budget changed very little (Lubitz & Riley, 1993). Lubitz and Riley also note that the proportion of Medicare payments made in the last 60 days of life in 1976 and 1988 was also virtually identical, suggesting no increase in heroic (and perhaps unjustified) efforts to stave off death.

An update of Medicare expenditures in the last year of life shows little change (Hogan, Lunney, Gabel, & Lynn, 2001). About 5% of Medicare enrollees continue to die each year. Not surprisingly, decedents continue to be older, more frail and disabled, and more diseased than survivors. Based on Medicare claims, the typical Medicare decedent has about four major disease conditions at the time of death, compared to only one disease condition among survivors. Some three-quarters of decedents have heart disease; one-third cancer, stroke, chronic obstructive pulmonary disease, or pneumonia/influenza; and more than a quarter dementia.

Suppose now that we match these decedents to survivors with the same disease profiles. Hogan and colleagues (2001) determined that decedents' costs were about 50% higher than those of a survivor cohort matched by age and disease diagnoses, and about 30% higher than those of a survivor cohort matched on age, diagnoses, and a hospitalization during the year. This important finding suggests that the high costs of the last year of life are mostly a function of the high disease burden that precedes dying, "Much of what has been labeled the 'high cost of dying' is just the cost of caring for severe illness and functional impairment. Decedents' costs are, roughly speaking, not much different from those of others with similarly complex medical needs" (Hogan et al., 2001, p. 194). This approach also suggests that Medicare data of this sort may be useful in identifying groups at high risk of dying.

Decedents are also more likely to use nursing home care and hence incur high Medicaid costs. Nearly 40% of decedents had some nursing home care in their last year of life. In fact, 22% of decedents were full-time nursing home residents in the year of death, and the remainder had short-term or part-year residence in nursing homes (Hogan et al., 2001).

Analysis of Medicare costs also reveals interesting variation consistent with results reported earlier and in chapter 2. Decedents who die at younger ages (65-74) are more likely to be male, to die of cancer, and to have higher costs. Older ages at death were associated with a greater prevalence of dementia and nursing home use, with attendant Medicaid expenditures. Women were more prevalent in this group.

Hogan and colleagues (2001) also report an important racial difference in Medicare expenditures in the last year of life. End-of-life care costs were higher for minorities and for people living in high poverty areas. Medicare spending per capita for minority decedents was 28% higher compared to non-minorities, and 43% higher in high poverty areas compared to low poverty areas. Part of the difference can be attributed to the poorer health of minorities and low-income groups at the end of life. For example, 7% of minority decedents had end-stage renal disease covered in the End-Stage Renal Disease (ESRD) program, a costly death (see the organ failure trajectory described above), compared to only 2% in the remainder of the Medicare decedent population. But costs for minority decedents in the last year of life remained about 20% higher even with exclusion of decedents in ESRD program.

Reasons for the greater expense of dying among minorities remain unclear. Reports also suggest that family members of minority and low-income decedents are more likely to request life-sustaining technologies. A sense of exclusion from medical care earlier in life may be at work here, as well as broader differences in culture and expectations regarding medical care. This question merits further research.

Finally, one large change is the increasing use of hospice. Hogan and colleagues (2001) report an increase in hospice care use from 11% in 1994 to 19% in 1998. In 1998, more than half of Medicare cancer decedents used hospice. This is welcome but suggests that hospice remains underutilized in non-cancer deaths and should be higher in cancer deaths as well.

These data speak to medical care costs. Medical care costs increase with the approach of death and decline as people die at later ages. Controlling heroic measures to stave off death and curtailing use of life-sustaining technologies, or rationing medical care by age, as suggested by Callahan (1987) and others, is not likely to save money. As we have seen, medical care for the oldest old is already at least implicitly rationed and these deaths in any case are not the largest source of expenses at the end of life. What is expensive about old age—and not likely to be affected by any sort of Medicare cost control—is the custodial care needs of older people (Scitovsky, 1994), a topic discussed below.

TERMINAL DROP

What sorts of changes mark the point when people begin to die? If we start with a group that has died and work backward to examine changes in health before death, can we identify a point when decline begins?

Finally, how much of the negative changes in health that we see in late life can be attributed to pre-death decline?

Inquiry in this area has led to the suggestion of a period of "terminal drop" before death (Kleinmeier, 1962). However, in practice it is hard to date the start of this period of terminal decline, since this inquiry requires prospective follow-up in a cohort of people who have died. Wilson and colleagues (in press) reported the results of such a study and determined that cognitive decline began, on average, about four years before death. This study involved the Religious Orders cohort, a group of highly-educated nuns and priests. People in the cohort who did not die showed almost no change in cognitive performance over the same period.

More generally, little research has been conducted on changes prior to the last year of life. This is an important and neglected area.

SUMMARY

Causes of Death. Death certificates distinguish between "underlying" or "primary" causes of death and "contributory" causes. "Underlying causes" indicate proximal or immediate conditions that led to the death, while "contributory causes" indicate more distal or remote causes, that is, longstanding chronic conditions that may have played a role in the death. While underlying cause information in death certificates agrees well with hospital records, the validity of cause-of-death information is less sure for deaths outside of medical settings. More generally, because dying in late life almost always includes frailty, multiple diseases, and additional intervening medical events, it is often difficult to identify the cause of death. Once we move beyond simple counts of total or cause-specific mortality to measurement of mortality as a sequence of events over a potentially long period, we are forced to recognize that it is often difficult to state when dying begins and what someone actually died of.

Death Rates by Age, Race, and Sex. The death rate per 100,000 is about 50 at age 10 and increases to 100 at age 20, 500 at age 40, 1,000 at age 60, and over 10,000 at age 80. Within this strong association between age and mortality risk we find considerable variation by race and gender, with white women showing the lowest rates and black men the highest.

Three broad patterns can be identified for the association between age and mortality:

- A j-shaped pattern, evident for heart disease, many of the cancers, stroke, pneumonia, liver, and chronic obstructive pulmonary disease (COPD), in which death is high in the perinatal period, lowest in childhood, and steadily increases over the remainder of the life span;
- A variant of the j-shaped pattern, in which mortality from some of the cancers and liver disease appears to reach a plateau in the 6th decade and perhaps declines at older ages;
- A final pattern in which mortality rises very quickly and reaches its peak among younger people. Mortality from unintentional injuries, motor vehicle accidents, homicide, and suicide is highest for young people and reaches its peak at about age 20. Mortality from these causes may continue to increase over the life span (unintentional injuries), remain more or less flat (motor vehicle accidents, suicide, firearm suicide), or decline (homicide, firearm homicide).

Declining Mortality. The age-adjusted death rate for the United States shows that annual mortality has declined by half over the century, from about 1,100 to less than 500 per 100,000 people. For example, in 1950 the death rate per 100,000 men was 5,000 at age 65–74, 10,000 at age 75–84, and 20,000 at age 85+. By 1998, these rates were 4,000, 7,500, and about 19,000, respectively. The declining rate of mortality continues, resulting in fewer years of life lost to disease across the lifespan.

Rank Order of Causes of Death. In 1999, 1,797,451 people aged 65+ died. The ten leading causes of death were much the same as in 1980, with heart disease, cancer, and stroke again accounting for the preponderance of deaths (63.8% of all deaths). Alzheimer's disease was a leading cause of death in 1999, reflecting new awareness of the disease as a cause of death.

Socioeconomic Status and Mortality in Late Life. Education is an important predictor of mortality risk in older people as in younger people. Men and women each face lower mortality risk with increasing education. An education gradient applies across the entire range of education but becomes most pronounced with completion of high school and more advanced schooling. The protective effect of education is attenuated at older ages. For example, relative to men with high school education, young men with 16+ years of school face a mortality risk of 0.67, while men aged 65+ with 16+ years of school face a mortality risk of 0.76. Given the great significance of education for mortality risk and the increasingly educated older population, we can expect

postponement of mortality from this factor alone, apart from improvements in medical care.

Declines in Cause-Specific Mortality by Birth Cohort. Cohort plots
show that cause-specific mortality is truly declining for some (but, of
course, not all) of the major diseases of late life. The results imply that
deaths from these conditions are being postponed to later ages, either
because people contract the disease at later ages or because they are
living longer with it.

Specifying Different Trajectories of Dying. Analysis of Medicare claims
suggests four broad trajectories of dying:

• A short but expensive death, typical of deaths from cancer. This
trajectory accounts for about a quarter of American deaths and
has a mean cost of $31,000 in the last year of life.
• A protracted period of disability, with dementia and severe physical frailty at the time of death. This trajectory accounts for about
half the deaths of older people and carries a mean cost of $25,000
in the last year of life.
• Deaths due to organ failure. About 20% of deaths follow this
pattern, which carries a cost of $37,000 in the last year of life.
• Sudden, unexpected deaths characterized by little medical care
contact in the last year of life. This trajectory accounts for 7% of
deaths and is the least expensive, with a mean cost of $2,000 in
the last year of life.

Costs at the End of Life. Medicare costs are strongly associated with
time until death and only weakly with age. For example, for people
aged 75 who were 5 years from death, annual Medicare costs were
$3,000. These costs rise to $13,500 for people of the same age in the
last year of life. Medical care costs also decline with older age, especially in the last year of life. Medicare costs in the last year of life were
$13,500 per enrollee for people aged 75, $10,700 for people aged
85, and $7,000 for people aged 95. In fact, medical care costs in the
oldest age groups are lower even 3–4 years before death.

Increasing longevity may actually result in a decrease in Medicare
expenditures. Increasing longevity, if accompanied by delays in late-life
morbidity and disability, should postpone the period of high health-care
costs associated with the end of life. In pushing death to later and later
ages, we also push the last year of life to later ages, when frailty and
implicit rationing make dying less expensive. Evidence for increasing
longevity is indisputable, and evidence for decreasing morbidity and
disability is accumulating. It is therefore possible and perhaps even

likely that progress in keeping people alive to older ages will lower medical care costs in the last year of life, the major source of expense to Medicare. These costs have remained constant at about 30% of Medicare's budget.

Mapping Trajectories of Dying. Trajectories of dying can be mapped according to the flow of people through the health care system or through changes typical of the last year of life. Of the 1,966,000 deaths of non-institutionalized older people tracked in 1990 (6.7% of the total non-institutionalized population), about 60% died in hospitals, another 22% after nursing home placements, and the remainder in home settings, with or without hospice care. The home care-hospice component is growing, which, when coupled with other evidence, suggests increasing quality of life in the last year of life. Studies of the last year of life suggest that most people experience good quality of life as they approach death, and changes in the last decade suggest that dying people are more likely to be highly functional and remain home up to the point of death.

"Terminal Drop." It is still unclear when terminal changes begin in the period before death. One suggestion, based on cognitive decline, is that the period of "terminal drop" begins about 4 years before death. In general, while much is known about the last year of life, little is known about the longer period before death, when changes presaging death may have already begun.

5

Physical Function: Disability

Disability is the central outcome for public health and aging. Given the increasing prevalence of chronic disease with older ages and the development of senescent changes that lead to frailty, older people are at risk of dropping below the thresholds of physical and cognitive ability required for safe, independent, and efficient completion of everyday self-maintenance tasks. These self-maintenance tasks include the basic "activities of daily living": bathing, dressing, grooming, feeding oneself, getting to and using the toilet, and moving between bed and chair. This definition limits disability to reported difficulty in tasks of daily living linked to health conditions. We examine the different elements of the definition and their rationale below. When compensatory mechanisms (such as environmental modification) are unavailable or no longer suffice for completion of tasks that have become difficult, people become *dependent* on assistance from others or on assistive equipment to complete these tasks. Difficulty and dependence define important gradations of disability (Gill & Kurland, 2003).

As expected, difficulty is more prevalent than dependence: 22% of community-resident older adults in the U.S. aged 65+ report difficulty with at least one activity of daily living (ADL), but fewer than 10% receive assistance with an ADL. Some of the people reporting difficulty could profit from assistance; likewise, some (but most likely a very small number) receive assistance in the absence of true difficulty. The first group is over-challenged, the second under-challenged, and each condition may have adverse consequences (Lawton 1972).

In what sense can disability be understood as a model for aging, or alternatively, in what sense can aging be considered a model for disability? To the extent that loss of physical, cognitive, and affective or social function is a feature of both, understanding the process of change and adaptation in one may shed light on the other. Moreover, insofar as aging allows expression of senescence, it must be considered a source of disability in itself. In this sense, it would be useful to model aging and disability together. This is a key challenge for thinking about public health and the second 50 years of life (Crews & Smith, 2003).

THREE MODELS OF DISABILITY

Models of disability share common features but give different weight to the role of environment and excess morbidity or disadvantage (i.e., "handicap") in the expression of deficits related to impairments in physical and cognitive function. These models also differ in how wide they draw the net around the outcome of interest. Is the outcome disability in the narrow sense, that is, self-reports of difficulty with ADL tasks due to a health problem? Or is the outcome more general limitations in activity and restrictions in social participation? If the latter, disability prevalence will be much higher, for it is possible to experience activity limitations or restriction in participation without having ADL deficits. By contrast, someone with ADL disability is likely to experience activity limitations or restriction in social participation unless environmental modification or some other adaptation has been made. This reflects the hierarchical relationship between ADL and more advanced tasks (see below). With the broader definition of disability, the possibilities for intervention may also be greater, which may reduce prevalence estimates.

Model 1: Original WHO Formulation

The original WHO model was presented in the *International Classification of Impairment, Disability, and Handicap* (1981), an effort to catalogue defects in anatomic structure or physiologic function (impairment), limitations in roles as a result of impairment (disability), and excess morbidity attached to impairment because of social stigma (handicap). The relationship among the three key concepts is shown in Figure 5.1.

Aside from the distinction between disability and handicap, a key insight of the early WHO model was recognition that individuals with an impairment can be handicapped in the absence of disability. That is, individuals with an impairment can be discriminated against (denied employment, excluded from social life, denied opportunities for schooling) even though they are not disabled, that is, even though they are able to work, attend social functions, and succeed in school. This is indicated by the lack of overlap between "handicap" and "disability" in

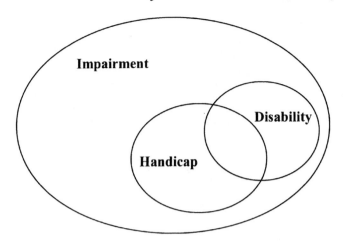

FIGURE 5.1 Initial WHO Model of Impairment, Disability, and Handicap.

Based on *International Classification of Impairment, Handicap, and Disability, World Health Organization.*

the Venn diagram of Figure 5.1. While stigmatization and exclusion of people because of impairment would be inappropriate in any case, the WHO model recognized that handicap could actually *cause excess morbidity* and, in fact, *create disability* in people who actually could competently perform valued roles. This was an important insight for the sociology of disability, which was given an even more prominent place in the revised WHO Model, discussed below.

Model 2: Disablement Process (Guralnik, Fried, Simunsick, Kasper & Lafferty, 1995; Patrick & Peach, 1989; Verbrugge & Jette, 1994)

The disablement model differs from the WHO approach in asserting a strict four-part temporal and causal sequence. It is shown in Figure 5.2, with representative examples in Table 5.1.

In the disablement model, *pathology* (e.g., sarcopenia) first leads to *impairment* (e.g., lower extremity weakness evident in manual muscle testing). When lower extremity weakness crosses some threshold, *functional limitation* becomes evident, measurable perhaps in gait speeds below age-and gender-appropriate norms. When gait speed in turn drops below the minimum speed required to cross at a signaled

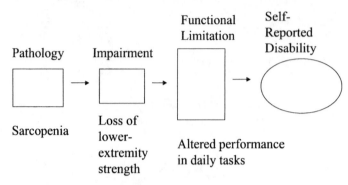

FIGURE 5.2 Basic Disablement Model.

intersection, a person is likely to report difficulty or a need for help crossing the street, that is, *disability.*

Note that disability is limited to (1) *self-reported* difficulty or need for assistance, (2) a *need* rather than use or receipt of assistance, and (3) difficulty or need due to impairment, that is, a problem with one's *health.*

The first condition makes disability a matter of subjective evaluation, as it should be: people with functional limitation who have successfully adapted by changing environments or by compensating through use of preserved abilities are likely not to report difficulty and are appropriately considered non-disabled. On the other hand, someone who uses personal assistance or equipment to complete ADL tasks would be considered disabled in this view, because use of assistance implies difficulty with tasks. We recognize, however, that people do complete ADL tasks using assistance and in this way maintain independence

TABLE 5.1 Elements of Disablement Model, with Representative Examples

Pathology	Impairment	Functional Limitation	Disability
Sarcopenia	Loss of strength	Slow gait speed	Difficulty crossing street
Ataxia	Loss of balance	Tandem stand <10 sec	Difficulty with stairs
Mild cognitive impairment	Memory < age/educ norm	Inefficient, unsafe cooking	Difficulty with meals

despite difficulty. They use assistance as a form of tertiary prevention to limit the effects of disability.

The second condition, the stress on need rather than use, is important because it gives due recognition to unmet need. Only some of the elders with a need for assistance receive such assistance, so that restricting disability to the group actually receiving assistance would severely underestimate disability.

Finally, the third condition requires that self-reports of disability be due to health conditions rather than an environmental restriction, personal motivation, or other non-health sources of task restriction. This distinction may be hard to maintain in some cases, as environmental restrictions can also be considered legitimate targets for public health interventions, and disease may affect motivation (as in the case of depression).

Additional disablement sequences are shown in Table 5.1 for two neurologic pathologies. Ataxia (brain pathology) leads to balance disorders (impairment), eventually affecting timed gait speed (functional limitation), and finally leading to reports of difficulty or need for a cane to navigate indoor mobility. Similarly, memory loss (brain pathology) affects cognitive performance (visible in memory test scores below age- and education-appropriate norms, impairment), leading to inefficient or unsafe operation of a stove when cooking (functional limitation), and finally to recognition of difficulty, need for help, or cessation of meal preparation tasks.

Note a potential confusion in terminology between this model and the earlier WHO model. "Impairment" in the WHO formulation is divided into two elements in this model, "pathology" and "impairment," with the latter limited to direct, measurable effects of pathology. These effects may be diffuse and not obvious to people, such as performance on a memory test below an age norm. Similarly, "disability" in the WHO model is also broken into two components, "functional limitation" and "disability." (The use of identical terms for different concepts in both cases is unfortunate.) Functional limitation involves progression of impairment to the point where skills or abilities required to complete daily tasks (such as gait speed or the ability to hold a tandem stand for 10 seconds) are affected. "Disability" in the disablement model explicitly involves self-reports of difficulty or need for assistance to perform daily tasks because of functional limitation.

The disablement model does not make direct reference to handicap, though clearly social and environmental factors affect this sequence. For example, changing the timing of traffic lights or even changing the time one goes out to do errands might prevent slow gait speed, a functional limitation, from producing disability. Rehabilitation or exercise to promote leg strength, or use of a motorized scooter, could break the link between impairment and functional limitation. Below, we present elaborations of the model that accommodate environmental and compensatory interventions.

One advantage of the model is the solid tradition of measurement behind it. For example, even in people who do not report mobility problems, weakness in lower extremity strength predicts future mortality and incident disability in the activities of daily living (ADL) (Guralnik et al., 1995a). Likewise, people who do not report difficulty in ADL but report they have changed the way they perform these tasks have slower gait speeds and poorer grip strength (Fried et al., 1996). We describe this approach in more detail below.

The disablement model makes disability an outcome and uses a fairly narrow definition of disability. This approach has been criticized for neglecting other components of daily life, such as non-ADL activity and general participation in social life, which can be preserved even with severe ADL disability, and which may be more important to personal identity and self-worth than independence in ADL. These are given prominence in the third model of disability, discussed below.

Critics of the disablement approach assert that in making disability an outcome, the experience of people who use personal assistance or assistive technologies to perform daily activities is devalued (Crews & Smith 2003). We do not think so. Take the example of the 92–year-old woman described in chapter 1. She used a walker, required 24–hours-a-day personal assistance for ADL, and took ten different medicines for six chronic conditions. Her ADL dependence was complete, yet she scored quite high on measures of activity and social participation, and she considered every day quite satisfying and interesting. By any account this is successful aging, yet she also sought ways to reduce her ADL dependency. For understanding her need for assistance, the etiology of this need, and potential points for intervention, it is useful to model disability explicitly, even if narrowly defined.

Model 3: Revised WHO Model

An alternative indicator of disability, described in the WHO *International Classification of Functioning, Disability, and Health* (ICF), stresses "activity limitation" and "participation restriction," rather than disability, and explicitly includes environmental factors in assessing the impact of health conditions (WHO, 2001). The model is shown in Figure 5.3.

"Disability is characterized as the outcome or result of a complex relationship between an individual's health condition and personal factors, and of the external factors that represent the circumstances in which the individual lives" (WHO, 2001, p. 17).

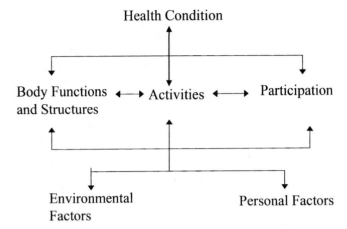

FIGURE 5.3 Revised WHO Model of Disability: International Classification of Functioning and Activities.

WHO, *International Classification of Functioning, Disability, and Health,* WHO 2001: 18.

The revised WHO model demotes disability in the narrow sense as an outcome; in fact, the term disappears from the model. Instead, in this approach pathology causes a cascade of events: impairment, activity limitation, and restriction in participation, where all three are related in complex ways. At the same time, personal and environmental factors are given equal weight as causal factors affecting this complex of outcomes. In this model, all of these effects and relationships are considered "disability."

Thus, the revised WHO model is a "social model of disability"; disability is not an attribute of the individual but rather a feature of person-environment relationships. This approach sees the issue mainly as a socially created problem, and basically as a matter of the full integration of individuals into society (WHO, 2001). The disablement approach, by contrast, is essentially a "medical model," in which disability is a problem of the person caused by a health condition. "Disability management" in the disablement approach requires appropriate medical care and alteration of the environment, as much as possible, to minimize negative consequences of the medical condition.

Which approach is superior? The question is probably inappropriate because the revised WHO model is not meant to describe disablement, but rather to inspire more extensive integration of environmental and personal factors into the management of impairing conditions. While the disablement model suggests clinical strategies, the revised WHO model suggests political action. As the authors state, if "disability is not an attribute of the individual, but rather a complex collection of conditions, many of which are created by the social environment," then "the management of [disability] requires social action, and it is the collective responsibility of society at large to make the environmental modifications necessary for the full participation of people with disabilities in all areas of social life" (WHO, 2001, p. 20).

Our approach is to stress the disablement model, since it offers an immediate and productive research strategy, with clear clinical and public heath applications. However, it is also worth keeping in mind the revised WHO model, since environmental modification and other compensatory strategies are central to the disability experience and indeed can define the nature of disability in some cases as much as impairing conditions do.

DEFINING AND MEASURING DISABILITY: CENTRALITY OF THE ACTIVITIES OF DAILY LIVING

Disability in late life is the central outcome of chronic disease. Chronic disease can also cause symptoms or functional limitations short of disability, an increased risk of hospitalization and death, a need for regular medications and physician visits to monitor indicators of disease progression or therapy, dependency on people or equipment in daily self-maintenance activities, depression and anxiety, and changes in self-image and sense of control. All of these outcomes are appropriate targets for public health inquiry, but disability is central because it is implicated in each of the alternative outcomes.

Verbrugge and Patrick (1995) define chronic conditions as "long-term diseases, injuries with long sequelae, and enduring structural, sensory, and communicative disorders." They add, "their defining aspect is duration. Once they are past certain symptomatic or diagnostic thresholds, chronic conditions are essentially permanent features for the rest of life. Medical and personal regimens can sometimes control but can rarely cure them" (p. 173). These conditions may cause difficulty or make it impossible for people to learn, go to school, work, play sports, travel, participate in conversation, drive, or complete the basic tasks required for independent living, such as eating, bathing, dressing, grooming, using the toilet, or moving between a bed and a chair. These, as we have seen earlier, are the "activities of daily living" (Katz et al., 1963) or "personal self-maintenance activities" (Lawton & Brody, 1969), which over time have picked up the modifier of "basic" or "physical" ADL (hence BADL and PADL) to distinguish them from more complex household tasks usually considered "instrumental activities of daily living" (IADL).

In public health and aging, we mostly focus on the activities of daily living or personal self-maintenance activities. We do so, first of all, because of a public health tradition in which ADL competencies were typically considered the primary sphere of activity in old age, on par with attending school for children and working or running a household for adults (Sullivan, 1966). While older adults do not work or attend school at rates anywhere near those of younger people, an increasing proportion do; we may want to rethink this rationale for the focus on ADL. (Indeed, the early Sullivan [1966] classification also considered housework the primary sphere of activity for adult women under age 65.)

There are much better reasons for the focus on ADL as the central indicator of disability in older adults. First, *ADL are the basic and universal competencies of adulthood.* An adult who does not bathe or use the toilet reliably is likely to be incompetent mentally or physically. Our first reaction is to shun this person and consider a referral to adult protective services. This gives an indication that loss of ADL competencies is a severe threat not just to social participation and safety, but also to adulthood as we understand it, and hence self-worth. (However, note that there is some variability by culture in the degree to which this sort of independence is considered central to adulthood [Albert & Cattell, 1994].) Loss of ADL competency, then, represents a major milestone in the progression of chronic disease.

A second reason is *the universality of ADL. All people need to accomplish ADL tasks; people perform these tasks on all or most days.* Thus, all older people can be asked if they have difficulty bathing or dressing or using the toilet. The tasks are not gender-specific, optional, or subject to variation in lifestyle. This is not the case with other competencies, such as the instrumental (sometimes called "intermediate") activities of daily living (IADL). The IADL are household competencies, which typically include managing finances, going shopping, doing housework, doing laundry, using the telephone, and taking medications. The need, desire, and training to perform IADL tasks vary by gender, education, health status, lifestyle, and culture. The same applies to the so-called advanced ADL, such as using a microwave oven, programming a VCR, or using a computer, and to any of the more general lists of activities that have been proposed as indicators of adult competencies.

A third reason for the focus on ADL is their hierarchical nature. *ADL differ in task complexity, and hence in motor and cognitive demand, and as a result appear to be gained and lost in a generally consistent (but not necessarily fixed) order.* Early on, Katz and colleagues (1963) suggested that the order in which ADL tasks are acquired in childhood development (first, feeding and transfer; later, toileting and dressing; last, bathing) is the reverse of the order in which they are lost in chronic disease (so that the first lost is bathing, the most complex of the tasks), as well as the order in which they are regained in recovery from stroke or brain injury (so that the last competency reacquired is again bathing). For this reason, Katz considered the ADL a measure of "primary sociobiologic function." His early research showed that the disability status of almost all elders in a skilled care setting adhered to this rough hierarchy of preservation and loss of task ability, which formed a Guttman scale. That is, people who were unable to do just one task from this set of tasks almost always had lost the ability to bathe. Likewise, people who could not dress themselves independently were also very likely to have trouble bathing independently. People who could perform only one task independently from the set of ADL were likely to have retained the ability to feed themselves. In fact, a simulation study has shown that a number of alternative patterns, mostly relating to the order of the most primitive of the ADL tasks, form equally good hierarchical scales (Lazirides, Rudberg, Furner, & Cassel, 1994). However, it is well to remember that Katz and his colleagues (who developed the measure in the late 1950s and early 1960s) did not have access to sophisticated modeling software and yet their clinical judgment regarding the scalability of the items was essentially accurate.

It is worth mentioning as well that a number of changes in task items have been introduced since Katz first proposed the measure. The original Katz items included bathing, dressing, toileting ("going to the toilet room for bowel and urine elimination; cleaning self after elimination, and arranging clothes"), transfer, continence (ability to control urination and bowel movements), and feeding. Current measures of ADL competency include only one toileting item, and have added indoor mobility and personal grooming. Also, the original Katz scale items had very detailed descriptors for categories of ability. Each item was assessed on a three-point scale, with quite detailed scale values. For example, the middle scale point for dressing was "gets clothes and gets dressed without assistance except for assistance in tying shoes." Current versions use a single underlying measure for all ADL tasks: either level of difficulty (none, some, a lot) or need for help (none, sometimes, all the time).

A last point involves the source of information about ADL. While the ADL items have been selected to rule out "does not apply" or "don't know" responses (since the tasks are both basic and universal), cognitive impairment prevents a small proportion of the young-old (about 6% of people under aged 75) and a much larger proportion of the old-old (about 20% of people aged 75+ and perhaps 50% of people residing in nursing homes) from answering the questions. For information about the ADL status of these more disabled respondents, re-

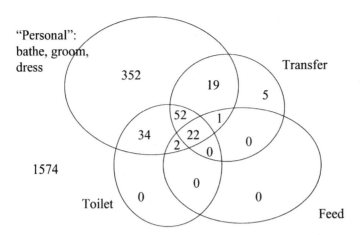

FIGURE 5.4 Distribution of ADL Disability: Washington Heights-Inwood Columbia Aging Project.
Source: Washington Heights-Inwood Community Aging Project, 1992 Baseline.

searchers and clinicians must rely on proxy reports, that is, information from family or service providers, or observed performance. But for people able to report on ADL status, it is their judgment that defines disability. As in the case of quality of life measures (see chapter 8), this seems appropriate: who better than the person at hand is better able to report on the degree of difficulty he or she faces in performing daily tasks (Gill & Feinstein, 1994)? In fact, studies comparing patient and proxy reports of patient ADL status show only moderate levels of agreement, and if patient factors affect accuracy (i.e., denial, loss of insight, wish for a more intense level of services), so do proxy factors (i.e., degree of contact with patient, mental health, perceived burden as caregiver) (Magaziner, Simonsick, Kashner, & Hebel, 1988).

Still, even with these limitations, the ADL hierarchy is highly robust. For example, the Venn diagram shown in Figure 5.4 demonstrates that in a sample of more than 2000 elders *none* had difficulty with feeding or toileting without also having difficulty in bathing, grooming, or dressing.

DIFFICULTIES IN THE MEASUREMENT OF DISABILITY IN OLDER ADULTS

The centrality of basic ADL (BADL) and IADL as measures of disability is clear, but measuring disability in even these most basic tasks is not simple. Kovar and Lawton (1994) describe many issues to be considered in obtaining reports of disability. These include:

1. Deciding which activities should be assessed ("the number of possible IADL tasks seems almost limitless")
2. Ceiling effects ("the ADL/IADL scales do best at identifying the most-disabled minority")
3. Problems with the standardization of question formats to control for interpretation of environmental effects ("estimates of functioning reflect an unknown mix of personal disability and contextual constraint")
4. Effect of emphasizing different components of disability in question formats ("dependence" vs. "difficulty" vs. "limitation") or combining them (Gill, Robison & Tinetti 1997)
5. Effect of proxy reporting (proxy respondents are more likely to report disability than self-respondents but may be the only source of information for people with severe impairment)
6. Relevance of cultural differences ("socially or culturally assigned roles are obvious conditioners of IADL task performance and, conceivably, capability")
7. Cognitive factors in interpreting questions ("help from another person" can mean ongoing help, occasional help, or indirect help, that is, purchasing an assistive device).

These measurement challenges may be responsible for the different prevalence estimates of ADL disability evident in national surveys. Wiener, Hanley, Clark and Van Nostrand (1990) went through the major national probability surveys of disability in the 1980s and found substantial variation in the number of ADL queried, whether "disability" in an ADL required a specified period of duration, and whether distinctions were made between need for assistance and receipt of personal assistance, use of special equipment, and stand-by help. Table 5.2 shows results from their effort.

The prevalence of receiving help with any ADL ranges from 5.0% (1984 Supplement on Aging) to 7.8% (1982 and 1984 National Long-Term Care Surveys). Given the common definition of "receives help from another person," these differences are impressive. This variability applies to disability in all the ADL, both those with relatively high prevalence, such as bathing (4.6% to 6.3%), and those with low prevalence, such as eating (0.7% to 2.5%).

Given this variability, it is also impressive that self-and proxy-reports of disability have been shown to be related to concurrent health indicators and have proven to be reliable predictors of health outcomes in longitudinal studies. For example, in the National Long-Term Care

TABLE 5.2 Activity of Daily Living Disabilities among the Noninstitutionalized Elderly Age 65 and Over, by Survey and Type of Activity (in thousands)

	1982 NLTCS	1984 NLTCS	1984 SOA	1984 SIPP	1987 NMES
Total aged 65 and over noninstitutionalized elderly population (millions)	25,440	26,481	26,268	26,422	27,909
One or more ADL problems	1,992	2,062	1,318	1,538[a]	2,250
	(7.8)	(7.8)	(5.0)	(5.8)	(8.1)
Bathing	1,609	1,660	1,211	1,459[a]	1,926
	(6.3)	(6.3)	(4.6)	(5.5)	(6.9)
Dressing	1,072	1,063	771	—[b]	1,228
	(4.2)	(4.0)	(2.9)	(4.4)	
Transferring	1,072	1,072	675	699	977
	(4.2)	(4.0)	(2.6)	(2.6)	(3.5)
Toileting	857	880	619	n.a.[d]	670
	(3.4)	(3.3)	(2.4)	(2.4)	
Eating	624	618	183		
	(2.5)	(2.3)	(0.7)		

Note: Numbers in parentheses indicate percentages.

[a]Excluded toileting.

[b]Combines bathing, dressing, eating and personal hygiene in one question.

[c]Cell size too small for reliable estimate.

[d]not asked.

Source: Weiner, Hanley, Clark, & Van Nostrand (1990).

Survey (NLTCS), baseline IADL/BADL status was associated with risk of increasing disability, nursing home admission, and mortality over five years in a reassuring "dose-response" relationship. Among nondisabled elders, 5.7% died in this period, compared to 19.5% among the moderately disabled (1-2 BADL) and 39.2% among the severely disabled (5–6 BADL) (Manton, Corder, & Stallard, 1993). It should be noted that the NLTCS only enrolled older adults with "chronic disability," which was defined as an IADL or BADL limitation for at least three months prior to the interview.

Self-reported ADL disability in the NLTCS also predicted later transitions in disability, including admission to skilled care facilities, as shown in Table 5.3 (Manton, 1992). These two-year transition probabilities are very valuable for understanding the complex dynamics of disability and recovery, even over fairly short periods.

TABLE 5.3 Transition Proportions by Age Group

Status and age (years) in 1982	IADL Nondisabled	only	1-2 ADLs	3-4 ADLs	5 ADLs	Institutionalized	Deceased
Status in 1984							
Nondisabled							
65+	79.1	4.6	3.2	1.1	1.0	1.9	9.2
65174	86.0	3.6	1.9	0.8	0.6	0.7	6.3
75-84	70.1	6.2	4.9	1.4	1.5	3.1	12.8
85+	42.3	7.5	9.3	2.8	3.2	9.7	25.2
IADL only							
65+	11.6	39.1	19.4	4.8	4.1	5.7	15.3
65-74	16.4	45.3	16.4	3.7	3.3	3.1	11.7
75-84	9.4	34.8	21.2	5.7	4.4	7.5	17.1
85+	1.7	30.2	24.1	6.0	6.0	9.5	22.4
1-2 ADLs							
65+	6.5	13.8	33.2	12.2	6.3	7.6	20.6
65-74	8.8	17.5	35.7	12.1	5.3	4.6	16.0
75-84	5.6	13.4	33.5	11.4	5.2	7.7	23.2
85+	3.7	7.6	27.7	13.7	10.1	13.2	24.0
3-4 ADLs							
65+	4.1	4.0	16.8	22.1	19.2	10.0	23.9
65-74	6.7	5.4	22.7	25.7	16.0	4.2	19.3
75-84	2.7	3.5	16.5	20.9	20.0	12.1	24.4
85+	2.1	2.1	7.4	17.9	23.2	16.3	31.1
5-6 ADLs							
65+	3.2	4.5	7.4	8.5	29.9	9.8	36.8
65-74	5.2	6.9	8.8	9.6	31.1	7.2	31.1
75-84	2.9	4.4	7.0	8.6	30.5	10.7	35.9
85+	0.4	0.9	5.7	6.6	26.9	12.3	47.1
Institutionalized							
65+	2.5	1.1	1.0	1.1	1.1	52.9	40.5
65-74	4.4	1.9	1.9	2.2	1.4	58.4	29.9
75-84	3.1	1.4	1.4	0.9	1.2	54.4	37.6
85+	1.1	0.4	0.1	0.7	0.7	48.8	48.1

Source: 1982 and 1984 National Long-term Care Surveys.

These results from the 1982 and 1984 NLTCS show very strongly how disability status predicts new, or incident, disability. Take, for example, people without ADL disability in 1982. Two years later, 79.1% of these people continued to be free of ADL disability, 4.6% experienced disability in an IADL, 5.3% experienced an ADL disability, 1.9% entered nursing homes, and 9.2% died. In other words, within two years about 20% of that non-disabled population declined, either dying or developing new disabilities. Already in 1982 it is possible to identify features that distinguish those who will progress to disability and death by 1984, and those who will remain free of disability. We examine these factors below. It is also clear that people who die or go into nursing homes in this relatively short period must differ from people whose progress toward disability is more gradual. The former likely experienced catastrophic illness, while the latter experienced continuing, but more indolent, progression of chronic disease (Ferrucci, Guralnik, et al., 1996).

If we turn now to people with ADL disability in 1982, say, those with mild (1-2 ADL) disability, we see that this group faces a far greater risk of additional, new disability. Of people with 1-2 ADL disabilities in 1982, only a third remained in this state by 1984. Nearly half these people declined in the 2–year period: 18.5% acquired additional ADL disabilities, 7.6% were institutionalized, and 20.6% died. On the other hand, about 20% showed improvement in disability profiles, including 6.5% who reported no ADL disability 2 years after the initial survey. The different outcomes suggest heterogeneity in this group of people with mild ADL disability. One important goal of public health and aging is to identify features of older people that allow reasonable predictions about risk and suggest interventions for people with these risk profiles. Still, having 1-2 ADL disabilities is clearly a strong predictor of increasing disability.

Finally, if we examine the most disabled group, people in institutions in 1982, it is apparent that the likelihood of regained abilities is very low. Within 2 years, 52.9% will remain institutionalized and 40.5% will die. Fewer than 7% will leave the institution.

Thus, ADL status is a powerful predictor of disability and health transitions, a point we will return to below. The likelihood of improvement and the rapidity of decline suggest important differences in risk at baseline and the likelihood of different disease trajectories.

Despite these impressive features of self-reported ADL for public health and aging, it is also important to recognize that imprecision in these disability measures is also apparent, especially when it comes to high-functioning elders. In the less disabled population recruited for the Assets and Health Dynamics among the Oldest Old study (AHEAD), the correlation between IADL/BADL indices and concurrent and prospective indicators of health is less impressive. Rodgers and Miller (1997, Table 9) report a correlation of 0.42 between BADL and number of health conditions, but no correlation with other health indicators (number of doctor visits, number of nights hospitalized, number of prescriptions, risk of nursing home admission) exceeded 0.30. An analysis using disability items from the Supplement on Aging (SOA) to the National Health Interview Survey and NLTCS items (fielded in subsets of AHEAD respondents) confirmed this rather low pattern of correlation (Rodgers & Miller, 1997, Tables 10,11,16). Thus, standard disability report measures are not as strongly related to indicators of health, and are therefore less informative, in less disabled older adults. For these elders, we need to develop more sensitive indicators.

MORBIDITY AND DISABILITY

Some of the common chronic conditions of late life, such as arthritis and visual and hearing impairment are not fatal but produce severe disability over long periods of time; others, such as ischemic heart disease, chronic obstructive pulmonary disease, diabetes mellitus, and malignant neoplasms, are fatal but nonetheless also produce substantial disability over potentially long periods of time. Verbrugge and Patrick (1995) have analyzed disability associated with the seven conditions, as well as other indicators of disease burden, such as visits to physicians, hospital stays, and death.

The most prevalent chronic conditions for older men in the 1980's, in rank order, were arthritis, hearing impairment, hypertension, ischemic heart disease, chronic obstructive pulmonary disease, chronic sinusitis, visual impairment, cataracts, diabetes, and arteriosclerosis. For women, these conditions were arthritis, hypertension, hearing impairment, cataracts, chronic sinusitis, chronic obstructive pulmonary disease, ischemic heart disease, varicose veins, orthopedic impairments involving the back, diabetes, and visual impairment.

Table 5.4 examines seven of these most prevalent conditions, along with cancer. Verbrugge and Patrick (1995) examined the target conditions in three large U.S. national probability surveys: the National Health Interview Survey, the National Medical Ambulatory Care Survey, and the National Hospital Discharge Survey.

Table 5.4 shows that arthritis is the most prevalent chronic condition in both men and women aged 65+: over a third of men (382.6 per 1000) and over half of women (544.1 per 1000) reported that they had been diagnosed with arthritis. Hearing impairment and ischemic heart disease were second and third (with some switching of places) for both men and women. This rank order is not very different for people aged 45–64, though prevalence is lower for each condition (for example, the prevalence of arthritis is 253.8 for men [about a quarter] and 338.9 for women [about a third] in this younger age group). Table 5.4 shows, not surprisingly, that nonfatal conditions are more common than fatal conditions (not surprisingly because prevalence reflects both the incidence of disease and how long people survive with it). Thus, cancer does not appear in the top 10 chronic conditions because of its usually high and rapid case fatality.

TABLE 5.4 Prevalence of Chronic Disease and Disability Burden

	Men, 65+ Prevalence	Limitation	Impact: Limitation/ Prevalence	Women, 65+ Prevalence	Limitation	Impact: Limitation/ Prevalence
Arthritis	382.6	74.7	19.5	554.1	144.1	26.0
Hearing Impairment	362.4	28.5	7.9	268.1	20.4	7.6
Ischemic Heart Dis	179.0	48.1	26.9	120.7	39.7	32.9
COPD	166.7	43.0	25.8	125.6	21.4	17.0
Visual Impairment	103.8	40.5	39.0	91.4	44.2	48.4
Diabetes	90.8	27.4	30.2	98.8	37.6	38.1
Cancer	52.1	21.4	41.1	38.1	13.5	35.4

After Verbrugge & Patrick, 1995.

Table entries are cases per 1000 (prevalence), cases of human assistance for ADL or IADL disability per 1000 (limitation), and percentage of people with the condition who receive human assistance for ADL or IADL disability (impact).

Note: We have corrected one entry in Verbrugge & Patrick, Table 5 (arthritis impact for women). Note, too, that the limitation column appears to apply to people age 65+ (not 70+, as stated in their paper).

Table 5–4 also shows the association between chronic conditions and the prevalence of activity limitation for people aged 65+, defined as inability to perform ADL and IADL *and* receipt of assistance to perform these tasks. These estimates of disability, then, represent a low-end figure. With inclusion of people reporting difficulty, perhaps without receipt of any assistance, disability associated with particular chronic conditions will be much higher. Remember too that people often have more than one chronic condition. The disability associated with a particular condition includes a mix of disability specific to the disease and disability that is part of a potentially broader set of conditions that includes the particular condition. The "Limitation" column shown in the table is the number of people (per 1000) with disability due to the particular chronic condition (Verbrugge & Patrick, 1995). The "Impact" column is the ratio of limitation to prevalence and can be interpreted as the proportion of disease cases associated with use of personal assistance for ADL or IADL support.

Table 5.4 shows that 74.7 of every 1000 men aged 65+ with arthritis, and 144.1 of every 1000 women, receive personal assistance with ADL or IADL. For these men, the proportion of arthritis cases associated with personal assistance is 19.5% (74.7/382.6). For these women, the proportion is 26.0% (144.1/554.1). Thus, arthritis is more likely to be associated with severe disability in women than in men. Otherwise stated, women with arthritis are about one-third more likely than men to be disabled by arthritis (odds ratio of 1.33 (26.0/19.5). In fact, the risk of disability given these particular chronic conditions is higher for women than men for all but cancer and COPD, that is, for the three nonfatal conditions and a number of the fatal conditions as well.

Verbrugge and Patrick's (1995) derivation of this impact factor, which might be called a "case disability rate," is very valuable, as it offers a measure of disability volume conditioned on chronic disease status. By this measure, given the many chronic conditions typical of late life, it turns out that cancer and visual impairment are the conditions most heavily associated with disability. At younger ages, ischemic heart disease and cancer have this distinction.

MORBIDITY AND PATHWAYS TO DISABLEMENT

For prevention of disability progression and frailty in older adults, a good target is the older adult with mild-to-moderate disability. Put in terms of the disablement model proposed above, it is important to measure *functional limitation* antecedent to disability, and to identify factors associated with reports of disability among individuals who demonstrate a range of limitation in the abilities or skills needed to undertake daily activities. "Functional limitation" antecedent to disability in IADL/BADL is represented by deficits in motor and cognitive skills used in performing daily activities. These skill elements (such as sequencing steps in a task, organizing a workspace, or maintaining bodily alignment) have been well examined in occupational therapy research and have been defined, with clear scoring criteria, as in, for example, the *Assessment of Motor and Process Skills* (AMPS) (Fisher 1997).

Relationship between Antecedent Skill Elements and Disability

What is the relationship between the motor and cognitive skills used in performing daily activities (functional limitation) and IADL/BADL disability? A first investigation in this area involved the relationship between leg strength and gait speed. Buchner (1991; Buchner, Larson, Wagner, Koepsell & de Lateur, 1996) found that the relationship between leg strength, measured in an exercise machine test, and gait speed was nonlinear. In such a non-linear relationship (or flattened S-

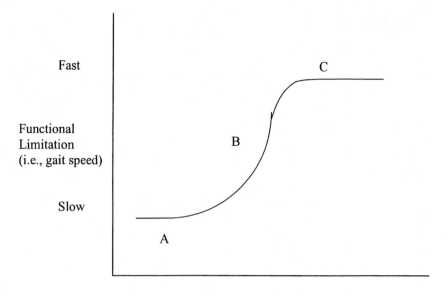

FIGURE 5.5 Hypothetical Relationship Between Functional Limitation and Disability.

Source: After Buchner, Larson, Wagner, Koepsell, & de Lateur, 1996.

shaped curve), three regions are defined, as shown hypothetically in Figure 5.5. The figure relates gait speed, (a measure of functional limitation), to independence or efficiency in bathing (a measure of disability). When leg strength is extremely low, people are essentially unable to walk or stand, and disability in bathing is complete. The curve is flat (region A), indicating that until gait speed exceeds a certain minimum (despite some minor improvements), disability in bathing will not change. In other words, there is a threshold of leg strength or gait speed required for bathing. Once this threshold is crossed, gait speed and independence in bathing are directly related, as shown in region B, so that each additional unit of leg strength or gait speed is associated with a proportional gain in independence or efficiency in bathing. Once leg strength or gait speed exceeds a certain level again, a second threshold is crossed, defining the beginning of region C. At this point, additional gait speed or leg strength does not translate into greater bathing efficiency. Given the biomechanical and ergonomic properties of the task, individuals are already performing as efficiently as possible, and any additional leg strength contributes to physiological reserve but does not affect the speed or efficiency of bathing. Above this threshold, increments in strength or skill are not associated with reduction in disability but only with increased reserve (Buchner, 1991; Sonn, Frandin & Grimby, 1995).

Identification of these thresholds is important, as they indicate the point on a continuum of ability, physical or cognitive, when functional limitation translates into disability or, more simply, at what point reduction in underlying skills or competencies finally disables someone. The thresholds also help set goals for intervention and rehabilitation. For example, a clinical trial seeking to prevent or reduce disability by improving strength would not show benefit if targeted to individuals in region C of the curve. These individuals are already beyond the threshold where improvements in strength will affect performance of daily tasks. Similarly, individuals in region A are unlikely to show improvement in disability even with some improvement in underlying abilities. Only with large improvement in these abilities could we expect to see reduction in disability. By contrast, people along region B of the curve would be the best target for such a trial. In this group, even small changes in underlying functional abilities can be expected to translate into increases in independence and efficiency.

Buchner and colleagues (1997) have shown the relevance of these considerations in a clinical trial of exercise to reduce the incidence of falls. The trial was part of the FICSIT initiative, "Frailty and Injuries: Cooperative Studies of Intervention Techniques." The study recruited elders with extensive functional limitation; all were unable to do an eight-step tandem gait test without errors, and all were below the 50th percentile in knee extensor strength based on norms for weight and height. A program of endurance and strength training led to increases in isokinetic strength and aerobic capacity, but no improvements in gait speed or balance. This lack of consistent benefit (reduction in measures of impairment, no benefit in measures of functional limitation) already suggests that selection criteria for the study were too stringent. People recruited for the study were likely near or within region A of the curve shown in Figure 5.5, so that improvement in underlying functional abilities may not lead to improvement in disability status. Indeed, in this study 1–year fall rates in the intervention group were 42%, better than the control group rate of 60%, but no different than the risk of falls typical of older people living in the community (Tinetti, Speechley & Ginter, 1988). Buchner and colleagues (1997) concluded that the eligibility criteria selected a sample on the verge of substantial decline, and exercise prevented this decline. A more efficient study would have selected a less impaired sample.

The nonlinear relationship between underlying ability and disability status has been established for a number of indicators. Jette, Assman, Rooks, Harris, and Crawford (1998) reported nonlinear relationships between balance and gait speed, and between gait speed and IADL/ BADL measures. In multivariate analyses, the association between impairment (balance and strength measures) and disability (reported IADL/ BADL) was attenuated when gait (functional limitation) was included in regression models, suggesting that functional limitations play an intermediary role. A causal interpretation of this cross-sectional finding is that impairments in strength or balance need to be severe enough to affect mobility before an individual reports disability in IADL or ADL. This would serve as important confirmation of the disablement model, described above. Other studies have reported similar findings (Cress et al.,1995; Ferrucci, Guralnik, Buchner, et al., 1997; Judge, Schechtman, Cress 1996; Rantanen et al. 1998; Rantanen, Guralnik, Sakari-Rantala, et al. 1999).

The nonlinear relationship between underlying ability and disability status also appears to hold for cognitive status and reported disability. Figure 5.6 is a scatterplot of disability status by number of errors on a cognitive screening measure, derived from a sample of caregivers to

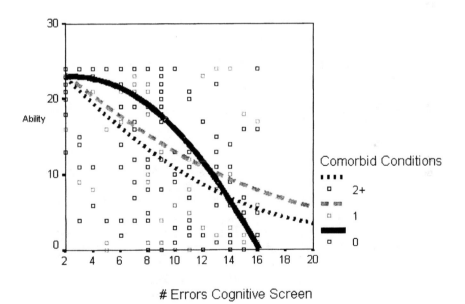

FIGURE 5.6 Relation Between Disability and Cognitive Status.
Source: Washington Heights-Inwood Community Aging Project, 1992 Baseline.

elders diagnosed with Alzheimer's disease. Caregivers reported on disability status in the elder. Scores ranged from 24 (best score: independent all the time in all 12 tasks assessed) to 0 (worst score: dependent all the time in all 12 tasks). Elders completed a 15–item cognitive screening test, which included items from a series of brief cognitive status tests (CARE-Diagnostic Screen: Gurland et al., 1995). These items assess a person's orientation, short-term memory, attention, and language ability. The scatterplot stratifies by number of comorbid conditions to better isolate the effect of cognitive deficit on reported disability.

The least-squares regression lines shown in Figure 5.6 were derived using a curvilinear regression model. The R^2 for the model in subjects without other comorbid conditions (thick line, n=78) increased from 0.41 to 0.52 with introduction of a quadratic term, suggesting that the nonlinear curvilinear model offers a better fit. By contrast, in the two groups with other concurrent disease, linear models provided an adequate fit. Subjects with cognitive impairment in the absence of other comorbid disease are not likely to report disability until they make 5+ errors on the cognitive screen. This relationship should be compared to that of subjects with cognitive deficit and 1 or 2+ comorbid conditions. They report greater disability at every level of cognitive ability. We conclude that the relationship between cognitive impairment and disability may follow that demonstrated for physical indicators and disability.

Measurement of Antecedent Skill Elements Relevant for Disablement

Elicitation of IADL/BADL status usually involves self-reports of difficulty or need for assistance in a global sense; for example, "By yourself, that is, without help from another person or special equipment, do you have any difficulty with meal preparation?" To assess underlying abilities or skills, by contrast, we need to measure functional limitation. For this effort, assessment tools from occupational therapy are useful. In the Assessment of Motor and Process Skills (AMPS) test, mentioned earlier, occupational therapists obtain *performance-based ratings of specific motor and cognitive skills* used in completing two tasks from a pre-specified list of 54 IADL/BADL tasks (Fisher, 1997). An occupational therapist, having undergone a 5–day training program in the AMPS, makes the ratings. Each of the motor and cognitive or "process" skills, drawn from extensive experience in occupational therapy with a variety of patient populations, is rated on a 4–point scale (competent, questionable, ineffective, deficit). The skills (and domains) are shown in Table 5.5.

TABLE 5.5 Assessment of Motor and Process Skills

AMPS Motor Skills: *Posture*: Stabilizes, Aligns, Positions; *Mobility*: Walks, Reaches, Bends; *Coordination*: Coordinates, Manipulates, Flows; *Strength and Effort*: Moves, Transports, Lifts, Calibrates, Grips; *Energy*: Endures
AMPS Cognitive/Process Skills: *Energy*: Paces, Attends; *Using Knowledge*: Chooses, Uses, Handles, Heeds, Inquires; *Temporal Organization*: Initiates, Continues, Sequences, Terminates; *Space and Objects*: Searches/ Locates, Gathers, Organizes, Restores, Navigates; *Adaptation*: Notices/ Responds, Accommodates, Adjusts, Benefits

An important advantage of the AMPS is its use of a many-faceted Rasch measurement model. The Rasch model has been used to (1) calibrate difficulty levels for the 54 tasks, (2) establish difficulty levels for ratings of each skill item, and (3) combine these skill ratings and task difficulty ratings to establish a single score for respondents on separate motor and cognitive/process skill dimensions. The equating of AMPS tasks, linked by common skill items, makes it possible to compare the ability of respondents who perform *different* sets of tasks. In addition, the many-faceted Rasch model is used to calibrate raters on the same scales, so that rater "severity" is incorporated into AMPS scoring software. This software is required for converting the raw skill ratings to logit scores on the motor and cognitive/process dimensions. The logit is the logarithm of the odds of obtaining a given skill item score when a person of a given ability is observed performing a given task.

IADL/BADL tasks vary in difficulty, as reflected in the logit scores for AMPS tasks on the motor and cognitive/process dimensions. For example, on the motor dimension "eating a meal" is the easiest task and "vacuuming" the hardest. On the cognitive/process dimension, the easiest item is "tying shoes," and the hardest "making eggs, toast, and espresso coffee." The AMPS tasks all involve meal preparation, household work, or dressing/grooming. The tasks reflect relevant cultural diversity in IADL/BADL tasks (e.g., variation in the kinds of foods prepared), since they were normed for a Spanish-and English-speaking population. Also, the AMPS procedure takes account of individual variation (i.e., expectations regarding neatness, etc.); the occupational therapist and respondent establish a clear contract regarding what is involved in completing the task, and respondents are scored relative to this expectation.

Fisher (1997) reports that a cognitive/process skill score of 1.0 logit, and a motor skill score of 2.0 logit, are 1 sd below the mean for community-resident older adults. These scores have been associated with clinician ratings of IADL/BADL difficulty. For example, discriminant analyses using these cutoff scores were quite accurate in classifying elders according to disease state and residence status: 97% of nondisabled older adults had cognitive/process scores greater than 1.0, and 92% of demented subjects had scores less than 1.0 (Fisher, 1997). These scores serve then as thresholds for likely disability.

An advantage of this approach is its explicit focus on the skill elements elders use *to get tasks done,* as observed in home settings using prespecified but ecologically valid tasks. In this way it differs from existing IADL or BADL performance tests (e.g., Myers, et al., 1993; Loewenstein et al, 1992; Muharin et al., 1991; Karagiozis, et al., 1998), which are limited to only a few tasks, require subjects to perform tasks they may not do in normal activity, and do not yield measures of ability or skill that are involved in all IADL/BADL tasks.

As part of a pilot study of self-reported IADL/BADL disability, we interviewed elders with mild-to-moderate disability, as defined by self-report of at least one but no more than three domains (upper extremity tasks, lower extremity tasks, IADL, and BADL). We randomly chose 10 for a repeat interview that included the AMPS occupational assessment conducted by an AMPS-certified occupational therapist (OT). Nine completed the home assessment (and in a third of the cases, we supplied props necessary for the task, e.g., bread and filling for a sandwich). For comparison, we conducted three AMPS assessments of inpatients in our rehabilitation unit, using the hospital "ADL kitchen." Table 5.6 shows the feasibility of in-home AMPS assessment. The assessments are acceptable, appropriate AMPS task are identified, and AMPS scores accord with expectations of disability based on cognitive status and self-reported disability. Subjects with cognitive impairment but who did not meet criteria for dementia (C3, C5, C7) scored below cutoff scores on the cognitive/process dimension, as did all three subjects on the rehabilitation unit. Subjects with disability in two or more domains were likely to score below the AMPS motor dimension cutoff score. Subject C4 scored extremely high on both motor and cognitive/process domains, consistent with his lifestyle (he drives, cares for a foster grandson, travels to Florida); in fact, he reported no disability in the home visit (as opposed to the prior interview, in which he reported upper extremity disability). Subject C7 is an especially interesting case. Her cognitive status clearly interfered with IADL/BADL competencies: in pouring milk into her coffee, for example, she failed to open the spout of the milk carton, forgot to return items to storage spaces, and could not remember all the elements of the task she was supposed to perform. Her cognitive/process skill score (-0.6) was well below the AMPS cutoff.

These results suggest the utility of measurement of underlying skills and competencies to better understand disablement. Standard perfor-

TABLE 5.6 AMPS Pilot

Sex, Age	AMPS Tasks Performed	Cognitive Status	Domains Disability, #	AMPS: Motor/ Cognitive- Process Logit Core
C1. F, 88	Prepare oatmeal; Mop	Normal	2	a
C2. M, 92	Vacuuming; Get foods from refrigerator	Normal	3	1.7*/1.6
C3. F, 78	Make bed; Fold laundry	MCI/QD*	3	−0.4*/O.7*
C4. M, 80	Make sandwich; Fold laundry	Normal	1	3.1/1.7
C5. F, 89	Pour juice; Make sandwich	MCI/QD	2	1.2*/0.8*
C6. F, 79	Make bed; Prepare instant soup	Normal	2	a
C7. F, 81	Set table; Prepare coffee and toast	MCI/QD	3	1.0 /−0.6*
C8. F, 77	Prepare coffee and toast; Make sandwich	Normal	2	a
C9. F, 83	Sweep kitchen floor; Cook vegetables	Normal	2	0.9*/1.0
11. M, 75	Make sandwich	unk	4	0. 3*/0. 9*
12. F, 75	Make bed	unk	4	−1.9*/0.4*
13. F, 71	Make sandwich	unk	4	−0.6*/−0.1*

Note: C, WHICAP (Washington Heights-Inwood Community Aging Project) resident; I, rehabilitation unit inpatient; a, OT trained made ratings but AMPS rater-specific calibration software not yet available at time of interview; *MCI/QD, nondemented but mild impairment or questionable dementia; asterisk indicates score below AMPS cutoff (motor 2. 0, cognitive/ process 1.0). #Disability domains: Women's Health and Aging study categories.

mance-based assessments are inadequate for reasons suggested earlier, but tools from ergonomic studies and occupational therapy are available and can be used in natural environments. These are likely to provide key insights on risks for disability and ways to reduce such risks.

Risk Factors for Incident Disability

We have already seen that the presence of disability is a strong predictor of new, additional disability with the passage of time. This stands to reason: older people with ADL disability have chronic diseases that put them at risk, with progression of disease, for acquiring additional disabilities. It is also important to look at older people without ADL disability to identify risk factors for its onset in the near future. People likely to progress to ADL disability differ from non-progressors 2-5 years (and perhaps longer) before the onset of disability. Prospective cohort studies have proven very productive in this effort. In these studies, a group of people without disability at baseline is followed over some defined interval. Onset of disability is recorded at standard assessment intervals. We are thus able to identify incident cases and go back to baseline assessments to see how these people differ from people who never reached the disability endpoint. Typically, we examine a series of baseline risk factors and calculate the risk associated with a factor, independent of other risk factors that make up a person's profile. Features associated with the disability outcome are "risk factors"; features that reduce likelihood of incidence are called "protective factors." We calculate these risks using logistic regression models, or proportional hazards models if we wish to incorporate a time dimension into analyses (i.e., time to onset rather than simply onset).

The Established Populations for Epidemiologic Studies of the Elderly (EPESE), a prospective study of community-dwelling elderly, has proven very useful for this effort. For example, risk factors for incident mobility limitation over a 6–year period were identified in the Iowa, east Boston, and New Haven components of the project, stratified by gender (LeCroix, Levalle, Hecht, Grothaus, & Wagner, 1991). Socioeconomic features (age and income, and to a lesser extent, education) consistently predicted increased risk of mobility disability. For example, among men in east Boston, 21% over age 85 at baseline remained free of mobility disability compared to 66% in the group aged 65-74. Baseline chronic condition status also predicted mobility status over follow-up. The presence of a heart attack, stroke, diabetes, hypertension, angina, dyspnea, or leg pain at baseline each predicted greater likelihood of incident mobility disability. Finally, behavioral factors at baseline were also associated with risk of mobility deficit over follow-up. Frequent exercise and walking were protective factors; smoking increased the risk of incident mobility disability.

An analysis of the Supplement on Aging showed that risk factors for ADL disability and death differed in important ways (Boutt, Kane, Louis, Boult, & McCaffrey, 1994). Over 4 years of follow-up, some baseline factors were associated with both outcomes (age, education, social contact, cerebrovascular disease), some with ADL disability alone (arthritis), and some with mortality only (gender, cancer, obesity, diabetes, income, locus of control, volunteering). Other factors were not associated with either outcome (marital status, coronary artery disease, hypertension, race, exercise).

These findings vary somewhat between studies according to the demographic composition of the cohort, the length of follow-up, how attrition is handled, how risk factors are categorized, and how competing risks (for death and disability) are handled.

More recently, potential biomarkers for disability have been identified. For example, serum albumin level (g/L) is a risk factor for both incident disability and mortality. Within the EPESE cohort, serum albumin concentration and disability were strongly related at baseline. Moreover, at follow-up, greater serum albumin concentration was associated with a greater risk of mortality within categories of baseline disability status. A new set of biomarkers for function is currently under investigation, including C-reactive protein, IL-6, and other cytokines.

A last but perhaps most productive set of predictors of incident disability is functional limitation, which, consistent with the disablement model, represents preclinical disability (Fried et al., 1991). Guralnik and colleagues (Guralnik, Ferucci, Simonsick, Salive, & Wallace, 1995), again using the EPESE sample, have shown that scores on three simple measures of functional limitation are very effective predictors of future mobility and ADL disability. They established quartiles of performance based on sample distributions for the time it took respondents to walk eight meters, stand up five times from a chair, and hold progressively more complicated stances. Quartile of performance within each test strongly predicted risk of disability. For example, 33.3% of older people in the slowest quartile at baseline went on to develop ADL disability over four years, compared to 15.5%, 8.3%, and 6.2% in quartiles representing progressively faster walking speed.

The four levels within each of the three tests can be used to establish a "physical performance" score with a range of 3 (poorest performance on all three measures) to 12 (top quartiles of performance on all three measures). This composite measure, summarizing gait speed, lower extremity strength, and balance, ranged from 4-12 in the sample. That is, no community-dwelling elder scored in the poorest quartile of performance on all three measures at baseline. Over 80% of people with a score of 4 at baseline developed mobility and ADL disability over follow-up. This endpoint was met by about 60% of people with scores of 5-6, 40% with scores of 7, 30% for scores of 8-9, and less than 20% for people with scores 10 or greater. In logistic regression models, scores of 4-6 were associated with a fourfold increase in the risk of ADL disability and a fivefold increase in risk of mobility disability, compared to people with scores in the 10-12 range.

The EPESE data also show an important difference in disability risk by gender. Using the same physical performance scale, Guralnik and colleagues (1994) determined that women have poorer physical performance (or greater functional limitation) than men at every age. This relationship held even when groups were stratified by self-reports of disability status. Why women should perform more poorly on these measures is unclear. It is possible that men with poor physical performance are less likely to live in the community; they may be more likely to reside in nursing homes or die. More likely, women in late life really do have lower strength and balance skill, perhaps due to greater prevalence of osteoporosis and sarcopenia.

One negative aspect of the studies above is their limitation to physical predictors and relative neglect of cognitive status. In one large community-based cohort, Gill and colleagues have shown that the risk of incident ADL disability associated with quartiles of performance on the Mini-Mental State Exam (MMSE) was independent of physical performance status (Gill, Williams, Richardson, & Tinetti 1996). A second population-based study, reported by Moritz, Kasl, and Berkman, (1995), showed that poorer scores on a brief cognitive screening tool were associated with increased risk of persistent ADL limitations over three years of follow-up. These findings have been supported in other studies (Greiner, Snowdon, & Schmitt, 1996). Finally, Ganguli, Seaberg, Belle, Fischer, and Kuller, (1993) reported on the service needs of cognitively impaired elders, defining cognitive impairment as scores at or below the fifth percentile on at least one test of memory and one test of another cognitive domain. They determined that such cognitive impairment was strongly associated with increased risk of hospital admission over the prior sixth months, as well as increased use of home health services, social services, and prescription medications.

One limitation of these studies, however, is the absence of dementia diagnoses. These studies were unable to separate mild cognitive impairment and dementia as risk factors, and by not excluding demented subjects may have introduced unreliable (from demented elders: Østbye, Tyas, McDowell, & Koval, 1997) or potentially differential reporting (from proxies: Kelly-Hayes, Jette, Wolf, D'Augostino, & Odell, 1992; Rubenstein, Schairer, Wieland & Kane, 1984) of disability. We take up this issue in chapter 6.

TRENDS IN THE PREVALENCE OF DISABILITY

In an important review of a voluminous and complex literature Freedman, Martin, and Schoeni, (2002) have summarized trend data on the prevalence of disability in the United States. They restricted their review to datasets of the highest quality, seeking surveys that merited "good" ratings on a variety of criteria: sampling of independent, repeated cross-sections of older people, national population coverage, a time frame covering nearly or more than a decade, annual or five or more survey waves, identical assessment instruments with detailed inquiry about each ADL and IADL, minimal attrition, minimal missing data, and sample sizes large enough to detect 1-2% changes per year. Surveys that best met these criteria included the national Health Interview Survey (HIS) and National Long-Term Care Survey (NLTCS). Less optimal surveys by these criteria were also examined in this review. These included the Asset and Health Dynamics of the Oldest Old (AHEAD), the Medicare Current Beneficiary Survey (MCBS), National Mortality Follow-Back Study, Supplements on Aging to the HIS, and Survey of Income and Program Participation (SIPP).

In the HIS, the prevalence of any disability (ADL or IADL) declined from 22.7% in 1982 to 20.2% in 1993 (Crimmins, Saito, & Reynolds, 1997), and continued to decline to 19.3% in 1996 (Schoeni, Freedman, & Wallace, 2001). In the NLTCS, the prevalence of any disability declined from 24.9% in 1982 to 21.3% in 1994 (Manton et al., 1997), and again to 19.7% in 1999 (Manton & Gu, 2001). These prevalence estimates are adjusted for differences in the age and sex composition of the U.S. population over these periods. Based on evidence from the two surveys, disability prevalence in older people has declined about 1% per year over the past 15–20 years. Results from the MCBS confirm this decline in the 1990's (Freedman, Martin, & Schoeni, 2002).

The decline in disability is actually mostly driven by declines in high-level IADL disability, not ADL disability. IADL disability includes difficulty or need for help because of a health problem in household management tasks, such as shopping for small items, preparing a meal, using the telephone, taking medications, handling finances, or light cleaning. When disability prevalence trends are disaggregated by IADL and ADL disability, the HIS data suggest that the prevalence of ADL disability has remained rather flat over this time period, fluctuating between 6.4% and 8.4% (Freedman, Martin, & Schoeni, 2002). IADL disability, as estimated in the HIS, declined from 14.5% in 1982 to 13.8% in 1993, and again to 10.9% in 1996, a decline of 1.7% annually (Crimmins et al., 1997; Schoeni et al., 2001).

The NLTCS data, by contrast, suggest a decline in both ADL and IADL disability. Between 1982 and 1994, IADL disability prevalence declined from 13.1% to 11.9%, and ADL disability from 5.6% to 4.3% (Manton et al., 1997). These declines in prevalence appear to be accelerating for both types of disability. In 1999, the prevalence of IADL disability in the NLTCS was 10.6% and the prevalence of ADL disability 3.2%, suggesting declines of 1%-2% annually in both domains. The MCBS survey confirmed these trends for both ADL and IADL disability (Waidmann & Liu, 2000).

Measures of functional limitations identified in these surveys, such as self-reports of difficulty with mobility, cognitive dysfunction, and sensory deficits (hearing and vision), also mostly showed declines in prevalence over this period. These declines were of the same order, about 1%-2% annually. However, using AHEAD data Freedman, Hakan, and Martin (2001)-(2002) reported even sharper declines for severe cognitive deficit (8.6% in 1993 to 7.1% in 1998), a decline of nearly 3% per year. Similarly, using SIPP data, Freedman and Martin (1998, 1999) reported declines in the prevalence of self-reported difficulty with vision of similar magnitude (15.3% in 1984 to 11.6% in 1993).

Evidence for declines in the prevalence of disability in older adults in the United States, then, is impressive. These declines are mostly consistent across our best national surveys, extend across different kinds of disability, are roughly of the same magnitude, and demonstrate some measure of biological plausibility, since they are accompanied by declines in the prevalence of functional limitations that precede such disability. The declines appear to be accelerating, at least between the 1980s and 1990s; it is less clear if these trends will continue (Schoeni et al., 2001). The declines are evident as well in the population of older people living in skilled care facilities (Manton et al., 1997; Manton & Gu, 2001) and in the period before death (Liao et al., 2000). These last trends are especially reassuring. Disability in residents of skilled care facilities and in people facing the last year of life is, on the whole, quite severe, so a decline in disability here represents an important confirmation of this broad trend.

These declines in the prevalence of disability offer support for Fries's (1983) early hypothesis on the compression of morbidity as a reasonable goal for public health and aging. As discussed earlier (chapter 3), Fries suggested that disability in late life could be compressed into an increasingly shorter period of life. This "compression of morbidity" would take place if the age of onset of disability were postponed to a greater degree than increases in life expectancy. The result would be reductions in cumulative average lifetime disability, or otherwise said, an increase in active life expectancy. The evidence from these surveys of disability prevalence provides some support for Fries's claim. As he points out, "senior mortality rates are declining at about 1% per year and disability is declining about 2% per year [according to NCLTS estimates]" (Fries, 2002, p. 3164). To return to the basic model of cumulative survival and disability-free life expectancy presented in Chapter 2, these trends suggest that the disability-free life expectancy curve is moving outward and to the right at a faster rate than the survival curve. Or expressed in terms of incidence, age-specific disability is declining to a greater degree than age-specific mortality. Fries concludes, "Compression of morbidity is occurring nationally, and that certainly is good news" (Fries 2002, p. 3164).

On the other hand, the difference in the magnitude of disability across surveys and in reported declines in prevalence is less welcome. These differences suggest that we still have not solved the problems identified some time ago by Wiener and colleagues (1990) for measurement of ADL disability. Even slight differences in the formulation of survey items, response categories, and question order can lead to important differences in the interpretation of questions, and hence quite different prevalence estimates, as noted above. A difference of 1-2% in the prevalence of an ADL disability can mean as many as half million older people improperly classified. If we use these estimates for planning services, such error can be consequential.

Also, it must stressed that the reasons for this decline in disability over the past 20 years are not completely understood. Explanations advanced include improvement in primary prevention efforts, such as changes in lifestyle risk factors (education, expectations about health in later life) or health behaviors (obesity, exercise, smoking); benefits from secondary prevention (bone density screening, prostate-specific antigen testing, estrogen replacement, use of non-steroidal anti-inflammatory agents); or the success of tertiary prevention efforts, such as adoption of effective health promotion and disease management programs, or improvements in geriatric medical care. Or, as we have stressed earlier, the declines in disability in late life could be the result of broader changes over the entire life course, such as better pediatric care, improved sanitation and hygiene at every age, or declines in manual labor. Most likely, some combination of all these factors is at work, and a major task of public health and aging will be to dissect them and measure the relative contribution of each to the reduction of disability. Until causes for the decline are identified (and until interventions to manipulate these causes are tested), we will not know with certainty "whether such trends in disability are real, driven by improvements in the underlying health or social environment of older Americans, or simply a statistical artifact stemming from methodological and conceptual problems" (Schoeni et al., 2001, p. S217).

SOCIAL CONTEXTS OF DECLINING DISABILITY

In their review of trends in the prevalence of disability, Freedman and colleagues (2002) also examined the extent to which disparities in the risk of disability were unevenly distributed, that is, whether gaps in disability prevalence among socioeconomic groups were widening, narrowing, or were essentially unchanged within this broad 20–year trend of declining disability. Among older adults, disability prevalence is higher among women, non-whites, and the less educated, in addition to the oldest old; and evidence for declining disability prevalence in these more vulnerable groups would be important evidence for a broad "compression of morbidity" effect and a more general claim of progress in public health and aging. Also, recognition of persisting disparities would be useful for identifying obstacles to public health efforts in this area.

Disparities in Declines in Disability Prevalence by Age

Analyses of disability trend data in the National Health Interview Survey (HIS) suggest that disability is declining faster in the young-old than in the old-old, though these differences did not achieve statistical significance. Among older adults aged 70–79, disability declined 1.5% per year between 1982 and 1996. In 80–89 year-olds, disability prevalence declined 0.8% annually. Notably, the oldest of the old in the sample, people aged 90+, showed declines in disability comparable to those of the young-old, 1.3% annually (Schoeni et al., 2001). The relatively better picture among people who have reached extremely old ages is consistent with other trends identified for nonagenarians and centenarians, such as a deceleration of mortality risk (see chapter 2). The National Long-Term Care Survey (NLTCS) found greater annual reductions in disability for elders aged 85+ compared to younger elderly (Manton & Gu, 2001).

Data from the National Mortality Followback Survey suggest an important age difference in disability trends among people in the last year of life. Declines in disability in the last year of life were larger among people aged 85+, relative to people aged 65-84, in a comparison of the last year of life in 1986 and 1993 (Liao et al., 2000).

The narrowing of differences in disability by age was also evident for self-reported measures of functional limitation. For example, in the Survey of Income and Program Participation (SIPP), among people aged 80+ declines in difficulty reported for upper and lower extremity tasks were greater than declines evident in people aged 50-64 or 65-79 (Freedman & Martin, 1998; Freedman, Martin, & Schoeni, 2002).

Results from the HIS also point to the key role of marital status for these age effects. "Elderly persons who were currently married experienced improvements that were a full percentage point higher —1.7% versus 0.7%—than elderly persons who were not married" (Schoeni et al., 2001, p. 5214). Marriage, already acknowledged as a protective factor for mortality risk and many other health outcomes, appears to offer some benefit (or reflect some selection factor) relevant for reduction of disability.

Finally, geographic effects should also be acknowledged, though their significance is less clear. Older adults living in the Northeast and South show greater declines in disability over this period than elders in the West or Midwest.

Disparities in Declines in Disability Prevalence by Gender

Results from the HIS suggest no differences in declining disability among men and women (Crimmins et al., 1997; Schoeni et al., 2001). Disability declined 1.2% annually both in men and women. Other surveys suggest some advantage for women in declines in the prevalence of functional limitation and sensory impairment (SIPP, Freedman & Martin, 1998), and similar declines for reduction of severe cognitive impairment (AHEAD, Freedman, Hakan, & Martin, 2001).

Disparities in Declines in Disability Prevalence by Race

HIS data do not suggest widening of the gap in disability between whites and non-whites. In both groups, disability declined: 1.6% annually among whites and 1.3% annually among non-whites (Schoeni et al., 2001). Data from the National Long-Term Care Survey (NLTCS) suggest that the gap between blacks and non-blacks narrowed between 1989 and 1999, after widening in the 1980s (Manton & Gu, 2001). The gap in the prevalence of functional limitation, sensory impairment, and severe cognitive deficit between blacks and whites appears to be narrowing, as annual declines have been greater among blacks than whites in the 1990s.

Disparities in Declines in Disability Prevalence by Education

In the HIS, declines in the prevalence of disability were significantly greater in older people who had completed more years of school (Schoeni, Freedman & Wallace, 2001). The NLTCS did not show a consistent pattern (Manton & Gu, 2001). Similarly, educational attainment was not consistently related to declines in functional limitations, sensory deficit, or cognitive impairment (Freedman, Martin & Schoeni, 2002).

It is hard to draw firm conclusions about socioeconomic disparities and changes in the prevalence of disability from these stratified analyses. Whether a gap is narrowed depends, at least in part, on how far apart these groups are in the first place. Gaps are more easily "narrowed" if groups are far apart: in this instance, there is simply more room to improve. Perhaps the safest conclusion is: "Although none of the results . . . suggested that the gaps were widening between old and young, men and women, or whites and nonwhites, whether the gaps have narrowed or have remained stable for these groups over the last decade remains unclear" (Freedman, Martin, & Schoeni, 2002, p. 3146).

COMPENSATION AND USE OF PROSTHETIC TECHNOLOGIES TO REDUCE DISABILITY

The disablement model, proposed earlier, allows specification of compensatory processes and environmental modifications that prevent impairment and functional limitation from becoming disability. Environmental modifications, such as lengthening pedestrian intervals at signaled intersections or replacement of bathtubs with walk-in showers, reduce the impact of functional limitation, in this case slow gait speed and deficits in lower extremity strength. Effective environmental modifications essentially reduce task demand, so that otherwise disabling functional limitations do not disable. This sort of intervention in the disablement pathway is shown schematically in Figure 5.7.

Perhaps the first, most basic, and most common environmental modification is simply altering the frequency of a task or changing the way a task is performed. If a shoulder range-of-motion limitation makes it difficult for someone to wash his or her hair, the first response is likely to be a reduction in the frequency of hair washing or a change in bathing routine, such as washing hair only when someone is available

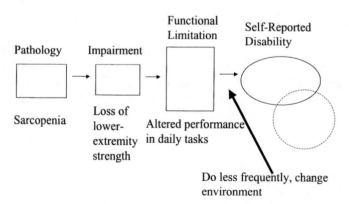

FIGURE 5.7 Disablement: Environmental Interventions.

to help. These are effective modifications for mild to moderately severe functional limitation. With progression of functional limitation, completing ADL tasks may become impossible without further modifications, either alteration of the physical environment (washing hair in the sink rather than shower, use of grab bar or bath stool, use of walk-in shower stall), or recourse to personal assistance (regular help getting into the tub, balance support, and personal assistance with application of shampoo).

One challenge for defining disability, already mentioned, is that people who have made successful adaptations of this sort may not report difficulty with the task. After all, they are successfully performing the task and have, to a great extent, overcome the functional limitation that caused this difficulty. Given the disablement model's stress on self-reported difficulty as a criterion for disability, these people are not disabled. But they do show poorer scores on measures of functional limitation and accordingly should be considered at risk for incident disability and need for services. For example, Fried et al., (1997) has shown that people reporting no difficulty with ADL but who also say they have reduced the frequency of these ADL tasks have lower grip strength, gait speed, dexterity, and balance scores.

Results from the Disability Supplement to the 1994-1995 National Health Interview Survey (HIS) offer important insights on the role of one type of environmental modification: use of assistive or prosthetic devices, relative to personal assistance (Verbrugge & Sevak, 2002). In the 1994-1995 HIS, the prevalence of ADL difficulty because of a health problem in people aged 55+ was 5.6% (bathing), 3.4% (dressing), 1.0% (eating), 3.2% (transfer), 2.7% (toileting), and 3.2% (indoor mobility). Among people reporting these disabilities, most received some kind of assistance: 89.9% (bathing), 85.2% (dressing), 83.6% (eating), 73.7% (transfer), 89.7% (toileting), and 84.8% (indoor mobility). Thus, between 10% (bathing, toileting) and about 26% (transfer) of people reporting difficulty with ADL received no assistance. Of people using assistance, some used only personal assistance, some only equipment, and some both types of assistance. The "equipment use alone" percentage showed wide variation: 22.2% (bathing), 2.0% (dressing), 4.2% (eating), 17.8% (transfer), 39.5% (toileting), and 42.5% (indoor mobility). This variation seems reasonable. For some ADL, assistive devices have long been available, such as canes, wheelchairs, commodes, indwelling catheters, bath chairs, and so forth. Assistive devices for other ADL, such as dressing or eating, are less well developed or accepted.

The 1994-1995 Disability Supplement to the HIS also asked respondents *receiving assistance* how much difficulty they had with tasks. This allows a measure of "difficulty reduction" according to type of assistance received. Verbrugge and Sevak (2002) show that equipment only or equipment with personal assistance is more likely to reduce difficulty than personal assistance alone. To explain this result, they point out "First, equipment is designed for the task, can be modified to suit the individual, and is generally on hand when needed.... Second, equipment maintains an individual's self-sufficiency. This can foster pride and keen perception of task improvements," (p.S376-377) This is an important result and suggests the need for further development of assistive devices. However, it is also worth recognizing the limits of equipment use in the case of cognitive disability, a major source of disability in late life (see chapter 6).

Environmental modification reduces task demand and in this way prevents disability. An alternative route to the prevention of disability is development of compensatory processes that increase a person's capabilities. Within the setting of functional limitation, a person's capacities can be increased through recruitment of remaining, relatively spared abilities. This compensatory process is shown schematically in Figure 5.9. This process is less well explored than environmental modification but is likely to be at least as important. It suggests far more extensive use of rehabilitative technologies to teach older people (and, indeed, anyone facing functional limitations) how to reorganize the way they do tasks by drawing on other remaining abilities.

As Figure 5.8 shows, compensation can be viewed as an intervention that interrupts the link between impairment and functional limitation. The older person with severe balance deficit (impairment) who still performs well in daily tasks, such as vacuuming or cooking, has presumably drawn on other faculties to prevent the balance disorder from

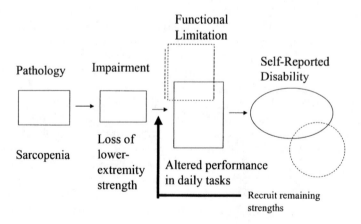

FIGURE 5.8 Disablement Model: Compensation.

disabling him in these daily tasks. We know very little about these processes, though efforts from kinesiology and neuroscience are underway to specify this effect. A simpler example is seen in the elder with mild cognitive impairment who uses other brain regions, visualized in functional MRI, to perform better than expected in certain memory tasks. This elder likely uses mnemonics or other strategies to perform the memory task and hence draws on other relatively spared domains of brain function.

With compensation, functional limitation and hence disability are altered. In fact, it is likely that older people facing disablement use both environmental modification to reduce task demand and compensatory processes to increase capability.

A Disability in Depth: Bathing

We can tie these insights on disability and efforts to mitigate the effects of functional limitation with a closer look at a particular disability. A good candidate is bathing. As we have seen, it is the most prevalent ADL disability and one that lends itself to environmental modification and use of compensatory processes.

In an ongoing study of nearly 200 older adults, all aged 70+, with mild to moderate disability (reported difficulty in 1-3 domains of upper extremity, lower extremity, IADL, and ADL function, but not all four), 9.5% reported that they had difficulty with bathing. These self-reports were quite stable. In the whole sample, less than 2% changed their self-report between a telephone interview and an in-home assessment. Respondents reported a variety of sources for their difficulty bathing, including fear of falling and concern about balance, pain, weakness, swollen legs (edema), and shortness of breath. People who reported difficulty bathing were more likely to report they had changed the frequency of bathing and the way they bathed. For example, of those reporting difficulty bathing, 87.5% said they had changed the way they bathe over the past 12 months. In people who did not report difficulty bathing, only 24.8% reported a change in the way they bathe. Thus, reports of difficulty and attempts to modify environments to mitigate difficulty go hand in hand.

If we look only at people who said they had no difficulty bathing, we find further evidence that environmental modification is a response to functional limitation. People who reported they had changed the way they bathe showed greater functional limitation than people who reported no change. Their grip strength was lower, their gait slower, and their performance on the Assessment of Motor and Process Skills (AMPS, the occupational therapy assessment described above) less efficient. We find this pattern even when we restrict the sample further to people who report they have not changed the frequency with which they bathe. People who have changed the way they bathe score more poorly on the measures, indicating greater functional limitation. Thus, environmental modification, indicated by changes in frequency and mode of performing the ADL, are clearly related to degree of functional limitation.

In the same sample, we also investigated one facet of compensation in the face of functional limitation. We established the poorest balance group by examining the distribution of scores on a series of progressively more difficult static stances. Those in the lowest tertile (or third) showed a great range of motor performance in the AMPS assessment. In fact, nearly half scored above the cutting score on the motor dimension, indicating an ability to live independently despite poor balance. Of those with poor balance but good motor performance 13.3% reported difficulty bathing. By contrast, nearly 40% of people with poor balance and poor motor performance reported difficulty bathing. Thus, some elders in the poor balance group were able to draw on other abilities to achieve reasonable motor performance despite balance deficit. These elders were also less likely to report bathing disability. We need to know more about this process.

HEALTH EXPECTANCY

Given a particular measure of disability, it is useful to determine the proportion of the life span people can expect to live without disability, and by extension the person-years lived by a particular birth cohort with and without disability. We can use the survival model proposed in chapter 3 to calculate this "disability-free life expectancy" (DFLE) or "active life expectancy" (ALE), or more simply "health expectancy" (or "health-adjusted life expectancy," HALE). Assuming we can define states of disability and their duration, we can construct disability-based survival curves, much like the mortality curves generated in the life table model. One difference between survival and disability as an endpoint is that mortality is an absorbing state, while disability may or may not be. That is, once people die they do not return to life. However, people can become disabled and then regain abilities even in late life, as we have already seen. Thus, more sophisticated models may be necessary, such as multistate life tables, for modeling disability-free survival.

Robine, Blanchet, and Dowd (1992) have shown that interest in DFLE or ALE measures first emerged in the 1960s and 1970s. Health researchers recognized that mortality as a health outcome did not provide information about the range of health status in a population. However, no single measure of morbidity was available to summarize health. Early researchers, such as Sanders (1964) and Sullivan (1971), recognized that the ability of individuals to fill expected roles could serve as a reasonable proxy for morbidity. Thus, Sullivan (1966) first proposed a very simple series of health states, "a unified concept of morbidity, based on disability," as shown in Figure 5.9. Each node in the figure (boxes marked with a thick border) represents a health state, and every American, he argued, could be assigned to one of these five states.

The health states were meant to be hierarchical and absorbing. People could either reside in the community or in an institution, the poorest state of health. If they resided in the community, they could either have a continuing mobility limitation (the second poorest state of health) or not. If they did not have a continuing mobility limitation, they were further differentiated according to whether they could perform the major activity for their age (school, work, housework, ADL) or not, the next health state in this model. If they had no serious major role or activity limitation, they were further divided into those who had a restriction in usual days of activity over the past 30 days and those who did not. Thus, the best health state in this model was defined as absence of restriction in the past 30 days, no serious limitation in the major role appropriate for one's age, no serious mobility limitation, and

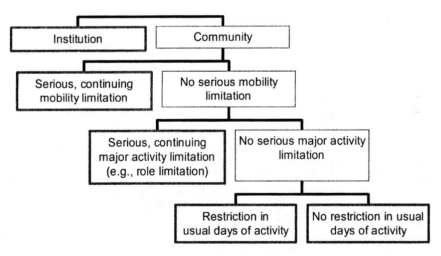

FIGURE 5.9 Unified Concept of Morbidity, Based on Disability.
After Sullivan, 1966.

TABLE 5.7 Disability-Free Life Expectancy: Sullivan Method, France, 1991, Females: Long-Term Disability

Age	Survivors	Years Lived in Interval	Disability Prevalence %	Non-Disability Years in Interval	Non-Disability Years, Cumulative	DFLE, yr
0	100,000	496,177	.0097	491,367	7,075,234	70.8
5	99,242	496,288	.0242	484,296	6,583,868	66.3
10	99,158	495,324	.0253	482,792	6,099,572	61.5
15	99,076	495,698	.0419	474,927	5,616,780	56.7
20	98,911	493,614	.0358	475,933	5,141,853	52.0
25	98,685	492,480	.0631	461,391	4,665,920	47.3
30	98,401	491,881	.0395	472,470	4,204,529	42.7
35	98,051	488,649	.0548	461,869	3,732,059	38.1
40	97,583	486,447	.0632	455,710	3,270,190	33.5
45	96,876	481,630	.0867	439,895	2,814,480	29.1
50	95,854	476,094	.1068	425,246	2,374,585	24.8
55	94,400	467,568	.1221	410,473	1,949,339	20.6
60	92,336	454,384	.1508	385,853	1,538,866	16.7
65	89,347	436,687	.1885	354,390	1,153,013	12.9
70	84,952	408,482	.2740	296,546	798,624	9.4
75	78,000	363,546	.3455	237,956	502,078	6.4
80	66,522	290,185	.4675	154,520	264,122	4.0
85	48,434	297,869	.6320	109,602	109,602	2.3

Source: REVES, World Health Report, WHO, 1995.

community residence. This approach has been extended in quality-of-life (QOL) research, which we take up in chapter 8. The central innovation in QOL research, as we will see, is assignment of numeric values to these health states.

Sullivan (1971) used these health states to calculate DFLE. The number of years lived by a cohort between successive ages is available from standard lifetables. He then applied the prevalence of disability (institutionalization, as well as permanent and temporary disability, as defined above) to the number of years lived by the cohort between each successive set of ages. The product of these years and the prevalence estimate for that age group is the number of years lived with disability between the two ages. Subtracting these from the total years lived in an interval yields the number of years lived without disability. The cumulative sum of these years through any given age, divided by the number of survivors who reach that age, gives the DFLE for that age. An example of the calculation is shown in Table 5.7, which gives DFLE estimates for women in France in 1991 (REVES, 1994).

As in the standard period lifetable, we begin with a birth cohort of 100,000. The mortality rate for each age interval is reflected in the "Survivors" column. For example, as shown in Table 5.7, using 1991 age-specific mortality rates, 78,000 women are projected to reach age 75, but only 66,522 are expected to survive to age 80, a 5–year mortality rate of 14.8%[(78,000 - 66,522)/78,000]. Because of this mortality risk, these 78,000 women lived a total of 363,546 (instead of 5 x 78,000, 390,000) years in the 5–year interval ("Years Lived in Interval"). The prevalence of long-term disability (restriction in major activity, or ADL) in this age interval, estimated from prevalence surveys, was 34.55% ("Disability Prevalence"). If we multiply this prevalence by the number of years lived by these women (363,546 x .3455), we obtain the number of years lived in disability within this age interval (125,605), and if we subtract this from the total number of years lived in the interval (363,546—125,605), we obtain the number of disability-free years lived by these women in this age interval, or 237,956 years ("Non-Disability Years in Interval," slight discrepancy due to rounding).

We complete this calculation for all age intervals. We then establish the cumulative total of these non-disability years across all age intervals. Thus, the total number of non-disabled years lived by the cohort, across all ages, was 7,075,234 years. Beginning from age 5, the cumulative sum of non-disabled years was 6,583,868 (7,075,234 - 491,367, the number of non-disability years contributed between ages 0 and 5). We complete this summation for all age groups. Finally, we divide this cumulative sum by the number of people entering each age interval. Thus, DFLE at birth for French women in 1991 was 70.8 years. Women surviving to age 75 could expect to live 6.4 more years with disability.

With mortality rates and prevalence data from a variety of disability indicators, disability-based survival curves can be constructed for a variety of health states. Key outcomes in public health and aging include active life expectancy (independence in ADL), dementia-free life expectancy, and a variety of service-use states, such as non-nursing home survival and survival without formal (paid) or informal home care. Time to these endpoints can be modeled as a series of nested survival curves (Manton, 1992). The area between the curves represents the number of person-years lived in these nested states of varying degrees of disability.

Disability-free life expectancy estimates can be compared to life expectancy to yield the proportion of life lived in disabled and non-disabled states, at birth and at later years, such as age 65. These proportions can be tracked over time to examine trends, or compared across countries to examine risks of disability in different health systems and environments, or compared across subgroups within a single country.

For example, in 1980, life expectancy for men in the United States was 70.1 years, and disability-free life expectancy 55.5 years, or 79.2% of the lifespan. Life expectancy for women was 77.6 and disability-free life expectancy 60.4, or 77.8% of the life span (Erickson, Wilson, & Shannon, 1995). Women live longer but live more years in disability, consistent with findings reported earlier on the risk of disability and greater functional impairment in late life. At age 65, life expectancy for men is 14.2 years and disability-free life expectancy 6.6 years, so that men can expect to live 46.5% of their remaining years with disability. For women, the comparable numbers were 18.4 and 8.9 years, indicating that 48.4% of remaining years are likely to be lived with disability. These differences have been established for groups defined by education (Haywood et al., 1999), income (Katz et al., 1983), and race (Guralnik, Land, Blazer, Fillenbaum, & Branch ,1993), all showing that social disadvantage is associated with greater risk of disability and fewer years of disability-free life expectancy. The European REVES group has collected these estimates for a variety of countries across a number of decades (see *http://euroreves.ined.fr/reves/database/tab1NO.html* for the North American estimates).

SUMMARY

Defining Disability. Older people are at risk of dropping below the thresholds of physical and cognitive ability required for safe, independent, and efficient completion of everyday self-maintenance tasks. These self-maintenance tasks include, first, the basic "activities of daily living" (ADL): bathing, dressing, grooming, feeding oneself, getting to and using the toilet, and moving between bed and chair. *Recognition of difficulty with these tasks, by the older person, because of a health problem, is disability.*

Models of disability. Models of disability share common features but give different weight to the role of environment and excess morbidity or disadvantage (i.e., "handicap") in the expression of deficits related to impairments in physical and cognitive function. The most useful model for aging and public health is the disablement model. In the disablement model, *pathology* (such as sarcopenia) first leads to *impairment* (e.g., lower extremity weakness evident in manual muscle testing). When lower extremity weakness crosses some threshold, *functional limitation* becomes evident, measurable perhaps in gait speeds below age- and gender-appropriate norms. When gait speed in turn drops below the minimum speed required to cross at a signaled intersection, a person is likely to report difficulty or a need for help crossing the street, that is, *disability*.

The disablement model uses a fairly narrow definition of disability. This approach has been criticized for neglecting other components of daily life, such as non-ADL activity and general participation in social life, which can be preserved even with severe ADL disability.

ADL are the central indicator of disability in older adults. This is so for three major reasons. First, ADL are the basic competencies of adulthood. A second reason is the universality of ADL: all people need to accomplish ADL tasks; and people perform these tasks on all or most days. Thus, all older people can be asked if they have difficulty bathing or dressing or using the toilet. The tasks are not gender-specific, optional, or subject to variation in lifestyle. A third reason for the focus on ADL is their hierarchical nature. ADL differ in task complexity, and hence in motor and cognitive demand, and as a result appear to be gained and lost in a generally consistent (but not necessarily fixed) order.

Difficulty of Measuring ADL Disability. Prevalence estimates for ADL disability vary across national surveys, likely because of differences in the way questions are posed, such as the number of ADL queried, whether "disability" in an ADL requires a specified period of duration, and whether distinctions are made between need for assistance and receipt of personal assistance, and use of special equipment or stand-by help. Despite the difficulty of measuring ADL disability, self-and proxy-reports of ADL have been shown to be related to concurrent health indicators and have proved to be reliable predictors of health outcomes and mortality in longitudinal studies. However, in less disabled older adults ADL measures are not as strongly related to indicators of health. For these elders, we need to develop more sensitive indicators.

Chronic Conditions and Disability. Arthritis remains the most common source of disability in both men and women. An estimated 74.7 of every 1000 men aged 65+ with arthritis, and 144.1 of every 1000 women, receive personal assistance with ADL or IADL. For older men, the proportion of arthritis cases associated with personal assistance is 19.5% (74.7/382.6). For older women, the proportion is 26.0% (144.1/554.1). Using this derived "case disability rate," cancer and visual impairment are the conditions most heavily associated with disability in late life.

Pathways to Disability. "Functional limitation" antecedent to disability is visible in deficits in the motor and cognitive skills used to perform daily activities. The relationship between underlying functional ability and disability appears to be nonlinear. Perhaps the most productive predictor of incident disability is functional limitation, which, consistent with the disablement model, represents preclinical disability. Scores on simple measures of functional limitation are very effective predictors of future mobility and ADL disability.

Declining Prevalence of Disability in the United States. The prevalence of any disability (ADL or IADL) declined from 22.7% in 1982 to 20.2% in 1993, and continued to decline to 19.3% in 1996 (National Center for Health Statistics, 2002). Based on evidence from a series of surveys, disability prevalence in older people has declined about 1% per year over the past 15–20 years. However, the decline in disability is actually mostly driven by declines in high-level IADL disability, not ADL disability.

Modifying Pathways to Disability. Environmental modification reduces task demand and in this way prevents disability. An alternative route to the prevention of disability is development of compensatory processes that increase a person's capabilities. This latter process is less well explored than environmental modification but is likely to be at least as important. It suggests far more extensive use of rehabilitative technologies to teach older people (and, indeed, anyone facing functional limitations) how to reorganize the way they do tasks by drawing on other remaining abilities.

Health Expectancy. Assuming we can define states of disability and their duration, we can construct disability-based survival curves, much like the mortality curves generated in the life table model. These estimates of disability-free life expectancy, or active life expectancy, are useful for calculating the proportion of life lived in disabled and nondisabled states, at birth and at later years. Research suggests that female, minority, low-income, and less educated elders live a greater proportion of the life span with disability.

6

Cognitive Function: Dementia

Alzheimer's disease and the other dementias are a major source of morbidity and disability in older people. The medical and custodial care needs of people suffering from the dementias are a major challenge to families, medical care, and every component of long-term care services, not to mention older people themselves, who perceive declining memory and are increasingly diagnosed with "mild cognitive impairment" without being told what this diagnosis means for risk of Alzheimer's (Albert, Talbert, Dienstag, Pelton, & Devanand, 2002). Since the risk of dementia is highly related to age, with the vast majority of people diagnosed at the oldest ages, dementia is a central problem in geriatric care. The strong association between age and risk of dementia also makes the study of cognitive deficit and its consequences a key element in the epidemiology of aging.

The Alzheimer's Association reports a prevalence of 4 million Americans with Alzheimer's disease (AD) in 2000, with a projected increase to 14 million in 2050 (Alzheimer's Association, 2000). About 10% of people aged 65+ and half those aged 85+ meet criteria for the disease. Survival with the disease from the point of diagnosis averages about 8 years, but evidence suggests a very long latency, with progressive cognitive decline over a period of 20 or more years before people come to medical attention and receive the diagnosis. In fact, many older people in the community meet criteria for AD but have not received a diagnosis (Ross et al., 1997)) and may not receive the diagnosis until quite late in the course of the disease (or may even die without ever receiving the diagnosis).

Families confronting the disease face the very difficult problem of deciding when driving should cease, when supervision is required for safety, when elders can no longer live alone, and when parents or spouses are no longer competent to handle money, take medications, or manage their lives independently. They will likely have to contend with the personality changes, psychiatric symptoms, and challenging behaviors typical of the more advanced stages of the disease. They may have to perform ADL care, manage custodial care staff hired to assist the elder, or more likely both sets of tasks, possibly at a distance. They may face the difficult decision to admit the Alzheimer's patient to a nursing home. Or, as is increasingly more common, older people themselves may choose residences (such as assisted living or continuing care retirement communities) that can accommodate Alzheimer's or nursing-home levels of care, should they need such services.

A central question for public health with respect to Alzheimer's disease is to ask if early diagnosis would make lives better for patients and families. A new array of technologies—from imaging and EEG to clinical chemistries and cognitive assessment, or some combination of all of the above—now offer increasingly early detection. Does early detection do any good? Does it translate into better use of existing therapies, more effective planning for the future, and reduction in the excess morbidity associated with the disease, such as falls, depression, car accidents, weight loss and dehydration, or self-neglect? At this point we cannot say.

The explosion of research in the area of Alzheimer's and other dementing diseases makes this realm difficult to summarize. We take up the following topics in this chapter: definitions of dementia, the question of normal memory decline and pathologic changes, including the significance of awareness of declining cognitive ability and early effects of cognitive decline on daily activities; estimates of the incidence and prevalence of AD; risk factors for AD (genetic and environmental, as well as concurrent medical status predictors); and outcomes for people with dementia.

WHAT IS DEMENTIA?

DSM-IV (*Diagnostic and Statistical Manual of Mental Disorders*, 2000) has established criteria for a dementia diagnosis. A person meets criteria for dementia if he or she has:

- *Memory impairment,* defined as an impaired ability to learn new information or recall previously learned information; and one or more of the following additional impairments in cognition:
- *Aphasia,* difficulty in language comprehension or production manifested in difficulty finding the right words, and marked by the presence of frequent word substitutions, breaking off in mid-sentence, and repetition;

- *Apraxia,* difficulty performing movements in response to verbal commands despite intact motor function;
- *Agnosia,* difficulty recognizing familiar faces, objects, places despite intact sensory function; or
- *Executive function deficits,* difficulty in planning or sequencing activity, or difficulty completing a task in the presence of interference from another task.

In addition, these cognitive deficits must be severe enough to cause significant impairment in social or occupational function and must represent a significant decline from a previous level of functioning.

For a person to be diagnosed with Alzheimer's disease, the course of this general cognitive disorder must, in addition, be characterized by gradual onset and continuing, progressive decline. The defect in cognition should not be attributable to other central nervous system conditions that cause progressive deficits in memory and cognition, such as cerebrovascular disease, Parkinson's disease, Huntington's disease, subdural hematoma, normal-pressure hydrocephalus, or brain tumor. Nor should the cognitive disorder be caused by systemic conditions that are known to cause dementia, such as hypothyroidism, vitamin B12 or folic acid deficiency, niacin deficiency, hypercalcemia, neurosyphilis, or HIV infection. Substance-induced conditions should also be excluded. Finally, the cognitive deficits should not occur exclusively during the course of delirium, an acute and temporary confusional state. Delirium, unlike dementia, is usually the result of a general medical condition, a medication reaction, or substance use, and resolves with treatment.

The distinction between dementia and delirium is important. Delirium is characterized by fluctuating disturbances in cognition, mood, attention, arousal and self-awareness. This clouding of consciousness and disorientation is acute, and will resolve with appropriate medical treatment. It is highly prevalent in some settings: 10–30% of hospitalized medical patients, and up to 80% of terminally ill patients in the last weeks of life, have been reported to have episodes of delirium (Inouye et al., 1999). It is also common in the nursing home. Delirium can affect a patient with dementia, and in these cases distinguishing between the two may be difficult.

The Alzheimer's Disease and Related Disorders Association (ADRDA) (McKhann et al., 1984) has developed additional criteria for diagnosing AD. A definitive AD diagnosis requires that clinical criteria for probable AD be met and, in addition, that histopathologic evidence from biopsy or autopsy be available. "Probable AD" is defined by the criteria listed above, but a diagnosis of "possible AD" can also be made on the basis of the dementia syndrome described above in "the presence of variations in the onset, presentation and clinical course" or in "the presence of a second systemic or brain disorder sufficient to cause the dementia but not considered to be the cause of the dementia."

The "possible AD" distinction is important because dementia can also be a feature of other neurodegenerative diseases, such as Parkinson's or vascular disease, and can also accompany stroke or trauma. In other adults, these diseases or effects from disease can co-occur. In such cases, the diagnosis of AD may depend on which came first; for example, if dementia precedes Parkinson's disease, it is reasonable to call this person an incident case of AD, with a further complication from Parkinson's. In other cases, the temporal sequence is less clear and a diagnosis of "possible AD" may be warranted.

When an elder is brought to medical attention because of memory disorders or progressive inability to manage independently in a household, the treating physician is likely to assess cognitive status with the Folstein Mini-Mental Status Exam (MMSE), a 30–point assessment of orientation, memory, attention, language, calculation, and visuospatial construction skills, typically used as a screening test. The MMSE is shown in Table 6.1. Current recommendations suggest that a score greater than 24 is considered normal, a score of 15-24 mild-to-moderate impairment, and a score less than 15 definite impairment. However, the test is not a diagnostic tool and should be considered only a first-line glimpse at cognitive function.

Properties of the MMSE have been intensively investigated. Performance on the measure is related to age and education, apart from dementia status, suggesting that these influences must be considered when interpreting scores on the test. In one effort, the MMSE was administered to over 18,000 adult participants selected in a probability sample within census tracts and households (Crum, Anthony, Bassett, & Folstein, 1993). Median MMSE scores ranged from 29 in people 18-24, to 27 in people aged 70-74, to 25 in people aged 80+. The median MMSE score was 29 in people with 9 or more years of school, 26 for people with 5-8 years, and 22 for people with 0-4 years. Because a score less than 24 is often taken as an indicator of possible dementia, education obviously needs to be taken into account in interpreting performance. The need for caution in applying cutoff scores in the MMSE is even clearer when we examine older people with low education. For people with 0-4 years of school, the median MMSE score for those under age 65 ranges from 22-25, but it is 21-22 in people aged 70-79 and 19-20 in people aged 80+. More recent research suggests that literacy may be as important as years of school for MMSE performance (Albert, & Teresi, 1999), and that quality of education should also be considered when interpreting education-referenced scores, especially among minorities (Manley, Jacobs, Touradji, Small, & Stern, 2002).

TABLE 6.1 Mini-Mental State Exam (MMSE)

This brief test of cognitive functions is useful in the screening for dementia and following its course over time. The maximum scores are shown in parentheses.

ORIENTATION:

Score Maximum

_____   _____   _____   _____   _____   ___ (5)
(year)   (season)   (date)   (day)   (month)

_____   _____   _____   _____   _____   ___ (5)
(state)   (county)   (city)   (hospital)   (floor or room)

REGISTRATION:

Have patient repeat 3 items   Number correct: ___ (3)
(e.g. "apple," "book," "coat") # of trials until correct_____

ATTENTION AND CALCULATION:

Serial 7's or spell "WORLD" backwards   Number correct: ___ (5)

RECALL: Ask for 3 items named above   Number correct: ___ (3)

LANGUAGE:

Name a pencil, watch   Number correct: ___ (2)

Repeat "No ifs, ands or buts" (1 point if correct)   ___ (1)

3-stage command: Score "1" for each step.

  "Take paper in left hand, fold in half, lay it in your lap."   ___ (3)

Read and obey: CLOSE YOUR EYES!   ___ (1)

Write a sentence: _____   ___ (1)

CONSTRUCTION: Copy the design below.   ___ (1)

                                      TOTAL: ___ (30)

Out of the maximum score of 30, 24 to 30 is considered normal. Scores of less than 24 increase the likelihood of dementia.

Adapted from M. F. Folstein, S. E. Folstei, P. R. McHugh (1975). Mini-mental state: a practical method for grading the cognitive state of patients for the clinician. J Psychiatr Res 12:196–198.

One way to grade the severity of dementia is through instruments such as the Clinical Dementia Rating, or CDR (Hughes, Berg, Danziger, Cohen, & Martin, 1982). The original scoring categories and criteria are shown in Table 6.2. The CDR involves six dimensions: three cognitive (memory, orientation, judgment and problem solving),

TABLE 6.2 Clinical Dementia Rating

	Impairment Level and CDR Score (0, 0.5, 1, 2, 3)				
	None 0	Questionable 0.5	Mild 1	Moderate 2	Severe 3
Memory	No memory loss or slight inconsistent forgetfulness	Consistent slight forgetfulness; partial recollection of events; "benign" forgetfulness	Moderate memory loss; more marked for recent events; defect interferes with everyday activities	Severe memory loss; only highly learned material retained; new material rapidly lost	Severe memory loss; only fragments remain
Orientation	Fully oriented	Fully oriented except for slight difficulty with time relationships	Moderate difficulty with time relationships; oriented for place at examination; may have geographic disorientation elsewhere	Severe difficulty with time relationships; usually disoriented to time, often to place	Oriented to person only
Judgment & Problem Solving	Solves everyday problems & handles business & financial affairs well; judgment good in relation to past performance	Slight impairment in solving problems, similarities, and differences	Moderate difficulty in handling problems, similarities, and differences; social judgment usually maintained	Severely impaired in handling problems, similarities, and differences; social judgment usually impaired	Unable to make judgments or solve problems
Community Affairs	Independent function at usual level in job, shopping, volunteer and social groups	Slight impairment in these activities	Unable to function independently at these activities although may still be	No pretense of independent function outside home; appears well	No pretense of independent function outside home; appears too

TABLE 6.2 (continued)

	Impairment Level and CDR Score (0, 0.5, 1, 2, 3)				
	None 0	Questionable 0.5	Mild 1	Moderate 2	Severe 3
			engaged in some; appears normal to casual inspection	enough to taken to functions outside a family home	ill to be taken to functions outside a family home
Home and Hobbies	Life at home, hobbies, and intellectual interests well maintained	Life at home, hobbies, and intellectual interests slightly impaired	Mild but definite impairment of function at home; more difficult chores abandoned; more complicated hobbies and interests abandoned	Only simple chores preserved; very restricted interests, poorly maintained	No significant function in home
Personal Care	Fully capable of self-care	Needs prompting	Needs prompting	Requires assistance in dressing, hygiene, keeping of personal effects	Requires much help with personal care; frequent incontinence

Source: http://www.adrc.wustl.edu/adrc/cdrGrid.html.

and three functional (home and hobbies, community affairs, and self-care). The original system allows a diagnosis of normal, "questionable," "mild," "moderate," and "severe" dementia. The CDR has also been expanded to include a "profound" and "terminal" level of severity (Dooneief, Marder, Tang, & Stern, 1996).

Scoring of the CDR requires a semi-structured interview with both the caregiver and patient. In particular, caregivers provide information that the clinician can use in his or her discussion with the patient to check a patient's level of insight on the extent of memory deficit. The University of Washington has prepared a series of training videotapes, that well illustrate variation in the severity of dementia. The tapes are very good teaching tools for rating severity but also for showing features of dementia, such as lack of insight, difficulty with verbal production and comprehension, retardation of motor activity, depression, and confabulation to mask memory difficulty. Students unfamiliar with dementia who view the tapes report how difficult, even excruciating, it is to see someone struggle with language and the simplest comprehension tasks (they also rush to defend patients from what they see as an overly probing clinician!)

Scoring of the CDR can take a number of forms. Clinicians can use it to formulate a global impression, or they can more formally assign severity according to the sum of box scores or some other algorithm for weighting dimensions in making an assignment.

The CDR score offers an important endpoint for studies of dementia progression or treatment efficacy. What proportion of patients with mild dementia (CDR 1), for example, progress to moderate or more severe dementia (CDR 2+) over a defined interval? Natural history studies of incident cohorts provide information of this sort, which is important for assessing the efficacy of a therapy in delaying progression. The risk of progression from mild to more advanced dementia in an incident AD cohort is about 6-10% per year (see below); thus, a reasonable goal for delay of disease progression would be a rate significantly lower than this.

An alternative to composite measures of cognition and function (such as the CDR) for assessing severity of dementia is use of cognitive measures alone. Neuropsychological assessment allows fairly fine differentiation of strengths and weaknesses in a variety of cognitive domains. Age-and education-based norms, in different languages, are now available for an increasingly wide range of tests. With so many tests, scored in so many different ways, however, it is often difficult to decide how best to use the measures. Should tests be aggregated according to the cognitive domain they have been designed to assess (such as memory, visuospatial skill, language, or executive function), or according to data reduction techniques (such as factor analysis). Assuming we combine tests, should we count the number of tests 1 or 2 standard deviations below norms to compute a "deficit score," or rather should we standardize scores and compute a sum of z-scores? After we have computed a composite measure, should we be concerned with variation in the clustering of test scores over time?

One factor-analytic study of neuropsychological test performance offers some reassurance for these questions. Mayeux and colleagues reported a stable and plausible factor structure for test performance in a sample of non-demented elders (Mayeux, Small, Tang, Tycko, & Stern, 2001). In this effort, three factors emerged:

Memory: Total recall, long-term recall, delayed recall, long-term storage, cued long-term recall, and total recall over six trials of the Selective Reminding Test (Buschke & Fuld, 1974)

Visuospatial/Cognitive Skill: Matching and recognition components of the Benton Visual Retention Test Benton, 1955), Rosen Drawing Test (Rosen, 1981), and Identities and Oddities of the Mattis Dementia Rating Scale (Mattis, 1976)

Language: Boston Naming Test (Kaplan, Goodglass, & Weintraub, 1983), Controlled Oral Word Association Test (Benton, 1967), and WAIS-R Similarities (Wechsler, 1981).

In this study, composite scores for each factor were computed and used to examine decline in cognitive performance over follow-up in a non-demented, community-dwelling cohort of elders drawn from Medicare enrollee files. The authors used the scores without reference to norms because the purpose of the study was not to establish impaired performance but rather to track change in different cognitive domains.

COGNITIVE DECLINE WITH AGE: DISTINCT FROM ALZHEIMER'S DISEASE?

Earlier, in chapter 1, we showed that people enter late life with different cognitive and health resources, along with differences in wealth and family support. Differences in the case of cognitive resources, or "cognitive reserve," are especially important. By age 65 or 70 any sample of non-demented older adults will show a wide range of performance on tests of memory and other cognitive domains. But older people scoring more poorly on measures of memory, for example, can be expected to reach the dementia endpoint, or "convert" to AD, sooner (adjusting for other differences) than older adults with better memory performance. This difference in cognitive resources at the beginning of

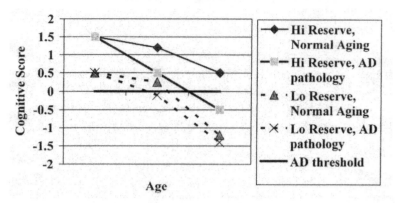

FIGURE 6.1 Cognitive Reserve, Normal Memory Decline, and AD Risk.

old age means some people are closer to the threshold of detectable dementia even when they are not very old, as shown schematically in Figure 6.1.

This figure shows that we must consider the decline in memory performance typical of aging and also ask whether the pathological process of AD is something separate from this decline. It shows two groups of elderly, one entering old age (for convenience, age 65) with high cognitive reserve (a score of 1.5 on a hypothetical cognitive score), the other entering old age with low reserve (cognitive score of 0.5). The two groups can have different trajectories according to whether memory changes in ways typical of "normal aging," or whether memory declines much more quickly as the result of a potentially distinct Alzheimer's pathologic process. The figure also includes an "Alzheimer's threshold," a cognitive score (for convenience, set at zero) that is associated with disability and clinical diagnosis.

If we look only at the decline in memory associated with normal memory (see below), we see that the high-reserve group does not reach the Alzheimer's threshold even as late as age 85. The low-threshold group, by contrast, crosses the dementia threshold shortly after age 75. Note that this difference would obtain even if the slope of memory decline in the two groups were equivalent, shown by parallel or nearly parallel lines. If we look instead at the declines in memory associated with the pathologic process, we see that the high reserve group now crosses the Alzheimer's threshold at about age 80 and the low reserve group at age 75 or so. Again, the slope of decline in the two groups could be equivalent, represented by parallel lines, or we might hypothesize an important interaction in which low reserve and the pathologic process together result in a steeper slope of decline.

The big question in this kind of inquiry is whether distinct slopes for normal and pathologic memory change in aging exist at all. Within the high or low reserve groups, we will find variation in rates of change. Do the changes in memory at either end of this range represent different underlying brain processes, or is a single process enough to account for this variation? More simply, are the declines typical of Alzheimer's just one end of the continuum of changes typical of aging?

Recent research suggests that memory declines typical of Alzheimer's disease may be distinct from normal aging. Mayeux and colleagues (2001) first identified a cohort of nearly 600 older people who never met criteria for dementia over 7 years, who were evaluated, on average, every 20 months. The mean age of the cohort was 75.9 at baseline, and 14.2% had one or more *APOE*-e4 alleles. The *APOE* gene is the only gene identified so far for Alzheimer's risk in older adults (as opposed to *PS1, APP,* and other genes associated with familial disease and much younger onset). The increased risk of AD associated with the e4 allele has been confirmed repeatedly in large prospective cohort studies (Maestre et al., 1995). Mayeux and colleagues (2001) followed this cohort to investigate the relationship between declines in cognitive performance and *APOE* status. Declines in cognitive domains in people without the e4 allele could plausibly identify normal age-related changes in cognition. People with the e4 allele, who have a higher risk of AD, could plausibly represent early AD and should show steeper declines in memory performance.

In this cohort, memory performance mostly declined over time; two-thirds had a negative slope on the composite memory measure, described earlier. Older age and lower education were each associated with poorer memory scores at baseline and at follow-up assessments. Individuals with an *APOE*-e4 allele had steeper declines in memory performance, suggesting early changes typical of Alzheimer's disease. This steeper slope was evident only in people with low education, or low cognitive reserve, suggesting an interaction between low reserve and the Alzheimer's pathologic process.

Notably, memory was the only cognitive domain that declined in this cohort of people who never met criteria for dementia. Visuospatial and language performance was stable across the 7 years of follow-up. Scores in the visuospatial and language domains were stable even in people with an *APOE* e4 allele.

These findings suggest that memory decline typical of aging can be separated from the pathologic aging typical of AD. They also suggest the sensitivity of the memory domain for identifying age-related changes and the risk of AD. In a second set of analyses, Mayeux and colleagues

(2001) also examined changes in the three domains in a separate group of 228 people who did not meet criteria for AD at baseline but progressed to AD over the follow-up period. These people showed significant declines with time in all three domains, showing a more generalized decline of cognition in people closer to the Alzheimer's threshold.

This study is valuable for showing that memory decline is common in a group of older people who do not develop AD over a long period, but also more pronounced (steeper, in terms of Figure 6.1) in a group with an AD risk factor who are still, however, far from the AD threshold. These elders showed declines in memory only. It stands to reason, then, that areas of the brain involved in memory, such as the entorhinal cortex of the hippocampus, should be different in younger people and older people without AD. Differences in anatomy would not be expected, since the older people in this case do not have AD and would not be expected to show the pathologic lesions (amyloid plaques, neuritic tangles) typical of the disease. However, differences in physiology might be expected, since presumably poorer memory must reflect differences in cellular processes. In fact, recent research suggests just such a difference, with older people selectively showing less MRI signal than younger people only in this region of the hippocampal formation (Small, Tsai, DeLaPaz, Mayeux, & Stern, 2002).

COGNITIVE DECLINE PRIOR TO FRANK DEMENTIA

Mild cognitive impairment (MCI) is typically defined by the following criteria: subjective complaints of memory problems and memory performance below age-and education-referenced norms, with normal performance in other cognitive domains and absence of impairment in the instrumental and basic activities of daily living (Peterson, 2000; Peterson, et al., 1997). Another definition of mild cognitive impairment is "questionable dementia," which involves both mild deficits in cognitive status and mild deficits in functional status. This state is recognized in the 0.5 category of the Clinical Dementia Rating (CDR) (Hughes et al., 1982). Still other alternative nosologies include "age-associated memory impairment," which involves defective memory performance relative to people under age 50 (Crook et al., 1986; Feher, Larrabee, Sudilovsky, & Crook, 1994) and "aging-associated cognitive decline," which involves defective performance in any cognitive domain, relative to age-matched elders (Levy, 1994; Richards, Touchon, Ledesert, & Ritchie, 1999). The different definitions all strive to establish an intermediate cognitive status: people with MCI do not meet criteria for dementia but show deficits in memory or other domains of cognition. These deficits are evident to elders and distressing enough to lead them and their families to seek medical attention.

Even within the domain of "questionable dementia" it is possible to make distinctions based on prognosis. Morris and colleagues (2001) partitioned MCI patients ascertained in a clinic setting into three groups: CDR 0.5 but likely demented, CDR 0.5 with likely progressive dementia ("incipient AD"), and CDR 0.5 with uncertain dementia. All three groups faced a high risk of developing Alzheimer's disease (CDR 1.0 or greater) over a 5–year follow-up period: 60.5% for the likely dementia group, 35.7% for the likely progressive dementia group, and 19.9% for the uncertain dementia group. These rates should be compared to a control group (CDR 0, no cognitive or functional impairment) over the same time period, in which the incidence of Alzheimer's disease was 6.8%. Given these results Morris and colleagues conclude that, "individuals currently characterized as having MCI progress steadily to greater stages of dementia severity at rates dependent on the level of cognitive impairment at entry" (p. 397). People in the three groups who died and came to autopsy had neuropathogical evidence of AD, again suggesting that MCI, at least when defined by CDR 0.5 criteria, is a dementia prodrome rather than a benign variant of aging.

The situation is less clear for patients who do not meet CDR 0.5 criteria but whose cognitive performance is lower than expected. Ritchie, Artero, and Touchen (2001) assessed mild cognitive impairment in a population-based rather than a clinic-based sample. Only 11.1% of patients progressed to dementia. Moreover, these people moved back and forth across the dementia threshold, changing diagnostic category at different assessments. With more restrictive definitions identifying greater cognitive impairment, 28.6% met the dementia endpoint over 3 years.

More generally, studies suggest that dementia incidence in elders who report cognitive complaints and demonstrate mild deficits in cognitive assessment is much higher than that for elders as a whole, 18% over 3 years, compared to perhaps 3-6% in the population of older adults as a whole (Ritchie et al., 2001). Consequently, mild cognitive impairment cannot be considered benign or a normal feature of healthy aging, and elders with mild cognitive impairment in this sense (i.e., complaints of memory impairment supported by neuropsychological performance >1 sd below age norms) are indeed at risk for developing Alzheimer's over a 3–to 5–year period.

Insight on Declining Cognitive Ability

Older adults with mild cognitive impairment (MCI) describe their difficulties with memory in this way:

"I do feel the difference. I can't retrieve words easily. I lose words. It will take me a few minutes . . . and it takes me a while to retrieve it. Sometimes I can't, and that's disturbing. And to think of walking into a room and forgetting why you walked in is a killer. It's strange. Or getting a list in my head, and not writing it down . . . and then forgetting what I want to do. That kind of thing. I'm sure it happened before, but not as frequently as now. It's happening more."

The woman reporting these memory problems met criteria for MCI. She had a Global Deterioration Score (GDS) of 3, as indicated by a score below age and education-adjusted norms on the Logical Memory II subscale of the Weschler Memory Scale; did not meet criteria for dementia, as indicated by a Mini-Mental State Exam [MMSE] score greater than or equal to 24; and did not report difficulty in daily occupational, self-care, home management, or community activities, as indicated by a Clinical Dementia Rating of 0.5.

Still, she was concerned that her memory problems might presage Alzheimer's disease. Mainly, she was concerned that she might be denying the extent of her problems, which she recognized as a feature of memory impairment and incipient Alzheimer's disease. She was also concerned that she was not pushing herself as hard as she might and that this circumscription of daily activities and interests might be the result of her memory deficit. Was she actually avoiding situations that would reveal her difficulty with memory? Her assessment and the new label of "MCI" did not help. She reported great frustration with the clinical label: "They said there was some memory loss, that it might not mean anything, and that they would like to re-evaluate me in a couple of years to see if it's progressing. [But] the significance of it is what I'm interested in, and [that] they didn't tell me" (Albert, Talbert, Petton, & Devanand, 2002).

Mild Cognitive Impairment and Disability

Aside from "questionable dementia," the other definitions of mild cognitive impairment, reviewed earlier, assume no impairments in instrumental (household management) or basic (personal self-maintenance) activities of daily living but leave open the possibility of deficits in higher-level functions, such as the ability to work, travel, participate in community affairs, or manage complex activities (such as driving to a new place, appearing in front of an audience, planning an event, participating in competitive games, or taking part in activities that involve some degree of risk from slow reaction times or poor judgment). Ritchie, Artero, and Touchon, (2001) point out that no guidelines have been given as to what constitutes activities of daily living restriction in MCI. Recent studies show that people with MCI who ultimately progress to Alzheimer's disease do show mild functional deficits (such as occasional need for help or need for cueing and supervision in activity) and reductions in physical activity before AD diagnosis (Friedland et al., 2001; Touchon & Ritchie. 1999).

In prior research, we have found that quite mild cognitive impairment is associated with less frequency and diversity of advanced functions (Albert et al., 1999), as indexed by the Pfeffer Functional Activities Questionnaire (Pfeffer, Kurosaki, Chance, & Filos, 1982). The Pfeffer scale records perceived difficulty with writing checks, assembling tax or business records, shopping alone, playing games of skill, making coffee or tea, preparing a balanced meal, keeping track of current events, paying attention and understanding while reading or watching a TV show, remembering to take medications and family occasions, and traveling out of the neighborhood. Close informants to people with "minimal cognitive impairment" reported that these elders had more difficulty in these tasks than a group with no cognitive impairment. In this study we considered individuals to have mild cognitive impairment if they were not demented (score of 23 or greater on the Mini-Mental State Exam), but had performance ≥ 1 SD below norms on one or more of a series of neuropsychological tests (recall of 2 out of 3 objects at 5 minutes, delayed recall in the six-trial Selective Reminding Test [SRT], or a Wechsler Adult Intelligence Scale [WAIS] performance IQ score > 15 points below the WAIS verbal IQ score).

We have also shown that a discrepancy measure indicating lack of awareness of functional deficits (i.e., greater informant- than self-reported functional deficits) predicted risk of Alzheimer's disease more efficiently than self or informant reports alone (Tabert et al., 2002). In these models, which controlled for sociodemographic differences and cognitive status, self-reports of functional status at baseline were not associated with the risk of an Alzheimer's diagnosis. By contrast, informant reports of deficits at baseline were a significant predictor of dementia over follow-up. A discrepancy of 1+ deficit in the Pfeffer scale, relative to those with no discrepancy, was associated with a four-fold increase in the risk of a future AD diagnosis. These findings support research by Tierney and colleagues (1996), who showed that informant- but not self-reported cognitive deficits (i.e., memory for lists, events, and names, finding one's way around home and neighborhood, and financial management) also predicted risk of AD.

Finally, recent research suggests that older adults meeting criteria for MCI performed worse than normal elderly on tasks involving fine and complex motor skills (mainly tests of manual dexterity) (Kluger et al., 1997). These findings suggest a gradient of motor as well as cognitive performance in which MCI patients again fall between normal elders and people who meet criteria for Alzheimer's disease.

The upshot of our research, as well as that of others, is that MCI affects high-level function, not basic self-care; that people with MCI are not fully aware of the extent of their functional impairment; and that families recognize functional deficits in people with MCI. Furthermore, functional deficit, as reported by families and *not* reported by elders, may be useful for identifying MCI patients with high likelihood of rapid progression to Alzheimer's disease (Albert, Tabert, Dienstag, Pelton, Devanand, 2002).

PREVALENCE AND INCIDENCE OF ALZHEIMER'S DISEASE

As mentioned earlier, the prevalence of dementia increases dramatically with age. Current estimates of the number of people with AD in the United States range from 1.09 to 4.58 million (Brookmeyer, Gray, & Kawas, 1998). Estimates from the U.S. General Accounting Office fall in the middle of this range. In this synthesis of 18 prevalence surveys, 1.9 million people aged 65+ were identified as meeting criteria for Alzheimer's in 1995. Prevalence rises to 2.1 million if we include possible or mixed cases, that is, cases marked by AD and some other source of dementia. If we restrict cases to moderate or more severe AD, the prevalence is 1.0 million with the narrow definition and 1.4 million if we include possible and mixed cases. All told, 5.7% of Americans aged 65+ had AD in 1995, with 3.3% meeting criteria for moderate or more severe AD (GAO, 1998).

By 2015, we can expect 4.6 million cases of AD using the narrow definition and 5.3 million if we include mixed cases. About a third of these cases will have moderate or more severe forms of AD.

Table 6.3 reports prevalence by age and gender for the U.S population aged 65+. The table shows that prevalence doubles every 5 years, both for men and women, reaching about 40% for people aged 95+. The proportion with moderate or more severe AD in the oldest age group reaches about 25%. The prevalence of AD is higher in women than men in every age group, with the gap widening at successively older ages. This gender disparity most likely reflects greater risk of AD for women, but this finding is controversial. Some prospective cohort studies have found a greater risk for women (Launer et al., 1999); others have not (Tang et al., 2001).

If prevalence doubles every 5 years, then delaying the disease by 5 years would reduce prevalence by half. This is an important public health goal. With this delay, dementia-free life expectancy would increase, a greater number of older adults would live their last years

TABLE 6.3 Prevalence of Alzheimer's Disease, United States, 1995

Age	Alzheimer's Disease-All		Alzheimer's Disease-Moderate+	
	Men	Women	Men	Women
65–69	0.6	0.8	0.3	0.6
70–74	1.3	1.7	0.6	1.1
75–79	2.7	3.5	1.1	2.3
80–84	5.6	7.1	2.3	4.4
85–89	11.1	13.8	4.4	8.6
90–94	20.8	25.2	8.5	15.8
95+	35.6	41.5	15.8	27.4

Table entries are percentages meeting criteria for any Alzheimer's or Alzheimer's disease, CDR 2+.

Source: United States General Accounting Office. *Report to the Secretary of Health and Human Services: Alzheimer's Disease, Eestimates of Prevalence in the United States.* (1998, January).

without the need for costly custodial care, and older people at these late ages would die of other causes. Such a delay would obviously have a major impact on disability in late life and the caregiving demands associated with such disability. In simulation studies using available data on population growth, Brookmeyer and colleagues (1998) suggest that a delay of even 1 year in the incidence of the disease would result in nearly 800,000 fewer prevalent cases over the next 50 years. A delay of 2 years would cut prevalence by 2 million cases.

A number of prospective cohort studies have examined the incidence of Alzheimer's disease. These studies are superior to retrospective studies that ask family proxies to date disease onset (i.e., "when did _____ first report memory problems or first go to the doctor because of difficulty with memory?" [Wolfson et al., 2001]). Retrospective studies do not allow formal diagnosis and are always subject to recall bias. Prospective studies begin with a dementia-free cohort and follow the cohort over multiple assessments to track onset of disease.

However, prospective cohort studies of AD are complicated not just by differences in the definition of the disease, but also by different approaches to establishing the date of onset. Even with a regular schedule of follow-up assessments, it is not possible to establish the date when a person first met criteria for the disease. Further, most studies do not have long follow-up or closely spaced assessment intervals. The result has been imprecision in the true date of diagnosis, which affects calculation of person-years of dementia-free follow-up. In the face of this problem, the EURODEM pooled analysis of AD incidence used a statistical adjustment: "To account for the fact that reliable data regarding when the dementia started is difficult to obtain, we used a statistical adjustment based on the patient's age and age-specific dementia rates" (Launer et al., 1999). A simpler approach, if multiple follow-up assessments are available, is to call the incidence date the date of the assessment when the respondent first met criteria for the diagnosis (Tang et al., 2001).

The incidence of AD is closely related to age. For people aged 65-74, annual incidence ranges from <0.5% to 1.3%. For people aged 75-84, the range is 1.5% to 4.0%, and for people aged 85+ it is 4.7% to 7.9% per year (Launer et al., 1999, Tang et al., 2001). Thus, for someone over age 85, the risk of meeting criteria AD for the first time is about 5-10% per year, a very high rate.

Even within age strata, the incidence of AD varies considerably among groups defined by race and ethnicity. In New York City, for example, incidence was considerably lower among whites than in minorities. African Americans and Hispanics were 2-3 times as likely to develop AD; thus, for example, the risk among whites aged 75-84 was 2.6% per year and 4.4% in minority groups (Tang, et al., 2001). This difference persisted even with adjustment for socioeconomic (education, literacy status, gender) and disease (hypertension, diabetes) factors. It also persisted when analyses were limited to people with the *APOE-e3* allele (Tang, 1998) to control for the effects of this genetic risk factor (see below). Thus, minority status is among the most important risk factors for AD. Given the increasing number of minority elderly in the U.S., this disparity has great public health significance.

These rates for AD incidence apply to the entire population at risk in any given year. If we restrict risk estimates to the group of older people who report memory complaints or demonstrate mild cognitive impairment, annual AD incidence is, of course, much higher. The risk of AD in these older adults is between 10% and 25% per year, depending on ascertainment site (community versus clinic) and the stringency of the definition of mild impairment (Peterson et al., 2001).

RISK FACTORS FOR ALZHEIMER'S DISEASE

Genetic Risk Factors

The role of genetic factors in the development of AD is an active research area but at this point is still underdeveloped. Only about 7% of early-onset AD (< age 65) and less than 1% of late-onset AD have been linked to mutations on particular genes (Whalley et al., 2000). Early-onset Alzheimer's disease has been linked to mutations on a number of genes (located on chromosomes 1, 14, and 21). Risk of late-onset AD is associated with the e4 allele of the *APOE* gene on chromosome 19. The mechanism for the APOE-AD relationship is not completely understood.

While mutations for early-onset AD have been identified, their relevance for late-onset AD, which represents the vast majority of cases, is unclear. For public health purposes, attention is centered on APOE, the apolipoprotein E gene, which produces a plasma protein involved in the transport of cholesterol and other hydrophobic molecules (Farrer et al., 1995). While some forms of apolipoprotein E have been linked to disorders of cholesterol metabolism and coronary heart disease (Saunders et al.,1993), this protein product has also been shown to raise the risk of AD. A number of studies have shown over-representation of the APOE-e4 allele in people with AD. Thirty-four to 65% of individuals with AD carry the *APOE* e4 allele, compared to only 24% to 31% of non-affected people of the same age (Jarvik et al., 1995; Myers et al., 1993; Roses, 1994). The number of *APOE* e4 alleles is associated with earlier age of onset (Corder et 1993). The *APOE* e2 allele, by contrast, may be protective against AD, but this finding has been challenged (Corder et al., 1994; Talbot et al., 1994; van Duijn et al., 1995).

Despite the association between *APOE* and AD, *APOE* testing is currently not recommended as a screening tool. A number of reasons have been advanced. First, the presence of an e4 allele is not necessary for the development of AD (35% to 50% of persons with AD do not carry an e4 allele) (Roses et al., 1994). Second, the AD diagnosis is not difficult to make, and the extra predictive power provided by genetic testing would not add a great deal to clinical tools. Third, no treatment beyond tertiary symptomatic therapies is available in any case, so that awareness of AD risk before disease onset would not have practical benefit. And, finally, discrimination or other untoward effects are possible with such information, reducing the possible gain further.

A task force investigating the issue concluded

Because most patients presenting to physicians with dementia have AD, the additional information gained by genotyping would be useful only if it reduced the necessity for other more expensive or invasive tests. Individuals homozygous for epsilon-4 are the most likely candidates for disease, but they comprise only 2% to 3% of the general population; [and] even among AD patients, only 15% to 20% have this genotype. Most symptomatic epsilon-4 homozygotes will in fact have AD, but any uncertainty will oblige the physician to exclude other forms of dementia. . . .Thus, although *APOE* genotype may be a risk factor for AD, it cannot yet be considered a useful predictive genetic test. (Farrer et al., 1995, p. 1629).

Socioeconomic Factors: Education, Lifelong Occupation, Cognitive Reserve

Earlier, we discussed lifelong cognitive resources as a predictor of Alzheimer's risk. The significance of cognitive resources early in the lifespan for such a late-life outcome has become increasingly clear in studies that have linked risk of AD in late life to childhood IQ (Whalley et al., 2000), educational accomplishment and leisure activities (Wilson & Scarmeas), occupational attainment and job demands (Stern et al., 1994), language skills in early adulthood (Snowdon et al., 1996), diversity of physical and cognitive engagement over the life span (Friedland et al., 1996; Albert et al., 1996), parental socioeconomic status, and literacy (Albert & Teresi, 1999; Manly et al., 2002).

The case of childhood cognitive ability and AD risk is revealing. In a Scottish case-control study involving a match-back to childhood IQ tests, Whalley and colleagues (2000) found that people who developed AD after age 65 had lower scores on this early measure of cognitive ability when compared to people who did not develop AD. Differences in Alzheimer's risk, then, were already apparent at age 11. Notably, people who developed *early-onset* AD did not differ from other elders on the childhood IQ measure, suggesting an important difference in mechanism between early-and late-onset AD.

What do these findings suggest? One interpretation is that cognitive ability is similar to grip strength: differences (in muscle fiber density, in neuronal integrity or number) already apparent at birth or in the perinatal period, and which develop or set limits on development over the life span, provide variable reserve against depletions that occur with aging. These resources put one closer or further away from the threshold of disability associated with the loss of physical and cognitive function that occurs over the life span. In this view, development of AD is not so much a disease as one kind of aging, and some kind of early strengthening of cognition to build up reserve would be an appropriate intervention. The association between a cognitive resource and AD risk, then, is not evidence of an independent risk factor (as it is usually portrayed), but rather identification of an early phase of the process that will ultimately result in AD.

Medical Morbidity: Hypertension and Vascular Disease, Diabetes, Bone Mineral Density Loss, Estrogen Deficiency, Depression

An increasing number of morbid conditions have been shown to increase the risk of Alzheimer's disease. These are considered secondary risks in that they do not represent the primary mechanism for development of AD. Yet they also offer avenues for reducing Alzheimer's risk and may indicate points in the pathway of Alzheimer's neurodegeneration that may be amenable to intervention. Findings for these morbid conditions in some cases remain controversial.

Hypertension, Stroke, Diabetes

Hypertension has been associated with cognitive performance, so it stands to reason that this condition might be associated with later risk of AD. However, one large prospective study failed to confirm this association (Posner et al., 2002). In this cohort, 731 of 1,259 subjects (58.1%), all free of AD at baseline, had a history of hypertension associated with diabetes, stroke, or heart disease. A history of hypertension was not associated with an increased risk for AD but did raise the risk of vascular dementia. The increased risk of vascular disease was evident only in respondents who had multiple morbidities. Respondents with hypertension and heart disease had a threefold increase in risk for vascular dementia, while respondents with hypertension and diabetes faced a sixfold increase in risk.

These results stand in contrast to results from the double-blind, placebo-controlled Systolic Hypertension in Europe (Syst-Eur) trial, in which randomized patients with hypertension were offered active study medication after the end of the trial for a further period of observation (Forette et al., 2002). In this add-on component, long-term antihypertensive therapy reduced the risk of dementia by 55%, from 7.4 to 3.3 cases per 1000 patient-years, a finding that remained after adjustment for sex, age, education, and entry blood pressure. In a "number needed to treat analysis," the trial showed that treatment of 1000 hypertension patients for 5 years would prevent 20 cases of dementia.

Whether through an AD or vascular dementia process, diabetes is now increasingly recognized as a risk factor for cognitive decline. In the Study of Osteoporotic Fractures, women with diabetes (n = 682) had lower baseline scores than women without diabetes on a variety of cognitive measures (Digit Symbol, Trials B, MMSE). These women also faced greater likelihood of cognitive decline in models that adjusted for age, education, depression, stroke, visual impairment, heart disease, hypertension, physical activity, estrogen use, and smoking (Gregg et al., 2000). But, again, other research has shown only a modest association between diabetes and risk of AD (Luchsinger, Tang, Stern, Shea, & Mayeux, 2001).

Bone Mineral Density Loss and Estrogen Deficiency

Animal models and preclinical studies suggest that estrogen use may promote the growth and survival of cholinergic neurons and may also decrease cerebral amyloid deposition. Given the reduction in estrogen production that follows menopause, estrogen supplementation in women is a plausible strategy for delaying the onset of Alzheimer's disease. Hope for this approach was strengthened by prospective studies that showed a lower incidence of AD in postmenopausal women who take estrogen compared to women who did not. In a group of 1124 elderly women who were initially free of Alzheimer's disease, Parkinson's disease, and stroke, the age at onset of Alzheimer's disease was significantly later in those women who had taken estrogen. Of the estrogen users, 5.8% were diagnosed, compared to 16.3% of non-users, even after adjustment for such differences as education, ethnic origin, and *APOE* genotype (Tang et al., 1996).

Even a well-planned prospective study with statistical adjustment cannot rule out selection factors that are confounded with estrogen use (such as better education, income, and more proactive health behaviors). For this effort, randomized controlled trials are required. Confidence in estrogen replacement as a *treatment* strategy has been shaken by a series of negative clinical trials. In a Cochrane Review, Hogervost, Yaffe, Richards, & Huppert, 2003 assessed five high-quality trials of estrogen use (selected from a review of all double-blind randomized controlled trials on the effect of estrogen, alone or in combination with progestin, for cognitive function in postmenopausal women with AD or other types of dementia). In this combined set of 210 women with AD, meta-analyses unfortunately showed no significant benefit.

The negative result for these treatment trials does not rule out a protective effect for estrogen as a *preventive* agent if given earlier to women who have not yet developed AD. Long-term prevention trials are currently underway to examine this potential benefit. However, expectations of success have been dampened by recent findings from the Heart and Estrogen/Progestin Replacement Study (HERS), a randomized, placebo-controlled trial involving 2763 women with coronary disease. Participants at 10 of the 20 HERS centers (n=517 estrogen, n=546 placebo) completed a cognitive function substudy. At about 4 years of follow-up, the groups did not significantly differ on a variety of cognitive tests (modified Mini-Mental Status Examination, Verbal Fluency, Boston Naming, Word List Memory, Word List Recall, and Trails B) (Grady, Yaffe et al., 2002). There was only a single cognitive assessment at the end of the trial and it did not examine incident Alzheimer's disease, so the question of the efficacy of estrogen replacement as a prevention strategy remains open. Still, these negative results are not reassuring. Combined with reports from the Women's Health Initiative of an increased risk of some cancers and stroke in women using estrogen replacement therapy (leading to early termination of the unopposed estrogen arm of the trial), estrogen replacement may not turn out to be useful as an anti-dementia agent. Meta-analyses suggest that "benefits of HRT include prevention of osteoporotic fractures and colorectal cancer, while prevention of dementia is uncertain.

Harms include CHD, stroke, thromboembolic events, breast cancer with 5 or more years of use, and cholecystitis" (Nelson, Humphrey, Nygren, Teutsch, & Allan, 2002, p. 872).

Yet other evidence suggests that estrogen may turn out to be critical for cognitive health and risk of AD after all. For example, bone mineral density (BMD) is a marker of cumulative estrogen exposure and has been associated with cognitive function in non-demented older women. (Yaffe, Browner, Cauley, Launer, & Harris, 1999). In the Study of Osteoporotic Fractures (n=8333 older community-dwelling women not taking estrogen), women with low baseline BMD had up to 8% worse baseline cognitive scores and up to 6% worse repeat cognitive scores. For women who declined 1 SD in hip or calcaneal BMD, the risk of cognitive deterioration (defined as the most extreme 10% of those who declined) increased by about a third, compared to women with stable BMD. The same was true for women who had vertebral fractures. These women had lower cognitive test scores at baseline and greater odds of cognitive deterioration similar to those who declined 1 standard deviation in BMD.

Thus, the relationship between estrogen and risk of AD remains unclear. Results from the Women's Health Initiative combined estrogen/progestin arm, as well as other prevention trials, should help clarify the issue.

Depression

Depressed mood may be an early sign of AD or a risk factor in its own right. Prospective studies cannot settle the issue but do suggest that non-demented older people with depressed mood face an increased risk of AD. In one cohort study (n=478 without dementia at baseline, mean of 2.5 years follow-up), depressed mood at baseline increased the risk of incident dementia nearly threefold. The effect persisted after adjustment for age, gender, education, language of assessment, and functional status (Devanand et al., 1996). The role of depression in subsequent cognitive decline has been confirmed (Yaffe, Blackwell et al., 1999). However, a definitive treatment trial, in which depression would be treated to see if response improves cognition or delays AD, remains to be completed.

OUTCOMES ASSOCIATED WITH ALZHEIMER'S DISEASE

Mortality

Table 6.4 presents U.S. mortality from AD by age and race strata in 1998. About 50,000 deaths per year are attributed to AD, making it the eighth most common cause of death in the U.S. Mortality from AD

TABLE 6.4 Mortality and Alzheimer's Disease, United States, 1998

		White		African-American	
	Total	Men	Women	Men	Women
45–54	0.1				
55–64	1.1	1.2	1.2		
65–74	10.4	10.6	11.1	7.4	8.1
75–84	70.0	69.3	74.8	50.2	59.2
85+	299.5	257.9	336.2	142.5	202.5

Table entries are deaths per 100,000, 1998.

Source: http://www.cdc.gov/nchs/datawh/statab/unpubd/mortabs/gmwk51.htm. United States General Accounting Office. *Report to the Secretary of Health and Human Services: Alzheimer's Disease, Eestimates of Prevalence in the United States.* (1998, January).

is exceedingly rare in people under age 65: less than 1/100,000 per year. But AD very quickly becomes a prominent cause of death at later ages. It is noted on death certificates in 10 (ages 65-74), 70 (aged 75-84), and 300 (aged 85+) of every 100,000 deaths. This is almost certainly an underestimate, since AD may be a contributory cause and may not appear on the death certificate, especially if the certificate is prepared by a funeral home director, coroner, or doctor unfamiliar with the patient. The lower attribution of mortality to AD among African Americans may represent greater likelihood of death certificates completed in this way.

Alzheimer's disease increases the risk of mortality. Compared to non-demented elderly matched for age, drawn from the same community, and similar in socioeconomic features, these elders face a mortality risk 2-3 times higher. Figure 6.2 presents Kaplan-Meier plots of time to death in three groups first assessed between 1989 and 1992 and followed for up to 10 years. These elders were recruited from a Medicare enrollee sample and AD registry, both in the Washington Heights-Inwood community, northern Manhattan, New York City.

Between 1989 and 1992, people met criteria for AD when they were first seen (*prevalent AD*), or developed AD sometime in this period (baseline visit non-demented, later visit over the follow-up period demented: *incident AD*), or never met criteria for AD over the entire follow-up period (*non-demented*). A convenient measure of mortality risk is to note the point in follow-up time when 50% of people in each of the three groups have died. As the figure shows, this point was reached in 5.2 years in the prevalent AD group, 7.0 years in the incident AD group, and 9.2 years in the non-demented group. While an impressive difference, this approach does not adjust for differences

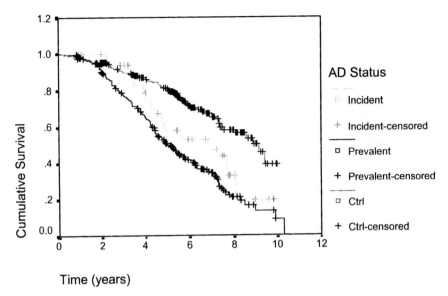

Time (years)

FIGURE 6.2 Survival by AD Status: Initial or Dementia CCD, 1989–1992.

in age or other factors, an important limitation, since age is related to AD risk, as we have already seen. To control for this confounding, proportional hazards models can be used to separate the effects of age and AD, as well as the influence of other factors. In such a model, we found that prevalent AD was associated with a twofold increase in mortality risk and incident AD a 1.7–fold increase, both highly significant effects.

Not surprisingly, survival with AD depends heavily on the age at diagnosis. Results from the Baltimore Longitudinal Study of Aging show that median survival after diagnosis ranged from 8.3 years in people aged 65 to 3.4 years for people aged 90. Comparing this survival to non-demented elders showed that AD reduces life span by about two-thirds for people diagnosed at age 65 and by about 39% for people diagnosed at age 90 (Brookmeyer, Corrada, Curriero, Kawas, 2002). These differences reflect the effect of competing risks of mortality, which increase at later ages.

Nursing Home Care

Alzheimer's disease is a major risk factor for nursing home placement. In the Washington Heights-Inwood, New York City sample, described above, we tracked nursing home admission up to 10 years of follow-up. This sample has the advantage of long follow-up and careful diagnostic assessment for AD, but is likely to be atypical for estimating the absolute rate of nursing home use because New York City offers an extensive alternative Medicaid-funded home care benefit. Also, this study enrolled a largely minority sample, and research has shown that minorities are less likely to use nursing homes than whites.

In the Washington Heights cohort, 8.8% of prevalent cases entered nursing homes, compared to 3.5% of people who never met criteria for AD. Incident cases were intermediate, with 5% entering nursing homes. With this background of relatively low rates of nursing home placement, it is still impressive to see that incident AD was associated with a large increase in the risk of nursing home admission. Using a time-dependent approach, in which the date of AD diagnosis is used as a predictor of time to nursing home placement, we found that incident AD was associated with an eightfold increase in risk in models that controlled for age, race-ethnicity, and education.

In other settings, nursing home placement is more frequent. Among participants in a clinical trial of selegiline and tocopherol, all with moderate dementia and living in the community, two-thirds of the 341 patients followed entered nursing homes over 2 years (Knopman et al., 1999). Dementia progression was the strongest predictor of placement, such that people progressing to severe dementia (CDR 3) were eight times as likely to enter nursing homes as people who remained moderately demented. Despite sociomedical determinants of nursing home placement (such as features of caregivers, e.g., caregiver burden; perceived skill or efficacy; presence of family support; and system-level features, such as availability of beds or alternative home-based services), nursing home placement remains an important outcome for assessing disease progression and treatment. To take these sociomedical factors into account, Stern and colleagues (1994) have developed a measure of "dependency" and "equivalent institutional care," that tracks need for services provided in institutional settings.

Hospitalization and Primary Care

Do people with Alzheimer's disease face an increased risk of hospitalization? This simple question is actually quite hard to answer. People with AD may enter the hospital for other reasons, and the Alzheimer's may not be recorded on the discharge diagnosis. Moreover, risk of hospitalization may be elevated in early stages of disease, when patients are likely to fall, fail to take medications, have a psychiatric admission, or decline with more severe stages of dementia. The most severely demented patients may reside in nursing homes, which provide medical care for many conditions, or may simply not be brought in for hospital care as part of a general strategy of less aggressive treatment. In addition, while use of Medicare billing records, which include *ICD-10* diagnoses of AD, can be used to establish hospital episodes and volume of costs, these sorts of analysis are prone to an observation bias, in which the most severe cases are over-represented (Newcomer et al., 1999). Since AD is also a terminal disease, it is hard to distinguish end-of-life care from AD care. Finally, the proper test would be a comparison between people with similar medical conditions and health status except for AD, but this comparison is difficult because AD may itself be associated with medical conditions, such as falls or injuries, wasting and dehydration, or pneumonia and infectious disease.

With these caveats, it is not surprising to see considerable variation in yearly rates of hospitalization in people with AD. The Consortium to Establish a Registry for Alzheimer's Disease (CERAD) reported a rate of 370 hospitalizations per 1,000 AD patients per year in a clinical cohort (Fillenbaum, Heyman, Peterson, Pieper, & Weiman, 2000). In a community cohort in New York City, the rate was 100 per 1,000 AD cases per year (Albert, Costa et al., 1999). What seems clear in any case is the elevation of this risk relative to matched elders without AD. In the New York sample, 10% of AD cases had a hospitalization in a year, compared to 6.8% among non-demented elders. In logistic regression models that control for differences in age, gender, education, number of comorbid conditions, and death in the follow-up period, severe AD (CDR 3+) was associated with an elevated risk of 2.3. This study has the advantage of a large population-based cohort in which hospitalizations were tracked with an innovative electronic medical record. This risk was comparable to the added risk associated with two comorbid conditions.

Primary care use and associated costs also appear to be elevated in AD. In the New York cohort, recently diagnosed people were more likely to have more medical care encounters than people without AD even 1-2 years before diagnosis (Albert, Glied, Andrews, Stern, & Mayeux, 2002). Other studies have not found excess primary care costs in the prodromal period (Liebson et al., 1999).

Disability and Psychiatric Morbidity

The hallmark of progressive dementia is increasing dependency in the activities of daily living (ADL) and an increase in both "negative" (apathy, withdrawal) and "positive" (agitation, aggression, delusions, hallucinations, wandering) psychopathologic symptoms. In the most severe stages of dementia, the prevalence of some symptoms declines (such as delusions), presumably because caregivers can no longer recognize these symptoms as patients become increasingly vegetative.

Cognitive performance in patients and ADL ratings from proxies (or from clinicians) are highly correlated in people with AD. For example, in one series of people with AD, correlations between the Blessed Memory-Concentration-Information test, a mental status measure similar to the MMSE, and IADL and ADL (personal self-maintenance scale) ratings were 0.83 and 0.78, respectively (Green, Mohs, Schmeidler, Aryan, & Davis, 1993). In this sample of 104 clinic patients with probable AD, PSMS (Physical Self-Maintenance Scale) scores were collected every 6 months and tracked for change. The PSMS items include toileting, feeding, dressing, grooming, indoor mobility, and bathing. These were scored on a scale of 0 (maximum difficulty) to 5 (no difficulty), so that total scores ranged from 6 to 30. In this sample, PSMS scores declined, on average, 2.44 points over 12 months, with a standard deviation of 3.87.

These numbers are important for gauging the clinical significance of changes in functional scales used in clinical trials in AD. A recent meta-analysis of the effect of cholinesterase inhibitors, the primary approved therapy for treatment of AD, showed a small but significant effect size of 0.1 sd favoring treatment. Using the standard deviation of 3.87, cited above, 0.1 sd is equivalent to 0.387, or about a 0.4 point change on the PSMS scale. Since the mean PSMS change over 12 months was 2.44, the 0.4 change is roughly equivalent to the decline patients can expect over a 2–month period (Trinh, Hoblyn, Mohanty, & Yaffe, 2003). Delaying decline by 2 months per year is a small but important benefit to patients and family caregivers.

A large trial of donepezil (Aricept) to assess preservation of ADL function in AD confirmed this benefit in an alternative way (Mohs et al., 2001). The trial sought to assess whether this cholinesterase inhibitor delayed "clinically evident decline in function," which was defined as progression to moderate or more severe levels of difficulty with particular ADL, or loss of 20% of instrumental ADL function, or onset of more advanced dementia, as assessed by the Clinical Dementia Rating (CDR). Of placebo patients, 56% met the endpoint, compared to 41% of donepezil patients. The median time at which patients met this endpoint was 208 days among placebo patients and 357 days in donepezil patients. The therapy, then, slowed progression by about 5 months in a 1–year period.

Cholinesterase inhibitors also showed benefit for the reduction in frequency of AD psychopathology. A meta-analysis showed that this class of therapies reduced Neuropsychiatric Inventory (NPI, Cummings, 1997) scores, on average, by nearly 2 points, an improvement in the frequency or severity of one psychiatric symptom (Trinh et al., 2003). Since the presence of psychiatric symptoms is an important predictor of nursing home placement, not to mention caregiver distress and burnout, these therapies offer an important benefit, at least in the short run.

Thus, at this point, AD cannot be prevented and disease progression remains relentless. Available therapies offer benefit mostly as a holding action, delaying time to severe disability and nursing home placement.

Family Caregiving

Families provide the vast majority of Alzheimer's care. While Alzheimer's patients are common in nursing homes, accounting for perhaps half the residents, these residents represent a minority of the Alzheimer's population. We have already mentioned that nursing home use has declined over the past decade in the U.S. (from 4.6% of older people in 1985 to 4.2% in 1995). Most people with AD are cared for at home, use a variety of in-home (home attendant, allied health) and out-of-home services (adult day care, acute rehab), and will enter nursing homes very late in the disease, if at all.

In fact, people residing in nursing homes are likely to be older and frailer than prior nursing home cohorts. They are also less likely to spend long periods of time in these institutions. The nursing home is becoming more of a short-stay rehabilitative or palliative care unit, funded by Medicare, than a long-term custodial residence (traditionally funded by Medicaid). The commonly cited estimate of a lifetime prevalence of 40% for nursing home residence (Kemper & Murtaugh, 1991), then, must be interpreted in this light.

How many people with Alzheimer's are cared for in the community? If we consider older people with three or more ADL disabilities, we have an imperfect but reasonable indicator of dementia in the community. About half of these people relied exclusively on family and friends for assistance in 1994, a decline from two-thirds in the 1980s (Feder, Komisar, Niefeld, 2001). This change reflects an expansion in financing for long-term care that occurred in the 1990s. Medicare spending for home health care grew from about $4 to $18 billion in the first half of the 1990s. Alzheimer's home care has benefited from this change. More recently, however, cost controls have been introduced into this health sector (Balanced Budget Act of 1997), which have reduced growth in Medicare-funded home care.

Estimates of the absolute number of family caregivers providing custodial care for older people, and also older people with Alzheimer's disease, are available in the 1996 panel of the Survey of Income and

Program Participation (SIPP). In 1998, 6.7 million family members were providing help to some 4.5 million older adults with disabilities (Alecxih, Zeruld, & Olearczyk, 2002). This estimate is slightly lower than the estimate of 7.1 million derived from the National Long-Term Care Survey. The SIPP allows estimates of particular features of Alzheimer's caregiving. In 1998, about 473,000 family members or friends were serving as primary caregivers to people diagnosed with Alzheimer's disease. These people were providing most of the non-paid support received by people with dementia living in the community and were nominated as the people most involved in such care. They spent an average of 48 hr/wk providing care and had been providing such care for a mean of 7 years. This compares to a mean of 24 hr/wk and a mean duration of 5 years for all non-paid caregivers in the community (Alecxih et al., 2000). Thus, Alzheimer's care is more demanding than standard care by this measure of caregiving intensity.

One investigation tracked hours of care provided to people with Alzheimer's according to severity of dementia and also over a period of nearly 2 years (Albert, Sano et al., 1998). Family caregivers reported that more than half the time they spent with these elders involved direct hands-on care, defined as help with ADL. Caregivers reported a mean of 7.2 hours per day of ADL care, or 50.4 hours per week. This report is quite close to the SIPP results, presented earlier. These informal, or non-paid, hours must be interpreted in light of the total hours of custodial care provided for these elders, which in this New York City sample were extensive. Total weekly hours were 56.7 for people with mild dementia, 81.2 for people with moderate dementia, and 112.0 for people with severe or greater dementia. Family contributions were 30.8 in mild dementia, 57.5 for people with moderate dementia, and 29.4 in severe dementia, suggesting substitution of formal for informal care in the most severe levels of dementia.

However, these cross-sectional findings can be deceiving. In longitudinal analyses, Albert, Sano, and colleagues (1998) found that caregivers did not, in fact, reduce the number of hours they provided as elders progressed to more advanced dementia. Rather, formal hours increased, suggesting that these caregivers were already providing the maximum of hours they could provide.

What are the tasks of families who provide care for elders with dementia? Family caregivers certainly provide help with ADL, but providing ADL support at home to a family member is not well described by ADL measures (Coon, Ovy, & Schluz, 2002). While the ADL/IADL measures tell us that someone has a particular care need, satisfying that need takes place in a complex environment. Take, for example, bathing. The ADL measure tells us that someone is dependent in bathing (Barrick, Rader, Hoeffer, & Sloan, 2002). It does not tell us the reason the person cannot bathe independently, which may involve impairments in mobility and balance, or limb weakness, or cognitive incapacity, or psychiatric disorder, or some combination of these deficits. As a result, the ADL measure does not tell us if the person is cooperative during bathing, whether she helps wash parts of her body once in the tub, or whether she needs supervision throughout the entire course of bathing or only when getting in and out of the tub. Yet these are the features that make caregiving for someone with bathing disability more or less difficult for families.

Thus, while a count of ADL/IADL needs will certainly be correlated with indicators of caregiving challenge (how many hours daily, reported burden and fatigue, risk of nursing home placement), these correlations will be low. Indeed, ADL status explains only a modest amount of the variance in caregiver reports of burden (Poulshock & Diemling, 1984).

The ADL/IADL measures also fail to capture the full context in which families provide care. What kinds of home modifications have family members made to facilitate caregiving? To return to our bathing example, providing bathing care will be easier if families have installed grab bars, or have a home with a walk-in shower or flexible shower head. Similarly, what kinds of care arrangements have families put in place to ensure such care if they work, or wish to travel, or are themselves weak or ill? These, too, will determine how challenging ADL/IADL care may be. These sorts of care management tasks are a critical part of the work of caregiving but are not considered in traditional ADL/IADL measures.

Thus, providing care is not simply the mirror image of the need for care, as expressed in ADL/IADL status (Albert, 2003; Kramer & Thompson, 2002). We have argued that ADL/IADL care should be subsumed within a wider, multi-domain formulation that gives adequate scope to *how people need ADL* care and *how caregivers develop environments for providing it.* This is especially salient in the case of care for people who suffer from cognitive disorders, such as AD.

Even if we limit ourselves to traditional ADL tasks, we quickly see that caregivers who provide such care mention many additional factors that make ADL care easy or difficult, manageable or unbearable. One is *timing*: whether care is required rarely, frequently but in predictable ways, or frequently in unpredictable, unexpected ways (Hoyman, Gonyea, & Montgomery, 1985). AD care is characterized by great unpredictability in the timing of ADL care because of poor sleep hygiene, psychiatric complications, incontinence, inability to communicate care preferences, and non-cooperation.

A glaring example of the central role of timing is night-time care; people who routinely need to be taken to the toilet at night, disrupting a caregiver's sleep, are clearly more challenging than people who can be taken to the toilet during the day and sleep through the night, though both equally need assistance in toileting (McCluskey, 2000). More generally, caregivers forced to adopt care receivers' schedules are likely to be most burdened, as they are most captive to caregiving.

A second dimension is *caregiver proximity* in the ADL task. Is it enough that a caregiver is in the house while someone eats a meal or bathes, or does the caregiver need to be in the same room standing by, or does she have to provide hands-on help? Stand-by help can be quite burdensome in that it limits caregivers to the home even if they do not have to provide hands-on help at all times. In fact, stand-by help in some cases may be more burdensome, as family members need to be available (and hence are prevented from doing other tasks) without a sense that they are providing care. This is a typical feature of caregiving to the mildly demented elder.

A third dimension is the *kind of effort* caregivers need to exert to see that the ADL need is met. Someone with a need for help in bathing may only require supervision, or coaxing and support, or complete guidance and direction. It is possible that coaxing and support in some cases may be more challenging than complete guidance and control. For example, taking someone to the toilet every two hours may be more burdensome than complete continence care involving disposable diapers (Albert, 1999).

Finally, it obviously matters whether care receivers participate, actively resist, or are passive as receivers of ADL care (Feinstein, Josephy, & Wells, 1986). Helping a person who is cooperative is far different from helping a person who is resisting assistance in bathing or eating. Unfortunately, care for the severely demented AD patient often incurs resistance.

The effects of providing care to a person with AD have been intensively studied. Marital discord and divorce, depression and anxiety, loss of employment, restriction of social life, invasion of privacy, impoverishment, and substance abuse have all been linked to caregiving stress. Buffering factors that mitigate these negative effects include support from family, religiosity, strong personal mastery and self-efficacy, satisfaction with caregiving, and strategies to reduce the burdensome nature of care.

Caregiving strain has also been linked to mortality risk, as suggested in the Caregiver Health Effects Study, a study of the bereavement experience of people who cared for spouses who died over follow-up (Schulz & Beach, 1999). Spouses who provided care and reported burden from caregiving were more likely to die than non-caregivers, but caregiving spouses who did not experience burden did not face an elevated risk. Schulz and Beach concluded that mental or emotional strain is an independent risk factor for mortality among elderly spousal caregivers.

End of Life Care

Family caregivers face difficult decisions related to end-of-life care of relatives in the last stages of the disease (Meier, 1999). Should patients with pneumonia be treated aggressively with IV antibiotics, transferred to hospital, and intubated or should they be treated symptomatically with analgesics, antipyretics, and oxygen? Should a demented patient refusing food or with swallowing difficulty be tube fed? Little is known about the ways families make these decisions.

Persons with advanced dementia suffer serious medical problems, such as pneumonia, urinary tract infections, and fever (Fabiszewski, Volicer, & Volicer, 1990; van der Steen, Ooms, van der Wal, & Ribbe, 2002). Research suggests a high prevalence of IV antibiotic use and invasive procedures (Ahronheim, Morrison, Baskin, Morris & Meier, 1996; Morrison & Siu, 2000). For example, despite the futility associated with aggressive care in end-stage dementia, Evers and colleagues (2002) found that more than 50% of the patients with dementia were treated with systemic antibiotics. Our own clinic series suggests similar trends. In a group of people with probable AD, 31% used IV antibiotics and 16% had feeding tubes placed in the 6 months before death.

It is still unclear why some families opt for use of life-sustaining technologies in the case of older people with profound or terminal AD. It may be that family caregivers who score high on measures of distress (depression, caregiver burden, lack of social support) are less likely to develop medical care goals that limit aggressive end-of-life care. These families may also be at greater risk of emergency room use of life-sustaining technologies. To our knowledge, no research has investigated this issue.

By contrast, AD patients may be less likely to be considered for life-sustaining technologies than other people with terminal conditions. The loss of cognitive ability and hence loss of personhood associated with disease may allow families to "let go" of people who are in the last stages of life.

Quality of Life in AD

One central problem for people with AD is their inability, in later stages of the disease, to report on subjective states: their perceptions of pain, satisfaction, comfort, enjoyment, contentment, anxiety, or well-being. Since quality of life assessment is unthinkable without a patient's reports of such states (see chapter 8), it would seem that assessment of quality of life in people with AD would be impossible. Severely affected patients (patients with Mini-Mental State Examination scores below 12 or patients with more than moderate cognitive impairment) cannot reliably complete self-report questionnaires. Yet it is clear even to the casual observer that people with AD have good and bad days, that facial expressions and body posture reliably communicate information about internal states, and that these perhaps primitive indicators of mood or well-being are associated with changes in environment (Albert & Logsdon, 2001). If we can perceive mood changes and illness behaviors in animals, we can certainly recognize such changes in people with dementia. Thus, the challenge in advanced AD is to identify indicators of internal states that reliably convey information about mood and well-being.

What domains or aspects of daily life are important to patients in the presence of severely compromised cognition and function? The domains included in current measures vary considerably. Among other domains, Rabins includes "awareness of self" and "response to surroundings" (Rabins, Kasper, Kleinman et al., 2001), and Brod, "aesthetic sense" and "feelings of belonging" (Brod, Stewart, Sands, 2001). Logsdon's QOL-AD measure includes items assessing "energy level" and "ability to do things for fun" (Logsdon, Gibbons, McCurry, et al., 1999).

These are patient or proxy reports and face a variety of limitations. Proxy reports about patient quality of life are correlated with caregivers' own mood or perceived caregiver burden. People can impute moods or symptoms based on their own status. Patients' self-reports will be reliable only up to a point, though some patients are evidently able to complete questionnaires with MMSE scores as low as 10 (Logsdon et al., 2001).

Behavioral observation measures avoid these limitations. The Apparent Affect Rating Scale (APS) (Lawton, 2001), Multidimensional Observational Scale (MOSES; Helmes, 1987), Discomfort Scale (Hurley, Volicer, Hanrahan, Houde, & Volicer, 1992), and other observer ratings capture negative and positive behaviors in real-time (Albert, 1997). "Behavior stream" technologies now allow clocking of the duration of mood or behavior states and the context in which patients express these states, such as "agitation during morning ADL care." Behavior stream measures are complicated by the need for extensive training of raters and limitation to institutional home settings.

One intermediate approach is to adapt behavior stream-like measures to proxy reporting. Albert and colleagues (Albert, Castillo-Castanada, Sano et al., 1996; Albert, Castillo-Castanada, Jacobs et al., 1999) asked proxies to report on affective states using APS items (i.e., facial expressions of the so-called "hot" affects: anger, anxiety, interest, pleasure) and patient activity over the prior two weeks (frequency of a series of in-home and out-of-home activities that could be completed with caregiving cueing and supervision). The measures were significantly correlated with dementia severity in both clinic and community samples (Albert, Castello-Castanada, Jacobs et al., 1999). This is important confirmation of the validity of the quality-of-life measures. Such measures should be correlated with stage of dementia (because dementia severity affects mood and opportunities for engagement) but should also show variance within stage (suggesting that there are other sources of pleasure or engagement relevant to dementia care).

This approach also is useful for specifying time to important quality-of-life milestones in the progression of AD. For example, in a group of people with moderate dementia at the start of follow-up, 50% were no longer leaving their homes within 20 months. In a group with mild dementia, this milestone was not reached until 30 months (Albert, Jacobs, Sano et al., 2001). This study was also able to show a hierarchy of QOL outcomes. Onset of home confinement preceded onset of null activity, which in turn preceded onset of null positive affect. Finally, this study showed that proxies identified states of pleasure even among patients with psychopathologic behaviors. This finding reminds us that we must pay attention to both positive and negative behaviors if we are to understand dementia adequately.

NON-ALZHEIMER'S DEMENTIAS

Vascular cognitive impairment (VCI), as opposed to Alzheimer's disease, is cognitive impairment related to cerebrovascular disease, such as stroke. VCI is mainly defined by neuroimaging, which allows further differentiation into subgroups that show cortical infarction, white matter changes, or some combination of the two. In cohort studies of incident dementia, such as the Cardiovascular Disease Study, about 70% of people meeting criteria for dementia can be classified as AD, another 10% VCI, 15% mixed AD and VCI, and the remaining 5% some other etiology (such as hydrocephalus, metabolic disorders, or Korsakoff's syndrome) (Lopez et al., 2003).

VCI is a risk factor for mortality. In a Mayo Clinic record linkage study, patients with vascular dementia had a greater risk of mortality than matched non-demented controls. Among VCI patients, dementia related to stroke was associated with the highest mortality risk. Patients without stroke but with imaging evidence of bilateral infarctions in gray matter structures had a lower mortality risk (Knopman, Rocca, Cha, Edland, & Kokmen, 2003).

Another source of dementia in the elderly is Parkinson's disease (PD). The Parkinson's Foundation has reviewed a series of prevalence and incidence studies of dementia in PD and found that about a quarter of all Parkinson's patients meet criteria for dementia. Demented PD patients are older but do not differ in the duration of the disease (Lieberman, 2002). The annual incidence of dementia in Parkinson's patients ranges from 2.7% (ages 55-64) to 13.7% (ages 70-79). Dementia risk in PD may vary according to whether patients have Lewy body inclusions in the brainstem or brain, or have Lewy bodies with Alzheimer's changes as well. Mortality risk in PD is related to the presence of dementia. Incident dementia in PD increases mortality risk even when the motor effects of PD are controlled (Levy et al., 2002).

SUMMARY

Families confronting dementing disease face the very difficult problem of deciding when driving should cease, when supervision is required for safety, when elders can no longer live alone, and when parents or spouses are no longer competent to handle money, take medications, or manage their lives independently. They will likely have to contend with personality changes, psychiatric symptoms, and challenging behaviors as people reach more advanced stages of disease. Caregivers may have to perform ADL care, manage custodial care staff hired to assist the elder, or more likely both sets of tasks, possibly at a distance. They may face the difficult decision to admit the Alzheimer's patient to a nursing home. Or, as is increasingly more common, older people themselves may choose residences (such as assisted living or continuing care retirement communities) that can accommodate Alzheimer's or nursing-home levels of care, should they need such services.

Definition of Dementia. A person meets criteria for dementia if he or she has memory impairment and one or more additional impairments in cognition, such as aphasia, apraxia, agnosia, or executive function deficits. These cognitive deficits must be severe enough to cause significant impairment in social or occupational function and must represent a significant decline from a previous level of functioning. For a person to be diagnosed with Alzheimer's disease, the course of this general cognitive disorder must, in addition, be characterized by gradual onset and continuing, progressive decline that is not attributable to other central nervous system conditions.

AD and Memory Decline in Aging. Research suggests that memory declines typical of Alzheimer's disease may be distinct from normal aging. In a nondemented cohort, declines in cognitive domains in people without the e4 allele, representing normal aging, were less pronounced than declines in people with the e4 allele, representing a likely early stage of AD.

Mild Cognitive Impairment. Mild cognitive impairment (MCI) is typically defined by subjective complaints of memory problems and memory performance below age-and education-referenced norms, with normal performance in other cognitive domains and absence of impairment in the instrumental and basic activities of daily living. Dementia incidence in elders who report cognitive complaints and demonstrate mild deficits in cognitive assessment is much higher than that for elders as a whole, 18% over 3 years, compared to perhaps 3-6% in the population of older adults as a whole. Consequently, mild cognitive impairment cannot be considered benign or a normal feature of healthy aging.

Prevalence and Incidence of Alzheimer's Disease. In a synthesis of prevalence surveys, the best estimate of AD prevalence is about 1.9 million people aged 65+ in 1995. Prevalence rises to 2.1 million if we include possible or mixed cases, that is, cases marked by AD and some other source of dementia. If we restrict cases to moderate or more severe AD, the prevalence is 1.0 million with the narrow definition and 1.4 million with inclusion of possible and mixed cases. All told, 5.7% of Americans aged 65+ had AD in 1995, with 3.3% meeting criteria for moderate or more severe AD.

By 2015, we can expect 4.6 million cases of AD using the narrow definition and 5.3 million if we include mixed cases. About a third of these cases will have moderate or more severe forms of AD.

The incidence of AD is closely related to age. For people aged 65-74, annual incidence ranges from <0.5% to 1.3%. For people aged 75-84, the range is 1.5% to 4.0%, and for people aged 85+ it is 4.7% to 7.9% per year. Minority status is among the most important risk factors for AD. Given the increasing number of minority elderly in the U.S., this disparity has great public health significance.

Risk Factors for Alzheimer's Disease. Only about 7% of early-onset AD (< age 65) and less than 1% of late-onset AD have been linked to mutations on particular genes. For late-onset AD, attention centers on the *APOE* gene. A number of studies have shown over-representation of the *APOE*-ε4 allele in people with AD. Despite this finding, the current recommendation is against use of APOE as a screening tool: "although *APOE* genotype may be a risk factor for AD, it cannot yet be considered a useful predictive genetic test."

The significance of cognitive resources early in the life span for dementia in late life has become increasingly clear in studies that have linked risk of AD to childhood IQ, educational accomplishment and leisure activities, occupational attainment and job demands, language skills in early adulthood, diversity of physical and cognitive engagement over the life span, parental socioeconomic status, and literacy. These findings suggest that cognitive ability is similar to grip strength: differences (in muscle fiber density, in neuronal integrity or number) already apparent at birth or in the perinatal period (and which develop or set limits on development over the life span) provide variable reserve against depletions that occur with aging. These resources put one closer or further away from the threshold of disability associated with the loss of physical and cognitive function that occurs over the life span.

A variety of medical conditions have been shown to increase the risk of AD, including hypertension and vascular disease, diabetes, loss in bone mineral density, estrogen deficiency, and depression.

The case of estrogen deficiency is instructive. An initial cohort study showed a benefit for estrogen replacement. In this study, 5.8% of estrogen users were diagnosed, compared to 16.3% of non-users, even after adjustment for differences in education, ethnic origin, and *APOE* genotype. However, confidence in estrogen replacement as a *treatment* strategy has been shaken by a series of negative clinical trials. The negative result for these treatment trials does not rule out a protective effect for estrogen as a *preventive* agent if given earlier to women who have not yet developed AD. However, expectations of success have been dampened by absence of differences in cognitive performance in a randomized trial using estrogen in nondemented women. Combined with reports from the Women's Health Initiative of an increased risk of some cancers and stroke in women using estrogen replacement therapy (leading to early termination of the unopposed estrogen arm of the trial), estrogen replacement may not turn out to be useful as an antidementia agent. Yet other evidence suggests that estrogen may turn out to be critical for cognitive health and risk of AD after all. For example, bone mineral density (BMD) is a marker of cumulative estrogen exposure and has been associated with cognitive function in nondemented older women. Thus, the relationship between estrogen and risk of AD remains unclear. Results from the Women's Health Initiative combined estrogen/progestin arm, as well as other prevention trials, should help clarify the issue.

Outcomes Associated with Alzheimer's Disease. Compared to nondemented elderly matched for age and comorbid disease, drawn from the same community, and similar in socioeconomic features, elders with AD face a mortality risk 2–3 times higher than elders with normal cognition.

AD is a key risk factor for nursing home admission. In one clinical trial series, two-thirds of people with moderate levels of dementia entered nursing homes over 2 years. Dementia progression was the strongest predictor of placement. People progressing to severe dementia were 8 times as likely to enter nursing homes as people who remained moderately demented.

AD is also associated with greater risk of acute medical care in the hospital, as well as general medical care in the community. In a New York City sample, 10% of AD cases had a hospitalization in a year, compared to 6.8% among nondemented elders. In logistic regression models that controlled for differences in age, gender, education, number of comorbid conditions, and death in the follow-up period, severe AD was associated with a twofold increase in risk of hospitalization.

Families provide the vast majority of Alzheimer's care. While Alzheimer's patients are common in nursing homes, accounting for perhaps half the residents, these residents represent a minority of the Alzheimer's population. Most people with AD are cared for at home, use a variety of in-home (home attendant, allied health) and out-of-home services (adult day care, acute rehab), and will enter nursing homes very late in the disease, if at all.

The effects of providing care to a person with AD have been intensively studied. Marital discord and divorce, depression and anxiety, loss of employment, restriction of social life, invasion of privacy, impoverishment, substance abuse, and mortality have all been linked to caregiving stress. Buffering factors that mitigate these negative effects include support from family, religiosity, strong personal mastery and self-efficacy, satisfaction with caregiving, and strategies to reduce the burden of providing care.

Family caregivers and clinicians face difficult decisions related to end-of-life care of relatives in the last stages of AD. Should patients with pneumonia be treated aggressively with IV antibiotics, transferred to hospital, and intubated; or should they be treated symptomatically with analgesics, antipyretics, and oxygen? Should a demented patient who refuses food or has difficulty swallowing be tube fed? Little is known about the ways families make these decisions, but evidence suggests that use of life-sustaining technologies is common in this terminal population.

Since quality of life (QOL) assessment is unthinkable without a patient's own reports of such states, it would seem that assessment of quality of life in people with AD would be impossible. Severely affected patients (patients with Mini-Mental State Examination scores below 12 or patients with more than moderate cognitive impairment) cannot reliably complete self-report questionnaires. Yet it is clear even to the casual observer that people with AD have good and bad days and that facial expressions and body posture reliably communicate information about internal states. QOL investigation of people with AD requires a judicious mix of patient, proxy, and observational measures. A useful QOL measure should be correlated with stage of dementia (because dementia severity affects mood and opportunities for engagement) but should also show variance within stage (suggesting that there are other sources of pleasure or engagement relevant to dementia care). In this way, QOL Investigation may be useful as a guide to clinical care and environmental modifications that will benefit patients and their families.

7

Affective Function: Suffering, Neglect, Isolation

Symptoms of poor mental health may be different in older than in younger people (Blazer, 2002). As we will see, older people are less likely to meet standard criteria for syndromal depression or anxiety disorders. Affective disorders are more likely to take the form of "subthreshold syndromes," symptom intensities and frequencies short of standard criteria for diagnoses of clinical disorders. Does this mean that older people are less depressed? Or should we draw the conclusion that depression needs to be redefined in this case because it is a different kind of clinical entity? The disability and excess morbidity associated with subthreshold disorders suggests the latter, as we will see below. These questions also suggest that we consider mental health in older adults within the broader context of emotional and social experience in old age.

BURDEN OF MENTAL ILLNESS

The first Surgeon General's Report on Mental Health (1999) begins with recognition of the immense burden of disability associated with mental illness throughout the world. In more developed countries ("established market economies"), for example, mental health disorders account for about 15% of all disease burden, more, in fact, than the burden associated with cancer (Murray & Lopez, 1996). The rank of these diseases in terms of the burden they produce is shown in Table 7.1. Mental illness is exceeded only by cardiovascular disease in years lost to disability and early mortality. Cancer follows, showing that diseases of mental health, because they begin early in life and persist over the life span, produce a greater volume of morbidity and disability.

TABLE 7.1 Disease Burden by Selected Illness Categories in Established Market Economies, 1990

	Percent of Total DALYs*
All cardiovascular conditions	18.6
All mental illness**	15.4
All malignant diseases (cancer)	15.0
All respiratory conditions	4.8
All alcohol use	4.7
All infectious and parasitic diseases	2.8
All drug use	1.5

*Disability-adjusted life year (DALY) is a measure that expresses years of life lost to premature death and years lived with a disability of specified severity and duration (Murray & Lopez, 1996).

**Disease burden associated with "mental illness" includes suicide.

Source: Murray & Lopez, 1996.

TABLE 7.2 Leading Sources of Disease Burden in Established Market Economies, 1990

		Total DALYs (millions)	Percent of Total
	All causes	98.7	
1	Ischemic heart disease	8.9	9.0
2	Unipolar major depression	6.7	6.8
3	Cardiovascular disease	5.0	5.0
4	Alcohol use	4.7	4.7
5	Road traffic accidents	4.3	4.4

Source: Murray & Lopez, 1996.

Clearly, treatment and prevention of mental disorders would go a long way toward the reduction of disease burden.

The burden of particular diseases involving mental health relative to total disease burden is shown in Table 7.2. The table shows that the equivalent of 98.7 million person-years were lost to disability or early mortality in the more developed countries in 1990. Unipolar depression, the most prevalent mental illness, accounted for 6.8% of this total burden. Burden associated with depressive disorders exceeded burden associated with cardiovascular disease (more narrowly defined than above), alcohol use, and road traffic accidents.

The measure of burden in these comparisons is the DALY, or disability-adjusted life year. This is a summation of years of healthy life lost to disability and early mortality. While the DALY is similar in principle to other measures of health expectancy, discussed in chapters 5 and 8, its calculation differs in an important way. It assigns weights to age, where these weights "reflect the relative importance of healthy life at different ages" (World Bank, 1995). These weights increase up to age 25 and then decline. They have also been designed to reflect the dependence of the young and elderly on working-age adults. One effect of this age-weighting factor in DALY calculations is the decrease in the contribution of old age disability to total years lost to disability. Be that as it may, the DALY approach to burden is useful for showing the great morbidity and disability associated with mental illness.

An alternative indicator of the severe burden of mental illness, especially depression, is visible in self-reports of disability from people with different chronic health conditions. The Medical Outcomes Study examined adult outpatients with a series of sentinel conditions (hypertension, myocardial infarction, arthritis, gastrointestinal disorders, and depression), who did not have other comorbidities (Wells et al., 1989). The impact of each condition on six health-related quality of life domains (physical function, role function, social function, mental health, self-perceived global health, and bodily pain) was assessed relative to a nationally representative sample of adults ascertained outside the clinic setting (see chapter 8). The differences in scores on each of the six domains, relative to the non-clinic sample, show important differences in disease impact. These findings are shown here in Figure 7.1.

The dotted line represents scores from the non-clinic sample, assigned a zero value for purposes on standardization. The figure shows that hypertension has little effect of reported function and well-being. People with the condition reported only poorer perceived health and a greater number of mental health symptoms, both in keeping with the disease label and the need to take medication (which may itself have a quality of life impact). Arthritis and GI disorders were roughly comparable in their effects on physical function, but GI orders were more burdensome on role, social function, and mental health domains, while arthritis was more burdensome in the bodily pain domain. Myocardial infarction had primarily physical effects, with very low scores in the physical and role performance domains.

Wells et al., (1989) point out the perhaps surprising result that outpatients meeting criteria for depression performed worse not just on the mental health measures, as expected, but looked very much like the myocardial infarction patients in their reports of physical function and role performance. He concluded, the functioning of depressed patients is comparable with or worse than that of patients with major chronic medical conditions.

Thus, the effect of mental disorders on daily life should not be underestimated. Below, we examine morbidity associated with depression

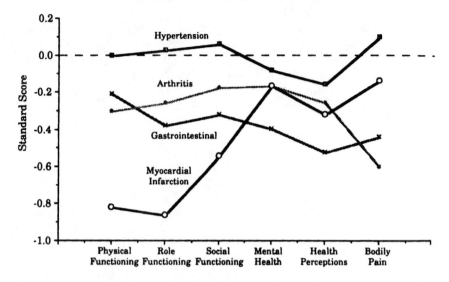

FIGURE 7.1 Health Profiles for Patients With Four Common Conditions From Medical Outcomes Study.

Note: the mean health scores for each chronic condition group and for the group with no chronic conditions are standardized. The difference between each chronic condition group and patients with no chronic conditions (deviation score) was divided by the standard deviation for the total sample for each health measure.

Source: Stewart et al., 1989. Reprinted, with permission, American Medical Association.

and the role of depressive disorders in increasing the risk of future mortality and disability.

PRESENTATION OF MENTAL HEALTH SYMPTOMS IN LATE LIFE

Mental health symptoms appear to change with older age. For example, in later life depressive disorders fulfilling diagnostic criteria are relatively rare; "subthreshold disorders" are more common. Subthreshold depression, for example, includes symptoms of depression that are not severe, frequent, or disruptive enough to be labeled as clinical depression. In practice, people are said to have subthreshold depression when they report symptoms on a depression self-report measure that fall below standard thresholds for defining likely depression. In the case of the Center for Epidemiologic Studies-Depression scale (CES-D), this would be a score above some minimum but below 16. In the case of the Geriatric Depression Scale (GDS) short form, this would be a score above 0 but below 10.

Rather than feeling depressed and reporting sadness or worthlessness, older people with depression may be more likely to report alternative clusters of symptoms, such as loss of interest in usual activities and somatic or cognitive symptoms, including fatigue, pain, sleep difficulties, and memory disorders. One study suggested that people at the oldest ages are more likely to report "delimited forms of distress," such as enervation, dysphoria, and sleep disturbances, rather than the more typical anhedonia typical of younger cohorts (Gallo, Rabins, & Anthony, 1999). A similar process appears to be at work for anxiety disorders, with greater likelihood of subthreshold anxiety disorders in later life.

Mossey, and Moss (2002) reported a study of 600 community-dwelling elders aged 70+ with a specific focus on subthreshold depression. They defined subthreshold depression using the CES-D (as well as additional questions assessing depressive symptoms) and found that 5.2% met criteria for depression and 22.2% for subthreshold depression. Not surprisingly, people who met criteria for depression scored more poorly on measures of physical, functional, and social health, and were also likely to have more physician visits (22, compared to 13 in the non-depressed group) and spend a greater number of days in the hospital (12 versus 5.2 in the non-depressed group) over the previous year. An important result of this study was a set of similar findings for the subthreshold depression group. Older adults with subthreshold depression scored more poorly in measures of health and were also likely to have a greater number of physician visits and hospital days than the non-depressed group. Mossey and Moss conclude that "with a prevalence of 22%, the public health burden of an even modest impact of sub-threshold depression on life quality and functioning of older individuals is substantial."

It is also worth asking about the persistence and effect of mental health symptoms in older people after a diagnosis of depression. The natural history of depression in older adults was examined in the Longitudinal Aging Study, a cohort of older adults recruited in Amsterdam (Beekman et al., 2002). Within this large cohort, 277 were identified as depressed at baseline and were followed for up to 6 years, with up to 14 assessments in this period. Elders were assessed with the Diagnostic Interview Schedule (DIS), a clinical interview that allows diagnosis of depression and its subtypes. Use of the clinical diagnostic interview with such extensive follow-up is rare, and allows insight on symptom duration, type of clinical course, and stability of diagnosis. In this group of older people who met criteria for depression at baseline, less than a quarter saw remission of their symptoms. On the whole, symptom levels remained high: 44% had an unfavorable but fluctuating course and 32% a continuing severe chronic course. Older people with sub-threshold disorders were at risk for progression to more severe forms of depression. In this community cohort, the natural history of late-life depression turned out to be poor, with persistence and increasing morbidity the most common outcome.

This brief review of research on the presentation of mental health symptoms in older adults suggests that symptom profiles in depression may be different than in younger adults, with less affective symptoms (i.e., feelings of worthlessness or sense that life is not worth living, crying, thoughts of suicide) and more somatic and cognitive symptoms. The result is a profile of symptoms short of the standard clinical syndrome. But subthreshold mental illness can also be consequential, with significant suffering, great health impact, and lost opportunities for productive aging. Clinical and service delivery staff who work with the elderly will need to recognize these differences if they are to provide effective care and referral.

Given the reduction in the most severe forms of depression and anxiety with age, one wants to know why symptoms of this sort decline and come to be replaced by more mild forms. Jorm, Christensen, Korten, Jacomb, and Henderson, (2000) suggest that "ageing is associated with an intrinsic reduction in susceptibility to anxiety and depression." They ask for caution in this conclusion, since we have few longitudinal studies covering the adult life span and therefore cannot yet reliably distinguish aging from cohort effects. If this difference in symptom expression turns out to be reliably associated with age, Jorm and colleagues suggest the reason may be decreased emotional responsiveness with age, increased emotional control, and a kind of "psychological immunization" to stressful experiences. Supporting the first of these hypotheses, Carstensen (1992) and Lawton, Parmelee, Katz, and Nesselroade, (1996) reported lower self-reported frequency of many affects in cross-sectional comparisons of young, middle-aged, and older adults. Carstenson (1992) has also demonstrated less interest in novel stimuli and greater social selectivity with age as a way of conserving psychological resources and promoting well-being. These findings provide some support for reduced emotional expression and greater emotional control in later life.

These last points deserve special emphasis because they show again the pervasive link between life span processes and health. Emotional life changes across the life span. As a consequence, the experience of depression may also change. Depression is not trivial in late life, but it may take on a less florid form because of changes in emotional make-up. If one talks to older people and asks about their emotions, one is likely to hear statements about the decline of emotion: "The highs are not so high anymore, but the lows are not so low either." In our research, we find that older people speak wistfully of their more intense emotional life at younger ages but also report a good deal of relief at getting off that treadmill.

PREVALENCE OF MENTAL ILLNESS AT OLDER AGES

As mentioned above, syndromal depression, that is, severity and duration of symptoms that meet criteria for clinical diagnosis, is less common among older people than younger people. This is apparent in population surveys that query respondents on symptoms of depression, such as the National Health Interview Survey, 2000 (HIS). "Severe psychological distress" in the HIS was measured according to the frequency of six distress symptoms over the past 30 days. The six items formed a scale with a range of 0-24 (so that each item was scored 0-4), and a score of 13 or greater was used to define severe distress.

As Figure 7.2 shows, less than 2% of people aged 65+ reported "serious psychological distress." In people aged 45-64, about 4% reported this level of distress, nearly twice as many. In the youngest age group, 18-44, the proportion was also higher, about 2.5%. Notably, in all age groups women were more likely to report severe psychological distress than men.

A common measure of depression in late life, as mentioned earlier, is the Geriatric Depression Scale, GDS (Yesavage, Brink et al., 1983). The short form is shown here in Table 7.3; bold answers indicate the presence of depressive symptoms. The items cover dysphoria, sadness or lack of enjoyment; anhedonia, or lack of interest in activities that are usually sought out; somatic symptoms associated with depression; and demoralization or existential suffering. "Yes" responses to the 15 items are summed. In the short-form of the GDS, scores greater than 5 suggest possible depression and warrant follow-up. Scores greater than 10 are very sensitive for detecting syndromal depression.

Depression is usually assessed using self-report instruments of this sort, rather than clinical diagnostic interviews that allow for true diagnoses. This should be kept in mind when interpreting the diverse prevalence estimates of depression in older adults.

What then is the prevalence of depression in older people? A key consideration is what sort of older person, frail or hale, community-resident or institutionalized, ascertained in a medical setting or not? Obviously, the prevalence of depression will be higher in people in medical settings or with extensive disability and chronic conditions than in a community sample of older people.

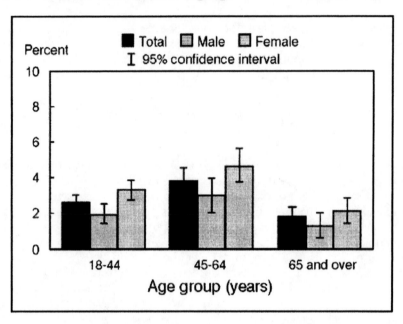

FIGURE 7.2 Percent of Adults Aged 18 Years and Over Who Experienced Serious Psychological Distress During the Past 30 Days, by Age Group and Sex: United States, January—June 2002.

Notes: Six psychological distress questions are included in the Sample Adult Core component. These questions ask how often a respondent experienced symptoms of psychological distress during the past 30 days. The response codes (0–4) of the six items for each person are summed to yield a scale with a 0–24 range. A value of 13 or more for this scale is used here to define serious psychological distress.

Data Source: Based on data collected from January through June in the Sample Adult Core component of the 2002 National Health Interview Survey.

In one community study of people aged 65+, the Alameda County Study, 6.6% of men and 10.1% of women showed symptoms of major depressive disorders. Once chronic conditions were controlled, the prevalence of depression of this severity did not increase with age. This is an important finding, consistent with what we have noted earlier. Depressive symptoms are much more closely associated with health status than with age. If the prevalence of depression appears to increase with age, it is entirely due to the increasing prevalence of chronic disease conditions with greater ages (Roberts, Kaplan, Shema, & Strawbridge, 1997).

Compare this 5-10% community prevalence to the much higher prevalence found in elderly outpatients. One study reported that 24%

TABLE 7.3 GDS Mood Scale: Short Form

Choose the best answer for how you have felt over the past week:
1. Are you basically satisfied with your life? YES / **NO**
2. Have you dropped many of your activities and interests? **YES** / NO
3. Do you feel that your life is empty? **YES** / NO
4. Do you often get bored? **YES** / NO
5. Are you in good spirits most of the time? YES / **NO**
6. Are you afraid that something bad is going to happen to you? **YES** /NO
7. Do you feel happy most of the time? YES / **NO**
8. Do you often feel helpless? **YES** / NO
9. Do you prefer to stay at home, rather than going out and doing new things? **YES** / NO
10. Do you feel you have more problems with memory than most? **YES** / NO
11. Do you think it is wonderful to be alive now? YES / **NO**
12. Do you feel pretty worthless the way you are now? **YES** / NO
13. Do you feel full of energy? YES / **NO**
14. Do you feel that your situation is hopeless? **YES** / NO
15. Do you think that most people are better off than you are? **YES** / NO

Answers in **bold** indicate depression. Although differing sensitivities and specificities have been obtained across studies, for clinical purposes a score > 5 points is suggestive of depression and should warrant a follow-up interview. Scores > 10 are almost always depression.

of an ambulatory care sample had clinically significant depressive symptoms. However, even here only 10% met criteria for major depressive disorder. Notably, only 1% of these people received treatment for a mental health problem (Borson et al., 1986).

The prevalence of depression in hospitalized and institutionalized older populations is even higher: 12-45% in the hospital, and 15-30% in skilled care facilities (Surgeon General's Report, 1999). Likewise, the prevalence of depression in community-resident patients with the chronic diseases of late life is also quite high: 15-20% in early Alzheimer's and perhaps 50% in Parkinson's disease.

MENTAL HEALTH IN A DISABLED OLDER POPULATION

The Women's Health and Aging Study, I, WHAS (Guralnik, Fried, Simonsick, Kasper, & Lafferty, 1995b) enrolled moderately to severely disabled women, representing the most disabled third of older women living in the community. Women were recruited from Medicare enrollee lists in the Baltimore, MD area. Mental health in the sample was assessed with a variety of indicators, including the Geriatric Depression Scale (Yesavage et al., 1983), anxiety indicators from the Hopkins Symptom Checklist (Derogatis, Lipman, Riskels, Uhlenhuth, & Covi, 1974), the Perceived Quality of Life scale (Patrick, Danis, Southerland, & Hong, 1988), and sense of control and efficacy from the Personal Mastery scale (Pearlin & Schooler, 1978). The sample of over 1000 women was divided into three age groups (65-74, 75-84, 85+) and three disability groups. Women had moderate disability (no ADL disability but difficulty in two of three domains: upper extremity, lower extremity, IADL), ADL disability without personal assistance, or ADL disability with personal assistance.

Table 7.4 presents the mental health of disabled women in WHAS, I. High levels of depressive symptoms, that is, symptomatology consistent with the clinical syndrome of major depression, were evident overall in 17.4% of the sample. Older people were less likely to report a high number of depressive symptoms: 14.3% of women aged 85+ vs. 18.6% of women aged 65-74. Disability, rather than age, was the stronger correlate. The proportion with symptomatology consistent with a diagnosis of depression was 13.1% in women with moderate disability, 16.4% in women with ADL disability not receiving help (mild ADL disability), and 29.3% in women with ADL disability who received personal assistance (more severe ADL disability).

Anxiety symptoms, unlike depression, increased with age: 2.8% in women aged 65-74, 4% in women aged 75-84, and 5.1% in women aged 85+. The relationship between disability and anxiety symptoms was less pronounced, increasing from 2.1% to 4.4% and 4.7% across severity categories.

Satisfaction with help received from family and friends was reported in about 80% of women, regardless of age or disability status (though note the gradient in satisfaction by severity of disability: 83.6%, 79.3%, and 74.8%). More pronounced are differences in the help these women feel they are able to provide to others. "Satisfaction with help provided to others" decreases from 84% in the moderately disabled, to 71.1% in women with mild ADL disability, to 56.2% in women with more severe ADL disability.

"Satisfaction with variety in life" was also more strongly related to disability than age: about a 20% difference between women with moderate disability (70%) and severe ADL disability (51.4%). But note also that half the women with severe ADL disability, and hence low scores on quality of life measures that emphasize function (see chapter 8), still report satisfaction with variety in daily life. Note, too, that "satisfaction with the meaning and purpose of your life" was stable across age and disability categories; about three-quarters of these women, whatever their age or level of disability, reported satisfaction in this area.

TABLE 7.4 Mental Health Indicators: Women's Health and Aging Study, I

	Age Group			Disability Status		
	65–74	75–84	85+	Moderate	ADL Disability: No Help	ADL Disability: Help
High level of depressive symptomatology, %[1]	18.6	17.3	14.3	13.1	16.4	29.3
High level of anxiety, %[2]	2.8	4.0	5.1	2.1	4.4	4.7
Satisfied with help received from family & friends, %[3]	79.1	81.1	78.2	83.6	79.3	74.8
Satisfied with help you give to family & friends, %[3]	77.6	70.1	68.0	84.0	71.1	56.2
Satisfied with amount of variety in your life, %[3]	65.9	62.1	62.3	70.0	63.6	51.4
Satisfied with the meaning and purpose of your life, %[3]	76.4	75.8	75.7	79.7	74.8	72.1
I can do just about anything I really set my mind to do, % Strongly agree[4]	48.6	45.1	44.4	51.4	45.2	40.2
I feel helpless in dealing with the problems of life, % Strongly agree[4]	8.8	10.3	12.3	9.3	6.8	20.0

"Moderate disability": self-reported difficulty in two of three domains: upper extremity, lower extremity, or IADL. Summarized from tables 8–1 through 8–5, Guralnik et al., 1995b.

[1]High level of depressive symptomatology: Score <greaterthan=>14, Geriatric Depression Scale, long form (Yesavage et al., 1983)

[2]High level of anxiety: maximum score ("extremely") on "felt nervous or shaky inside" during past week, Hopkins Symptom Checklist (Derogatis, et al., 1974).

[3]Items from Perceived Quality of Life scale (Patrick, et al., 1988).

[4]Items from Personal Mastery scale, (Pearlin & Schooler, 1978).

Finally, this sample of women on the whole reported relatively low self-efficacy. Less than half reported confidence they could accomplish "anything I really set my mind to do." On the other hand, a minority of respondents reported "helplessness": less than 10% in the less severe disability groups and 20% in women with the most severe ADL disability.

This inquiry suggests that disability has only a mild impact on mental health and general well-being. This is an important result. Most of the women in this sample were able to maintain mental equipoise despite disability. We should not underestimate the fundamental stability of mental health over the life span or the ability of older people to adapt to functional limitation and disability.

OUTCOMES ASSOCIATED WITH MENTAL ILLNESS IN LATE LIFE

Depression in late life has been associated with an increased risk of mortality. The central question in this association is whether depression is a feature of disease and for this reason is artifactually associated with mortality, or whether depression is itself an independent risk factor for early death.

An accumulating set of evidence supports the latter hypothesis. For example, in the Cardiovascular Health Study (CHS), Schulz and colleagues (2001) showed that baseline depressive symptoms were associated with 6–year all-cause mortality in older persons. The CHS consists of 5201 people aged 65+ from four communities across the U.S. This study found a higher mortality rate (23.9%) in people with high baseline depressive symptoms than in people with few depressive symptoms (17.7%). Depression in this study retained a significant association with mortality over 6 years of follow-up when controlling for sociodemographic factors, prevalent clinical disease, subclinical disease indicators at baseline, and biological or behavioral risk factors. In multivariate models that controlled for all of the factors, people with high depressive symptoms at baseline had a relative risk of 1.24 (95% CI, 1.06-1.46), about a 25% greater risk of mortality, compared to people with few or no depressive symptoms. Schulz and colleagues (2000) suggest that "motivational depletion," lack of attention to self-care and treatment adherence and a more general loss of the will to live, may be responsible for this greater risk of death. Other research has confirmed this association controlling as well for cognitive deficit (Rozzini, Frisoni, Sabatini, & Trabucchi, 2002).

A similar finding was reported by Unutzer, Patrick, Marmon, Simon, and Katon (2002). They found that older adults with the most severe depressive symptoms had a significant increase in mortality, again after adjusting for demographics, health risk behaviors, and chronic medical disorders. They point out that the increase in mortality due to depression was comparable to mortality associated with such chronic medical disorders as emphysema and heart disease.

Mortality from suicide in particular is also a consequence of depression in late life. Suicide risk is highest in younger people and in people aged 85+. In fact, recent reports suggest that the highest suicide risk appears to be in white men aged 85+. The suicide rate for this group is 21 per 100,000, nearly twice the national rate of 10.6 per 100,000 (CDC, 2003).

One of the strongest tests of the clinical relevance of depression in the case of older people is its role in predicting onset of disability. In a review of 78 high-quality reports involving longitudinal studies (Stuck et al., 1999), depression was a consistently strong predictor of incident disability in older people. Depression predicted onset of disability in two studies that controlled for the presence of chronic conditions, behavioral risk factors, and cognitive status (Bruce, Seeman, Merrill, & Blazer, 1994; Penninx, Leveille, Ferrucci, van Eik, & Guralnick, 1992). In one study, even the presence of depressive symptoms short of the severity or duration required for a diagnosis of depression ("subthreshold depression," described earlier) was a significant predictor of incident disability (Gallo, Rabins, Lyketsos, Tien, & Anthony, 1997). Finally, there is also evidence that depressive symptoms are related to loss of physical abilities, that is, to functional limitation, in the pathway toward disability (Pennix, et al., 1998); (see chapter 5).

These findings suggest that depression is a true cause of disability in older people, meeting many of the criteria for causality in epidemiology (Susser, 1997). It is temporally prior to development of disability, it affects a link in the pathway to disability, and it is a consistent finding in the literature across different age groups. Since treatment of depression is possible, this source of excess morbidity and disability should certainly be addressed in the care of the older person.

TREATMENT OF DEPRESSION IN LATE LIFE

We have already seen that depression is under-appreciated and under-treated in older people, as it is in younger people. The reasons for this neglect in late life are apparent from what we have already noted. A first reason has to do with the medical and psychosocial context of aging. Because most older people have a variety of medical conditions, it is tempting for physicians, families, and even the elder himself to assign symptoms of depression to these conditions. Similarly, it may be difficult in some cases to distinguish normal grief after loss of a spouse, for example, from depression.

A second reason for under recognition is the "softer" presentation of depressive symptoms in older people, described above, and the greater prevalence of subthreshold disorders rather than disease of accepted levels of clinical severity. The lack of affective symptoms in some cases, such as sadness, makes depression hard to diagnose for practitioners who do not have experience with geriatric mental health. The depressed elder may stress physical symptoms, reducing the likelihood of a mental health referral.

Finally, there is garden-variety ageism. Unfortunately, many providers and many elderly themselves still think that misery is normal in late life. After all, the reasoning goes, late life is the time of physical and mental health decline, so of course depression should be expected. This reasoning is absolutely fallacious, however, as we know from studies of patients at the end of life. Depression is more common in terminal patients but far from universal. Even in these patients risk of depression appears to reflect life long mental health more than illness and the dying process (Rabkin, Wagner, & Del Bene, 2000). And, most importantly, depression responds to treatment even in patients who are dying. Affective suffering should be considered a medical issue as significant as any other health indicator.

Treatment for depression in older people may rely on pharmacologic agents, psychosocial interventions, or a combination of the two. Response rates in older people appear to be comparable to those in younger people, as both age groups respond in about 80% of cases (Surgeon General, 1999). However, older people may take longer to respond to therapy and may face a greater risk of relapse.

NEGLECT AND ABUSE

Victimization of the elderly takes many forms and extends across a continuum of behavior. On one extreme of this continuum we might place neglect of the elderly, whether self-neglect or inattention to an elder's needs by others. On the other extreme, we might place active abuse and exploitation. Somewhere in the middle lies purposeful neglect designed to injure or coerce. These are often lumped within a single category of "mistreatment," which is defined differently across surveys. Adult Protective Services, municipal agencies that assess and intervene in the case of victimization of the elderly, define three forms of mistreatment (Lachs, Williams, O'Brien, Pillemer, & Charlson, 1998):

Abuse: Willful infliction of pain or mental anguish, or purposeful withholding of resources necessary to meet basic needs;

Neglect: Failure of an ·elder to satisfy basic needs (food, shelter, medication management, medical care) either because of incompetence in the elder or because another person charged with care for the elder fails to meet these needs (abandonment, poor custodial care);

Exploitation: Taking advantage of an elder to steal or dispossess the elder of money, wealth, or valued goods.

Over an 11-year period, the cumulative incidence of abuse in the New Haven component of the Established Populations for Epidemiologic Studies of the Elderly (EPESE) was 7.2% (202/2802). These 202 people came to the attention of the Connecticut Ombudsman and Elderly Protective Services. Of the 202, 44 were verified as cases of abuse, 120 were verified as cases of self-neglect, and 38 were non-verified allegations. Thus, the incidence of abuse over this 11-year period was 1.6% (44/2802) and self-neglect 4.3% (120/2802). If we take the total incidence of 7.2% and convert it to a yearly estimate, the annual incidence is about 6.5 cases per 1000 per year (.072/11 x 1000). We can compare this estimate to the 32 per 1000 reported in a random sample prevalence survey (Pillemer & Finkelhor, 1988). This suggests that about one in five cases of abuse, neglect, or exploitation comes to the attention of protective services.

A variety of research is now available on correlates of elder mistreatment. Using the merged EPESE-protective services data set described earlier, Lachs and colleagues (1998) have shown that elders referred to protective services were at an increased risk of mortality, a threefold increase in the case of abuse and nearly a two-fold increase in the case of self-neglect (Lachs, Williams, O'Brien, Pillemer & Charlson, 1998). This excess risk was calculated in models that adjusted for many predictors of mortality, including sociodemographic characteristics, chronic disease status, functional and cognitive status, social networks, and depressive symptoms.

Elders referred to protective services also faced an increased risk of nursing home placement. In the same EPESE cohort followed over 11 years, 31.8% of elders not referred to protective services were admitted to skilled care facilities. In elders referred to protective services for abuse, the rate was 52.3% and for elders referred for self-neglect, the rate was 69.2% (Lachs, Williams, O'Brien, & Pillemer, 2002).

What factors predispose elders to mistreatment? In the case of self-neglect, key risk factors are cognitive impairment and depression, though one study identified additional risk associated with living alone, poverty, male gender, and a particular profile of chronic conditions, such as stroke and hip fracture (Abrams, Lachs, McAvay, Keohane, & Bruce, 2002). The case of abuse involves both elder and family features. Elders with cognitive impairment and greater needs in care because of disability are more likely to be abused (and less likely to report it). Family caregivers with substance abuse problems, mental and physical health symptoms, lower socioeconomic status, and poor coping and caregiving skills are more likely to be abusers.

SOCIAL ISOLATION

One result of poor mental health is social isolation, which in turn is associated with poor outcomes in a variety of areas, including greater risk of suicide, poor medication management, inferior nutrition, over-use of laxatives and other over-the-counter medicines, and poor living environments (i.e., greater risk of exposure to extremes of heat and cold). The connection between comorbid disease, poor mental health, social isolation, and these additional negative outcomes has been called a "spiral of deterioration" (Alexopoulos et al., 2002).

Yet it also appears that social isolation in itself is a risk factor for poor outcomes. In one study, for example, poor health, physical disability, and social isolation were all independently associated with depression. Once controlling for these factors, the association between depressive symptoms and lower socioeconomic status was no longer significant, leading the authors to suggest that "money cannot buy happiness" in the elderly (West, Reed, & Gildengorin, 1998).

Social isolation and loneliness also increase the risk of nursing home admission, even when the effects of other predisposing factors (such as age, education, income, mental status, physical health, morale, and social contact) are controlled (Russell, Cutrona, de la Mora, & Wallace, 1997). Why should loneliness or social isolation predict nursing home admission? Russell and colleagues suggest that this association may indicate that some lonely and isolated older adults in their rural Iowa sample may have sought out nursing home admission as a strategy to gain social contact.

SUMMARY

Burden of Mental Illness. The effect of mental disorders on daily life should not be underestimated, in the young as in the old. By any measure, whether a national estimate of lost productivity or reports of daily symptoms, mental illness is as disabling as physical illness.

Presentation and Prevalence of Mental Health Symptoms in Late Life. Mental health symptoms appear to change with older age. In later life, depressive disorders fulfilling diagnostic criteria are relatively rare; "subthreshold disorders" are more common. Subthreshold depression, for example, includes symptoms of depression that are not severe, frequent, or disruptive enough to be labeled as clinical depression. In the National Health Interview Survey, 2000, less than 2% of people aged 65+ reported "serious psychological distress," less than half that reported by people aged 45-64. However, evidence is now available to suggest that subthreshold depression is a risk factor for poor outcomes, including declining function, increased disability, cognitive impairment, and death.

Mental Health in a Disabled Older Population. In the most disabled third of women, mental health is related to severity of disability, but mental health is, on the whole, good, with low rates of clinical and symptomatic depression. This speaks to adaptation in late life and psychological resiliency, and reminds us again that mental and physical health are separate but related spheres.

Outcomes Associated with Mental Illness in Late Life. The Cardiovascular Health Study showed that people with pronounced depressive symptoms were at risk for higher mortality (23.9% vs 17.7% in people with few depressive symptoms). This finding persisted when analyses controlled for other factors that increase mortality risk. Similar findings have been reported for depression, and risk of disability, cognitive decline, nursing home placement, suicide, and a host of other negative public health outcomes.

Treatment of Depression in Late Life. Evidence suggests that older people respond to treatment at rates comparable to younger people, though differences in metabolism, polypharmacy, and the presence of other chronic conditions complicate treatment. A major obstacle is an ageist expectation that affective suffering is a part of late age and frailty.

Neglect and Abuse. Despite difficulty in defining these domains, it is now clear that self-neglect is more common than outright abuse, that the most vulnerable elderly are most often victims, and that both forms of mistreatment have major public health consequences.

Social Isolation. Older people desire less novelty in social life than the young and may be more comfortable with a smaller set of friends. Yet isolation is a public health issue to the extent it is associated with medication misuse, poor nutrition, and greater risk of depression and suicide.

8

Aging, Public Health, and Application of the Quality of Life Paradigm

Research on "quality of life" actually involves two distinct domains, which unfortunately are not always clearly distinguished (Albert, 1997; Albert & Teresi 2002; Spilker & Revicki, 1999). One domain is *health-related quality of life,* or more simply, "health status assessment," which emerged from efforts to develop measures of disease impact that would be useful across a variety of clinical trial and program evaluation settings. The other is not a health impact measure but rather registers the effect of personal resources or environmental factors on daily experience. This might be called *non-health or environment-based quality of life.* This second set of measures emerged from efforts to identify community-level indicators of well-being and belongs to the "social indicators" or "social ecology" research tradition.

Maintaining this distinction is important. Health-related quality of life domains—patient reports of functional status, discomfort, pain, energy levels, social engagement—will track more closely with clinical measures of disease status than non-health-related QOL indicators, such as the capacity to form friendships, appreciate nature, or find satisfaction in spiritual or religious life. The latter are also quality of life domains, and severe health limitation will ultimately affect these as well, but they are less related to clinical indicators of health. Health-related QOL will therefore be correlated with clinical indicators, while non-health-related personal or environmental indicators of QOL may or may not be.

Recognizing this distinction eliminates much of the confusion about the "idiosyncrasy" or instability of QOL ratings (Leplege & Hunt, 1997). In this chapter, we briefly define the two quality-of-life fields and assess their relevance for research on public health and aging.

IDENTIFICATION OF QOL DOMAINS

Health-related QOL encompasses domains of life directly affected by changes in health. Jaeschke, Singer, and Guyatt, (1989) provide a good thumbnail test of whether a domain falls within the category of health-related QOL. They ask, if a patient is successfully treated by a physician, what aspects of his or her life are likely to improve? These are health-related QOL domains. Alternatively, if a patient reports changes in status that lead a care provider to seek a different medication or a change in a care environment, these changes are also likely to fall within the realm of health-related QOL (Berzon, Leplege, Lohr, Lenderking, & Wu, 1997).

What features of daily life or changes in status are likely to be medically relevant in this sense, and hence count as health-related QOL? Obvious candidates include *functional status* (i.e., disability, whether a patient is able to manage a household, use the telephone, or dress independently); *mental health, affective status, or emotional well-being* (i.e., depressive symptoms, positive affect); *social engagement* (i.e., involvement with others, engagement in activities); and *symptom states* (i.e., pain, shortness of breath, visual acuity, fatigue).

Non-health-related QOL domains, by contrast, include features of the natural and built environment (such as economic resources, housing, air and water quality, community stability, access to the arts and entertainment), as well as personal resources. These factors clearly affect quality of life but, unlike health-related QOL domains, are less likely to improve with appropriate medical care.

The two components of QOL differ in other ways as well. Non-health related QOL is more heterogeneous, with less consensus about the range of domains that should be included in the measure. For example, no one would suggest that severe abdominal pain is preferred to a runny nose; everyone would agree that the runny nose is associated with a better health-related QOL state. Research on ratings of the severity of health conditions is remarkably consistent across age groups and in cross-national research (Patrick, Sittampalam, Somerville, Carter, & Bergener, 1986), though people with disease conditions appear to rate their health-related QOL somewhat higher than non-patients asked to rate the same health state (Torrance, 1987). Consensus of this sort is harder to establish for spirituality, friendship, or access to the arts.

It is valuable to obtain information on both kinds of QOL, but health-related QOL is likely to be the more important measure for public health efforts involving older adults. First, older people are at risk for chronic conditions, and effective disease management in large part consists of finding treatments that minimize the QOL impact of disease. Second, measurement efforts for health-related QOL are further advanced than efforts related to non-health-related QOL. Finally, while housing, air quality, and other components of the environment are clearly important features of QOL, they are important mainly because of their effect on health and health-related QOL. On the other hand, Lawton (1991) reminds us that the two are sometimes hard to separate: successful treatment by a physician may improve one's capacity to make friends, for example.

As mentioned earlier, health-related QOL as a field of inquiry emerged from research on "health status." Early measures, such as the Sickness Impact Profile (SIP) (Bergner, Bobbitt, Pollard, Martin, & Gilson, 1976), sought to identify common domains affected by disease that would allow clinicians to gauge the impact of diverse clinical conditions. This goal was a major motivation for development of more recent measures as well, such as the Medical Outcomes Study (MOS) short-form QOL questionnaires (Stewart 1989) and FACT battery (Cella & Bonomi, 1996).

A key element of the SIP, and also of almost all QOL measures that have followed, is that patients themselves rate how impaired they are. This subjective element is the essential feature of health-related QOL, for who can better report on the QOL impact of a medical condition than the patient (Gill & Feinstein, 1994)? Indeed, health-related QOL is sometimes called "patient-reported outcomes" (PRO) to stress this subjective focus. The SIP identified 12 health-related QOL domains: ambulation, mobility, body care and movement, communication, alertness behavior, emotional behavior, social interaction, sleep and rest, eating, work, home management, and recreation. The MOS identified a different set of domains: health perception, pain, physical function, social function, mental health, role limitation from physical causes, and role limitation from mental health causes. Others, such as the Health Utilities Index (HUI), stress still different domains, in this case a "within the skin" approach to health status, that is, domains that are more closely connected to clinical conditions. Thus, the HUI Mark II measure includes sensation, mobility, emotion, cognition, self-care, pain, and fertility (Feeny, Furlong, Boyle & Torrance, 1996).

Apart from differences in the specification of QOL domains, the measures also differ in the ways they are used to derive a global health state or health-related QOL score. In the MOS, for example, domains are grouped according to their primarily "physical" or "mental" health basis, as established in factor analysis. Pain, physical function, and role limitation-physical form a "physical health component," mental health and role limitation-emotional a "mental health component." Scores within each set of domains are aggregated. Keeping the two separate as distinct indicators or dimensions of health-related QOL is appropriate because studies show that the correlation between mental and physical health is about 0.50, only a moderate correlation.

Other measures cross-walk health states and respondent-rated global reports to derive a single score. For example, the EuroQOL (Dolan, Gudex, Kind, & Williams, 1996) contains five domains (mobility, self-care, usual activity, pain/discomfort, and anxiety/depression), each with three levels. If each combination of the five domains were a true health state, even this simple 5–domain categorization would generate, 3^5 or 243 health states. Luckily, not all of these health states are possible (for example, it is impossible to be "confined to bed" on the mobility dimension and have "no problems with self-care" on the self-care dimension). After eliminating these empirically null states, a more manageable (but still large) number remain. Global scores can be assigned to the states by having respondents with the state rate their global health on a visual analogue scale (ranging from 0–100). More complicated generation of global scores from QOL domains is also possible. In the HUI, each domain is weighted, and global scores reflect the combination of domain weightings and levels reported for each domain.

Interest in assigning scores to subjective reports of health-related QOL draws on early research in psychophysics. Early on, psychologists noted that ratings of a subjective state (e.g., pain) corresponded to the intensity of a stimulus (e.g., increasingly cold temperature). These investigations suggested that subjective ratings were reliably associated with objective states. Thus, to return to our earlier example, people should give a higher score to "severe abdominal pain" on a measure of discomfort or interference with work than "runny nose." The challenge is to determine how much higher.

In fact, large-sample investigations have allowed researchers to estimate how much worse one state is relative to another. For example, suppose we establish two numeric anchors: 1.0 for the state of no symptoms/no daily limitations and 0.0 for death (recognizing, however, that some people consider certain health states, such as coma or intractable pain, as worse than death). Kaplan's Quality of Well-Being/General Health Policy Model (Kaplan & Anderson, 1996) subtracts 0.17 for the state of "runny nose"; thus, someone with a runny nose alone is at about 83% of optimal health. "Sick or upset stomach, vomiting" is associated with a subtraction score of –0.29; someone with this condition alone would therefore be at about 71% of optimal health. The difference between the two ratings is a measure of how much worse abdominal pain is than runny nose. These numerical ratings, derived from respondents who rated descriptions of a wide variety of health states, confirm our intuitions and establish the impact of one health state compared to another in terms of health-related QOL.

The underlying metric for these evaluations is abstract. It is essentially a measure of how preferred or "dispreferred" one health state is relative to another, in other words, a "utility." An alternative tradition in QOL measurement avoids specification of numeric values on such an underlying dimension. This tradition relies on naturally occurring indicators of morbidity or disability. Thus, Sullivan (1966), as we have seen in chapter 5, early on developed an index of morbidity, or health state, based on disability. Living arrangement (nursing home or community), severity of mobility impairment, ability to perform major age-appropriate roles (school, work, home maintenance, personal self-maintenance), and limitation in usual, daily activities formed a natural hierarchy of disability. This mutually exclusive classification generates five health-impact or QOL states, ranging from institutional residence at one end to community residence without disability or limitation in daily activities at the other.

Another approach, intermediate between these two, is to seek a single, common measure of health impact in terms of some other dimension of daily life. These dimensions include time use (Albert 2001; Moss & Lawton 1982), mood states (Larson, Zuzanek, & Mannell, 1985), or mental health stress (Testa & Simonson, 1996). The Behavioral Risk Factors Surveillance System (BRFSS) used by the Centers for Disease Control adopts this approach. It relies on reports of "not good health days," days when a component of health is adversely affected (Hennessey, Moriarty, Scherr, & Brackbill, 1994). Respondents are asked, "Thinking of the past 30 days, how many days were there when your physical health was not good?" Other questions ask about mental health, sleep, energy, anxiety, and related domains in the same format. This approach allows a conjoint measure of "healthy days" (30 minus the sum of "not good physical health days" and "not good mental health days") (Hennessey et al., 1994), which can serve as a global health-related QOL indicator. Thus, someone reporting 3 not good physical health and 4 not good mental health days would have a total of 7 not good days, or 23 healthy days. (Following BRFSS conventions, we adopt the conservative approach of a sum, allowing that the same day may have been a "not good" day in both physical and mental health.) Someone reporting this profile over the last month would have a global QOL score of 23/30 (0.77), or 77% of optimal health-related QOL.

The different approaches converge on a common central question. Can we determine *how much* better life is at a higher level of health than at a lower level? Or, more starkly, how much better than death a state of compromised health is? Patrick and Erickson (1993) rightly stress these questions when they define health-related QOL as "the *value* assigned to the duration of life, as modified by impairment" (p.

22, emphasis added). The goal of measurement of health-related QOL is first to define health states, that is, to develop measures that capture the impact of changes in health. The second goal is to assign plausible numeric indicators for such changes. While this second task may seem difficult, we should remember that people already implicitly assign values to these health changes. Every day people evaluate symptom states and make treatment decisions based on their judgment of the likely impact of treatment or non-treatment. The QOL paradigm attempts to formalize this process.

It is also worth noting what the QOL paradigm does not assess. Health-related QOL measures do not tell us what puts quality into life. They have the much more limited goal of establishing the effect of changes in health on everyday life. Nor do QOL measures tell us anything about the value of life, or what makes someone attached to living. We know that many people with very low scores on QOL measures find life satisfying and meaningful. For example, they may score very high on measures of mental health despite very severe limitations in physical status. Or they may even score poorly on physical and mental health measures and yet still express strong attachment to life. The QOL score only specifies the degree of *health impact*. It is not a measure of attachment to life or the perceived value of life.

As a final illustration of the position of QOL domains relative to other indicators of health, it is worth comparing clinical outcomes to health-related QOL outcomes. Take, for example, a randomized clinical trial in cancer therapy. Clinical outcomes for this trial would include survival time, disease-free survival time, tumor response, and perhaps treatment-associated toxicities (which together might be used to generate a "Q-Twist measure," time without symptoms or toxicity). By contrast, QOL outcomes for this trial would capture the effects of treatment and disease on someone's ability to function in everyday life, which might include productivity at work, independence in self-care tasks, emotional stability, and engagement in valued activities. Ware and Stewart (1992) summarize the differences this way: "Clinical measures of functioning do not characterize human functioning well. They reveal little about how well the individual functions in everyday life or how that person feels, both of which are affected by disease and treatment."

CLINICAL SIGNIFICANCE OF QOL MEASURES

How much must a QOL indicator change for us to be confident that an intervention has produced a meaningful improvement in patient status?

Lydick and Epstein (1993) remind us that this question is a problem for all clinical research, not just research in health-related QOL. They describe a therapy for benign prostatic hypertrophy that increased urine flow 3 ml/sec compared to urine flow in a placebo group. By itself, this effect is hard to interpret. Could this degree of change fall within normal variability? This question became clear only when an epidemiological study showed that urine flow rates decline 0.2–0.3 ml/ sec per year of life. A 3-ml/sec improvement is thus equivalent to about 15 years of "urinary aging." Thus, an improvement of 3 ml/sec is indeed a clinically meaningful change.

An alternative way to establish clinical significance in this case would have been to ask men with slower urine flow rates if urination is a problem for them. Do men with slower urine flow rates find urination more uncomfortable, more time consuming, or more embarrassing? Are men who differ by 3-ml/sec or more in urine flow more likely to report such problems? This would be an alternative indicator of clinical significance and may be required for definitive proof of clinical significance, even in the presence of age differences in urinary flow.

These thoughts suggest a view of clinical significance in terms of a "minimal clinically significant difference" (Jaeschke et al., 1989). This, as we stated above, is a change in patient-reported status that would lead a care provider to seek a different medication or a change in care environment. Otherwise stated, these are changes that would lead a clinician to make a change in patient management ("in the absence of troublesome side effects and excessive cost"). Again, patient behavior is a good guide here. If patients report such changes to a clinician, and the clinician is not impressed enough to alter management, patients are apt to go elsewhere.

To identify these minimal clinically significant differences, we can rely on distribution-based statistical tests or external criteria to anchor them. The basic distribution-based test to assess clinical significance is effect size. This examines the importance of a change by comparing the magnitude of the change in some measure to variability in the measure in a group at baseline, before implementation of the intervention. This ratio gives an indication of change over and above normal variation.

Anchor-based indicators are probably more useful for establishing the clinical significance of changes in QOL measures. The most obvious anchor is the patient's global rating of change in quality of life (Jaeschke et al., 1989). That is, do patients who report improvements of a certain magnitude in a particular QOL domain (for example, pain or fatigue) also report improvements in global quality of life or well-being? The minimal clinically significant difference in the pain or fatigue measure would be the score change associated with a difference in the global rating.

Other anchors include life events or mental health stress. These are perhaps most useful for measures of mental health. A mental health score difference of 3 points, for example, was shown to be equivalent to the effect of a major life event, such as losing a job. Testa and Simonson (1996) have generalized this approach.

But the best and most meaningful anchor for assessing changes in quality of life may be age. Given the pervasive effect of age on quality of life states because of senescence and the increasing prevalence of chronic conditions, age provides a natural metric for assessing the QOL effects of clinical interventions. If we know that an intervention improves quality of life by 5% on some scale, and also that a 5% difference is typical of two age strata (say, ages 75 and 80) for this measure, then the intervention is associated with a 5-year "reduction" in age. To establish clinical significance requires that we have QOL or clinical norms for different age groups, which are not always available. Still, age offers a natural scale for this sort of investigation, as we show below.

THE QUALITY OF LIFE PARADIGM IN AGING

Introduction of a quality-of-life focus in research on aging was pioneered by Katz and colleagues (1963) and Lawton (1969, 1991), with their focus on functional status and behavior, which is now universal in gerontology and geriatrics. Lawton summarized the QOL emphasis for care of older people very well when he wrote, "function and behavior, rather than diagnosis, should determine the service to be prescribed" (Lawton & Brody, 1969; p. 185). The common, final pathway of different diseases is their impact on functional ability and other domains of QOL; thus, the focus in later life should be development of strategies, both clinical and environmental, to minimize these effects and work with the strengths older people continue to retain.

However it is measured, health-related QOL declines with age. This is a central, inescapable consequence of the increased prevalence of chronic disease with greater age and the effects of senescent changes in many physiologic domains. Senescence, as we have seen, is evident in a variety of changes across biologic systems: for example, declines in working memory, psychomotor speed, touch sensibility, vision, and hearing; loss of skeletal muscle and strength; and reduction in joint range of motion. These changes affect health-related QOL: for example, pain in arthritic joints leads to circumscription of choice in daily activities, lower-extremity weakness means difficulty climbing stairs or standing up long enough to prepare a meal, and slowing of psychomotor skills may mean inability to drive safely. Older people adjust their daily lives to accommodate these decrements, and adjustment strategies may reduce the effects of such decrements on health-related QOL.

Still, cross-sectional studies show strong declines in health-related QOL with increasing age. The effect of age on the "healthy days" measure of the BRFSS, described above, is shown in Table 8.1. The mean number of days over the past month in which respondents reported problems with physical health increases monotonically with age, from 1.8 in the 18–24 year-old group to 6.2 in people aged 75+. Differences are small between the younger adjacent age strata (1.8 vs. 2.1 in people aged 18–24 and 25–44, respectively). These differences increase in later ages, from 3.5 in people aged 45–64, to 4.7 in people aged 65–74, and finally to 6.2 in the oldest age group.

Mental health shows the opposite trend, consistent with results from chapter 7. The youngest group reports the greatest number of "not good" mental health days, 3.4 out of the last 30 days, and this number declines with age until it reaches its low, 1.9, among people aged 75+.

The composite "healthy days" measure declines from 25.1 in the youngest age group to 23.0 in the oldest. Using the convention described above, these values represent global health-related QOL values of 83.7 and 76.7 on a scale of 0–100, a fairly small difference. As an indicator of clinical significance, people of all ages unable to work because of a health condition reported a mean of 10.7 healthy days, or 35.7 on the same transformed 0–100 scale.

An alternative indicator of the effect of age on health-related QOL is the "well year" equivalent developed by the National Center for

TABLE 8.1 Healthy Days by Age, Behavioral Risk Factors Surveillance System (BRFSS), 1993

Age Group	n	Good Health Days	Not Good Physical Health Days	Not Good Mental Health Days
18–24	4,279	25.1	1.8	3.4
25–44	19,756	25.2	2.1	3.1
45–64	11,445	24.6	3.5	2.8
65–74	4,975	24.2	4.7	1.9
75+	3,064	23.0	6.2	1.9

Data based on 21 states and District of Columbia. Not good days represent mean number of days in last 30 where component of health was "not good." "Good health days" is the subtraction of sum of not good physical and mental health days from 30, with the restriction that this sum cannot be negative.

Source: MMWR, May 27, 1994: 378.

Health Statistics to track progress toward the *Healthy People 2000* goal of increasing active life expectancy (Erickson et al., 1995). This measure uses two items from the National Health Interview Survey (HIS) to define health states. Self-ratings of health (excellent, very good, good, fair, poor) are cross-classified with self-reports of activity limitation (not limited, limited in some activity but not major activity, limited in major activity, unable to perform major activity, limited in IADL, and limited in ADL). Self-reported health serves as a subjective global summary of health, while self-rated activity limitation reflects a more clearly behavioral indicator of health and performance. The 5 × 6 cross-classification yields 30 health states, where the best health state is excellent health with no activity limitation, and the worst state poor health with ADL limitation.

Weaknesses of this approach are clear. The measure does not contain a true mental health component (except insofar as mental health figures in global ratings of health), and we lose information on the many domains that go into people's ratings of their health and participation in activity. Still, as a summary measure it offers the advantage of brevity, broad application, and availability from a large, well-conducted national survey. Every American can be assigned to one of the 30 states based on answers to the two questions. The distribution of the American population in 1990 across the 30 health states is shown in Table 8.2.

TABLE 8.2 Percent of Persons in the Civilian Noninstitutionalized U.S. Population, by Health State Defined in Terms of Activity Limitation and Perceived Health Status: National Health Interview Survey, 1990

| | Perceived Health Status | | | | |
| | | | | | |
Activity Limitation	Excellent	Very Good	Good	Fair	Poor
Not limited	38.1	26.3	18.2	3.3	0.3
Limited-other	0.6	1.1	1.8	1.3	0.4
Limited-major	0.5	0.7	1.3	0.7	0.2
Unable-major	0.1	0.2	0.5	0.6	0.5
Limited in IADL[1]	0.1	0.2	0.5	0.6	0.6
Limited in ADL[2]	<0.1	0.1	0.2	0.3	0.5

[1]IADL is instrumental activities of daily living.

[2]ADL is activities of daily living.

Source: National Health Interview Survey, Centers for Disease Control and Prevention, National Center for Health Statistics.

The largest proportion of Americans assigned themselves to the optimal health state of excellent health and no activity limitation, 38.1%. Another 26.3% and 18.2% assigned themselves to the no activity limitation category but with "very good" and "good" health, respectively. The next largest group, 3.3% assigned themselves to the no activity limitation category but with "fair" health. Thus, these four health states accounted for 85.9% of the American population. This distribution is welcome to the extent that it indicates high health-related QOL among a large majority of Americans. It is unwelcome, however, from a measurement point of view. It suggests that the "no activity limitation" anchor for this dimension does not differentiate QOL states well. That is, large proportions of people with vastly different ratings of health all endorse "no limitation" in activity. This suggests a ceiling effect in the activity limitation dimension, that is, need for additional differentiation of the state of "no activity limitation."

Note in Table 8.2 that each of the other health states contains less than 2%, and in most cases less than 1%, of the U.S. population. The worst health state, poor health and ADL limitation, is endorsed by just 0.5%. Since the HIS excludes institutional populations, this, as we have seen, is an underestimate of the proportion of people with low health-related QOL. Note, too, the off-diagonal cells (left-and rightmost corner cells of the table). A very small number, less than 0.1%, rate their health as excellent yet report maximum limitation in activity, that is, limitation in ADL. And 0.3% report poor health yet no limitation in activity. Are these QOL states possible, or should we assume error in people's answers? Can we imagine scenarios in which these answers would be plausible?

The small number who rate their health as excellent yet report maximum limitation in activity may include people with severe disability but non-progressive disease, such as the quadriplegic who relies on personal assistance but is able to work in an adapted environment. On the other hand, this person may also be among those reporting no activity limitation. The group reporting poor health yet no limitation in activity may represent people forced to be active despite their poor health, the "obligatorily active." Or this group may truly face no current limitation in activity but face a poor prognosis in the near future, such as persons recently diagnosed with cancer.

We can assess the effect of age on the likelihood of falling into one or another of these health states by re-examining Table 8.2, limiting the health state cross-classification to people in the oldest age groups. Table 8.3 is a similar table for people aged 85+. Remember that these older people are also community-resident, which is true for the HIS sample generally, and thus not representative of the oldest old (see below).

TABLE 8.3 National Center for Health Statistics: National Health Interview Survey. Population Aged 85+, 1990

	Excellent	Very Good	Good	Fair	Poor
Not Limited in Major Activity	7.0	11.7	16.4	6.3	2.0
Limited-Other Activity	1.9	2.6	4.7	4.1	1.0
IADL Disability	2.3	3.1	7.0	6.8	3.1
ADL Disability	1.2	1.6	4.9	5.8	6.5

Entries are proportion of non-institutionalized U.S. population, aged 85+, weighted to represent U.S. population.

Courtesy of Ronald Wilson, Office of Analysis, Epidemiology, and Health Promotion, National Center for Health Statistics.

We see a great migration to cells downward and to the right, reflecting an increased prevalence of poorer health-related QOL. In 1990, only 7% of the community-resident 85+ population fell within the optimal health-related QOL state. Almost as many, 6.5%, fell into the poorest QOL state. Note that the same ceiling effect is apparent in self-reports from the oldest-old: people with very different self-rated health states were still all able to endorse the "no activity limitation" category. Overall, among people aged 85+ all the health states were well populated. The modal health state was "no activity limitation-good health," rather than "no activity limitation-excellent health," which was the modal state in the population as a whole.

An important extension of the 30–state model was the assignment of QOL values or utilities to each state, shown here as Table 8.4. The optimal health state was assigned 1.0, the poorest state 0.10, reserving 0.0 for death. (Sensitivity analyses varying the 0.10 utility did not change differences between other states in large ways [Erickson, Wilson, & Shannon, 1995].) The values were established in the following way. First, a statistical technique was applied to determine differences between levels of the self-rated health and activity limitation dimensions. For this effort, correspondence analysis showed that levels of self-rated health and activity limitation were not equally spaced (for example, "very good," "good," and "fair" had values of 0.85, 0.70, and 0.30, respectively). Consistent with the utility estimation approach, these values specify numeric differences between states on a common scale of utility, how much more or less one state is preferred to another. Second, survey data were used to assign a value to one of the off-diagonal cells (use of the Health Utilities Index). Finally, the two sets of

TABLE 8.4 Values for Health States Defined in Terms of Activity Limitation and Perceived Health Status, 19??

| | Perceived Health Status | | | | |
	Excellent	Very Good	Good	Fair	Poor
Activity Limitation					
Not limited	1.00	0.92	0.84	0.63	0.47
Limited-other	0.87	0.79	0.72	0.52	0.38
Limited-major	0.81	0.74	0.67	0.48	0.34
Unable-major	0.68	0.62	0.55	0.38	0.25
Limited in IADL[1]	0.57	0.51	0.45	0.29	0.17
Limited in ADL[2]	0.47	0.41	0.36	0.21	0.10

[1]IADL is instrumental activities of daily living.

[2]ADL is activities of daily living.

Source: National Health Interview Survey, Centers for Disease Control and Prevention, National Center for Health Statistics.

values were combined in a multiplicative model to assign values to each joint state.

The final results, seen in Table 8.4, show that the state of excellent health/no activity limitation (1.0) is 0.08 units superior to the state of very good health/no activity limitation (0.92) and 0.19 units superior to the state of excellent health/limited in major activity. The latter difference suggests that disability at this level reduces health-related QOL by about 20%. Someone with "good heath" and limitation in his or her major activity is assigned a score of 0.67, or two-thirds of optimal health-related QOL.

These abstract values can be made more concrete if we view them as percentages of a full year of healthy life. For someone in the excellent health/no activity limitation state, which is assigned a utility of 1.0, a year of life is equivalent to a year of healthy life. For someone in the state of very good health/no activity limitation, with its utility score of 0.92, a year of life is equivalent to 0.92 years of healthy life (Erickson et al., 1995). Each year lived by someone in good health but with limitation in major activity (0.67) would be equivalent to 0.67 years of healthy life.

Each age group will have a distribution across the 30 health states and therefore a mean health-related QOL value. These values give a health-related QOL prevalence at each age and can accordingly be used in life table calculations to estimate a healthy life expectancy, on analogy with the disability-free life expectancy method of Sullivan (Sullivan, 1971). For the non-institutionalized population covered in the

HIS, mean QOL state values in 1990 were 0.77 for people age 65–70, 0.75 for age 70–75, 0.72 for age 75–80, 0.67 for age 80–85, and 0.60 for age 85+. People aged 40–45, by contrast, had a mean of 0.86 (Erickson et al., 1995).

To generate health-related QOL scores for age groups in the entire U.S. population, institutional populations must be included and values assigned to these groups, which include prisoners (mean value of 0.74: very good health, limited in major role), nursing home residents (mean value of 0.21: fair health, ADL limitation), long-term hospital residents (mean value of 0.45: good health, IADL limitation), residential care facilities (0.72), and the military (1.0). Including these populations (with these imputations of mean QOL state) lowers scores slightly in each of the older age groups. For the total U.S. population covered in 1990, mean QOL state values were 0.76 for people age 65–70, 0.74 for age 70–75, 0.70 for age 75–80, 0.63 for age 80–85, and 0.51 for age 85+.

These values are entered in the lifetable model to convert person-years lived by people in given age intervals to "healthy person-year" equivalents. Thus, people born in 1990 who reach age 85 contribute an additional 193,523 person-years to this birth cohort's total years of life before they die. However, because the mean QOL value for this age group is 0.51, these 193,523 person-years are equivalent to 98,697 (193,523 × 0.51) healthy years. Summing up these quality-adjusted years across all age groups yields the cumulative sum (T_x) we have seen in chapters 2 and 5. If we divide the cumulative sum at each age interval by the number of people entering this age interval, the result is healthy life expectancy, the quality-adjusted analogue to life expectancy.

In 1990, healthy life expectancy in the U.S. for men and women combined was 64.0 years and life expectancy 75.4 years. People born in 1990, then, had a "healthy proportion of life" expectancy of 84.9% (64/75.4), that is, about 85% of life in the state of optimal health, as defined above. This proportion of life remaining that can be expected to be lived in optimal health shrinks with advancing age: 68.5% at age 40–45, 57.2% at age 65–70, and 37.3% at age 85+.

Thus, the increasing prevalence of chronic conditions and senescent changes lowers mean QOL scores (by increasing the proportion of people in less optimal states), which means fewer years of healthy life in later age intervals and a smaller proportion of remaining years in healthy life. These trends differ by socioeconomic status. Healthy life expectancy at birth in 1990 was 65.0 among whites, 56.0 among African Americans, and 64.8 among Hispanics. The three groups had very different life expectancies: 76.1 for whites, 69.1 for African Americans, 79.1 for Hispanics. The proportion of total years in which individuals in each race-ethnicity group could expect to be in optimal health reflects both life expectancy and healthy life expectancy. This proportion was 85.4% for whites, 81.0% for African Americans, and 81.9% for Hispanics in 1990. These are significant findings, as they suggest the important public health goal of eliminating a health disparity and the need to improve the experience of all groups.

GENERALIZATION OF THE QUALITY-ADJUSTMENT PARADIGM

We have seen that health-related quality of life research depends on two key assumptions: specification of plausible, discrete health states, and assignment of numeric values to these states. The first assumption implies clear boundaries between health states and the ability to calculate survival in particular health states. The second implies reasonable consensus on how much worse one health state is relative to another. These distinctions can be difficult to draw for health states that are similar. Thus, if we return to Table 8.4, we note that adjacent health states sometimes differ by only a few units on the utility scale. This reflects our experience of being "indifferent" between states that are more or less equally good or bad.

If we accept these assumptions, the utility- or quality-adjusted life-year (QALY) can be a powerful tool for health services research. Let us examine a simple example. Table 8.5a presents data for a hypothetical individual who died at age 80. He occupied four health states during his life. From birth to age 60, his QOL state was valued at 1.0, optimal health. Thus, the healthy-year equivalent for this state of health was 60 years. At age 60, he suffered a heart attack, which prevented him from working, his major activity. The utility for this state was 0.80. He lived in this state for 5 years, resulting in a healthy-year equivalent of 4 years (0.80 × 5). At age 66 he suffered a second major health event. He was diagnosed with Parkinson's disease, forced to take a set of extensive medications, alter his daily activity (for example, limiting driving), and began to think himself as an old person in relatively poor health. The utility for this state was 0.60 and the duration of the state 10 years, resulting in a healthy-year equivalent of 6 years. Finally, at age 76 he was diagnosed with dementia secondary to Parkinson's disease. The QOL valuation for this state was 0.40 (see chapter 6), and he lived 5 years in the state before death, resulting in a healthy-year equivalent of only 2 years. If we sum down the columns in Table 8.5a, we see that he lived 80 years, but was in optimal health only 72 years.

Looking across the 80 years he lived, we see that the proportion of life in optimal health was 90% (72/80) (alternatively, his mean QOL

TABLE 8.5 Calculation of Years of Healthy Life (YHL)

a. Without Intervention

Age Span	Health State	Duration	HQOL Value	YHL
0–60	1	60	1.00	60
61–65	2	5	.80	4
66–75	3	10	.60	6
76–80	4	5	.40	2
Death				
		Σ 80		Σ 72

b. With Intervention

Age Span	Health State	Value	Duration	HQOL	YHL
0–60	1		60	1.00	60
61–65	2		5	.80	4
66–76	3a		11	.65	7.15
77–82	4a		6	.45	2.70
Death					
			Σ 82		Σ 73.85

value across the life span was 0.90). But note the very different picture in later life beginning at age 66. The proportion of life lived in optimal health from age 66 until death was only 53% (8/15), and his mean QOL state during this period was 0.53, quite low, equivalent, as we have seen, to the mean state for people age 85+.

If we look now at Table 8.5b, we can assess the effect of a health intervention using the same quality-adjusted model. In this simple model, some kind of health intervention, say, an effective disease management program for his Parkinson's disease, begins at age 66, state 3a. This program involves better pharmacotherapy (less adverse effects from his medication, easier dosing schedule and better adherence, better management of tremor and slowness). The QOL value for this state is 0.65, rather than 0.60 and he gains an additional year of life in this state because the drug therapy also delays onset of Parkinson's dementia. He lives in this state 11 years, the equivalent of 7.15 years in optimal health (11 × 0.65). He reaches the dementia milestone at age 77, but with excellent custodial care and perhaps moderation of dementia progression because of his prior drug therapy, the QOL state is valued at 0.45, rather than 0.40. He lives 6 years in this state for a healthy-year equivalent of 2.7 years (6 × 0.45).

With these interventions, the man lived 82 years, the equivalent of 73.85 years in optimal health. This is again 90% (73.85/82) of the life span in optimal health, no different than the prior model. Interventions often add years to life, which must be considered in calculated benefit. The true benefit is seen in the last years of life. From age 66, when the intervention was introduced, to death, he lived 17 years, the equivalent of 9.85 years in optimal health. Thus, the proportion of life lived in optimal health from age 66 on was 58% (9.85/17), an improvement of 5% over the non-intervention model. Through this intervention, our hypothetical individual lived an additional 2 years at a higher mean QOL (0.58 vs. 0.53).

Is this a large difference? Should we be impressed by a 5% improvement in mean QOL? This speaks to the issue of the clinical relevance of change in QOL scores, discussed above. A difference of 0.05 in mean QOL scores is equivalent to about a 5–year age difference in late life. For example, the mean QOL score for people aged 70–75 is 0.74 and for people aged 75–80 0.70. The intervention, then, brought about a change roughly equivalent in magnitude to the difference in QOL between people aged 70–75 and 75–80.

Even with this benefit measured on the scale of age, one can still ask if such an intervention is worth mounting. How does this benefit compare to the costs of implementing such a program? The quality-adjusted model can be used to develop a ratio of cost to utility helpful for answering such questions. In this effort we ask, "What does an extra year of healthy life cost?"

To answer this question, we need the cost of care with the intervention and the usual cost of care. Let's say that the cost of current, non-intervention care for this man was $5,000 a year, and the cost with the intervention $7,000 a year. These costs, incurred over the duration of the intervention, serve as the numerator for the cost-utility ratio. To return to the examples shown in Table 8.5[a and b], the numerator is (7000 × 17) minus (5000 × 15), that is, 17 years of life with the intervention ($119,000) versus 15 years of life without ($75,000), or $44,000. The denominator is the additional years of healthy life provided by the intervention. With the intervention, the man lived the equivalent of 9.85 years of healthy life or optimal health; without it, he lived only 8 years in this state. The difference, then, is 1.85 years. Given these values, the cost-utility ratio is 44,000/1.85, or $23,784. Thus, this program of effective disease management provides an additional year of healthy life at a cost of $23,784. (More complex calculations would include a discounting factor to control for the effect of inflation over long periods.)

Is this a good deal? Here one must compare this incremental cost to the cost of other interventions. In fact, this is a reasonable investment. It is comparable to the cost of an additional healthy life-year in hypertension management programs (Patrick & Erickson, 1993).

HEALTH-RELATED AND ENVIRONMENT-RELATED QOL IN OLD AGE

In contrast to health-related QOL, environmental or non-health QOL may remain high throughout life and may even improve with age. With retirement, for example, older people have greater leisure time; with children gone, houses paid for, and successful investments, they may have greater disposable income as well. As a result, older people have increased opportunities to develop interests and create satisfying environments. These freedoms and opportunities counterbalance declines in health-related QOL and may be responsible for the great resiliency older people show in the face of declining health and impending death. Since person-and environment-based QOL do not decline with age, older people may have advantages in building environments that promote QOL.

Lawton (1991) has expressed the relevance of non-health, environment-based QOL for old people very well. He asks, "Do frail people do better if they have a loved spouse, a fulfilling relationship with a child, an area of expertise that can be applied despite the illness, a sphere of life where autonomy can still be exercised, or an ideology that organizes the meaning of pain, suffering, life, and death?" (p. 8). The answer, of course, is yes. In the presence of declining health and declines in health-related quality of life, these factors may become even more important. They become the basis for continuing attachment to life but also play a role in effective adjustment to limitations in health and maximization of health-related QOL.

SUMMARY

Health-related and environment-based quality of life must be distinguished. Health-related quality of life is inexorably linked to age and shows clear declines across the life span, in keeping with senescent processes and increased susceptibility to chronic disease. Nonhealth or environment-based quality of life is not a health impact measure but rather registers the effect of personal resources or environmental factors on daily experience. The two come together in the ability of older people to modify environments in ways that limit the QOL impact of poor health.

Identification of QOL Domains. A good test of whether a domain falls within the category of health-related QOL is to ask what aspects of a person's life are likely to improve if a patient is successfully treated by a physician. These are health-related QOL domains, which typically include measures of physical, affective, and social function, along with symptom states.

Measuring QOL. Can we determine *how much* better life is at a higher level of health than at a lower level? Patrick & Erickson (1993) define health-related QOL as "the *value* assigned to the duration of life, as modified by impairment" (emphasis added). The goal of measurement of health-related QOL is to develop measures that capture the impact of changes in health and to assign plausible numeric indicators for such changes. While this second task may seem difficult, we should remember that people already implicitly assign values to these health changes. Every day people evaluate symptom states and make treatment decisions based on their judgment of the likely impact of treatment or nontreatment.

"Minimal clinically significant difference" in QOL. Clinical significance in self-reported QOL is identified by a change in patient-reported status that would lead a care provider to seek a different medication or a change in a care environment. Otherwise stated, these are changes that would lead a clinician to make a change in patient management. Patient behavior is a good guide here. If patients report such changes to a clinician, and the clinician is not impressed enough to alter management, patients are apt to go elsewhere.

Age as an Anchor for Assessing Change in Health-Related QOL. Given the pervasive effect of age on quality of life states because of senescence and the increasing prevalence of chronic conditions, age provides a natural metric for assessing the QOL effects of clinical interventions. Quality of life changes can be referenced to norms at different ages, allowing one to associate changes in a health-related QOL domain to age equivalents. Thus, increasing urine flow 3 ml/sec in men with benign prostatic hypertrophy is equivalent to lowering their "urinary age" 10–15 years.

Health-Related QOL and Healthy-Year Equivalents. In the *Healthy People 2000* "years of healthy life" measure, health states are defined by the cross-classification of self-rated health and reported activity limitation. These states are assigned QOL values on a 0–1.0 scale. Given one's QOL state and its assigned value, the number of years lived in this state can be converted to a "healthy years equivalent," or the number of years lived in optimal health. This is a quality-adjusted measure. Thus, 5 years of life in a health state with a value of 0.80 would be equivalent to 4 years of optimal health (5 × 0.80).

For the total U.S. population covered in 1990, mean QOL state values in 1990 were 0.76 for people age 65–70, 0.74 for age 70–75, 0.70 for age 75–80, 0.63 for age 80–85, and 0.51 for age 85+. The increasing prevalence of chronic conditions and senescent changes at later ages lowers mean QOL scores (by increasing the proportion of people in less optimal states), which means fewer years of healthy life in later age intervals, and a smaller proportion of remaining years in healthy life.

These trends differ by socioeconomic status. Healthy life expectancy at birth in 1990 was 65.0 among Whites, 56.0 among African Americans, and 64.8 among Hispanics. The three groups had very different life expectancies: 76.1 for Whites, 69.1 for African Americans, 79.1 for Hispanics. The proportion of total years in which individuals in each race-ethnicity group could expect to be in optimal health was 85.4% for whites, 81.0% for African-Americans, and 81.9% for Hispanics in 1990. This difference suggests the important public health goal of eliminating a health disparity and also the need to improve the experience of all groups.

Health-Related and Environment-Related QOL in Old Age. In contrast to health-related QOL, person-and environment-based QOL do not decline with age. Older people can use this to their advantage in building environments that promote QOL even in the presence of chronic conditions.

9

Emerging Applications of the Aging and Public Health Paradigm

In prior chapters we have stressed the heavy chronic disease burden associated with older age. About 80% of people aged 65+ have one or more chronic conditions, and 50% two or more. Nearly 20% have diabetes. Some 60% have arthritis. 6–10% have Alzheimer's disease, with AD prevalence increasing to nearly 50% in people aged 85+ (CDC, 2003). The number of Americans who will have to contend with disability due to chronic disease will triple by 2050 (Boult et al., 1996).

We have also stressed the severe disability and mortality burden associated with these chronic conditions. About 20% of older adults report difficulties with household and personal self-maintenance activities required for independent living. While this prevalence has declined in the last decades, declines have mainly been limited to early, mild IADL disability, not the basic ADL that require the most expensive long-term care services (Freedman, Martin, & Schoeni, 2002). Mortality continues to decline at each age as it is postponed to later ages, a clear public health victory, but the continuing, substantial proportion of the life span lived with disability (about 15% of the total life span, and nearly half the life span beyond age 65 [Erickson, Patrick, Shannon, 1995]) suggests that public health must now respond to the challenges created by this achievement (CDC, 2003).

Given this picture, prevention of physical and cognitive disability in late life is now increasingly recognized as an important public health goal. "To address the challenges posed by an aging population, public health agencies and community organizations worldwide should continue expanding their traditional scope from infectious diseases and maternal/child health to include health promotion in older adults, prevention

215

of disability, maintenance of capacity in those with frailties and disabilities, and enhancement of quality of life" (CDC, 2003 p. 104). We have argued that an adequate public health response to this challenge requires a life span approach to health and disease risk: recognition of the early-life origin of processes that increase the risk of chronic disease, frailty, and disability in late life; identification of behaviors in early and middle life that place a person at risk for poor outcomes in late life; and implementation of interventions in early and mid-life that will prevent or postpone disease that would otherwise develop in late life. This area of public health research and practice is still in its infancy.

However, a great deal of progress has been made in understanding the origin of frailty in late life, which may suggest ways to reduce the risk of physical and cognitive disability in people who have already entered old age. In this chapter we first examine progress in this area, beginning with recent advances in the biology of frailty, and then examine recent evidence regarding falls and preservation of independence. Evidence from clinical trials suggests that falls can be prevented through a multifactorial intervention. Likewise, recent trials suggest that independence can be preserved through physical and cognitive "pre-habilitation."

We then turn to two other major areas in which a public health perspective is likely to improve prospects in late life. These include promotion of chronic disease management for people with such conditions, and enhancement of custodial care for people who have already crossed the threshold into disability.

PREVENTING PHYSICAL AND COGNITIVE DISABILITY

Insights on the Biology of Frailty

An important finding from the Cardiovascular Health Study was the unexpected association between frailty and *preclinical* cardiovascular disease (CVD), apart from the expected relationship between frailty and disease. The frailty phenotype, discussed earlier in chapter 2, includes three or more of five clinical signs and symptoms: low strength ("weakness"), slow walking speed ("slowness"), low physical activity ("sedentariness"), unintentional weight loss ("shrinking"), and self-reported exhaustion ("lack of energy") (Fried, Tangen et al., 2001). A "pre-frail" group, or group at risk for frailty, was defined in this research by the presence of 1–2 of the signs and symptoms. Frailty represents clinically significant loss of physiologic reserve, a general slowing, shrinking, and weakening that indicate marginal functioning and high risk for disability, hospitalization, and mortality.

The prevalence of congestive heart failure was 1.8% in the non-frail group, 4.6% in the "pre-frail" group, and 14.0% in the frail group (Newman et al., 2001). Similar gradients in prevalence were seen for myocardial infarction, angina, and intermittent claudification (problems with peripheral circulation). Thus, as expected, CVD was more common in people with greater frailty (though a majority of the frail group did not have one of the cardiovascular diseases).

Importantly, in the group without cardiovascular disease, measures of preclinical or early disease followed the same pattern. Abnormal values for blood pressure, carotid stenosis (an indicator of stroke risk), ankle-arm brachial index (an indicator of peripheral vascular disease), ECG (a measure of cardiac function), and cerebral MRI (an indicator of vascular disease) were all related to frailty level. On all the measures, the intermediate frailty group was likely to have abnormal values relative to non-frail elders. Newman and colleagues (2001) conclude, "In those with no history of clinical CVD, measures of the extent of CVD measured noninvasively were also associated with frailty, suggesting that subclinical, as well as clinically manifest CVD, can have a substantial impact on the health of older adults," (p. 164).

Newman and colleagues (2001) suggest two possible mechanisms for the association between frailty and CVD indicators in people without frank CVD. One mechanism is end-organ damage, which decreases physiologic reserve and results in frailty. The noninvasive CVD indicators indicate abnormalities in the arterial tree, or defects in general cardiovascular integrity, which lead to damage in the heart, brain, and kidneys. In people without CVD, these defects have not yet led to frank disease but may still impair organ function. The result is a subclinical reduction in end organ reserve, which is manifest as frailty.

The second mechanism is actually a result of the body's success in avoiding acute cardiovascular events. People with extensive arterial plaques who avoid stroke or heart attack (for reasons unclear) still suffer inflammatory and thrombotic events in vessel walls. These states of chronic inflammation are visible in elevations in interleukin-6, fibrinogin, C-reactive protein, and tumor necrosis factor-alpha, and decreases in serum albumin. Inflammation accompanies the healing and remodeling of vessel walls that have been damaged by plaque or other processes. Chronic inflammatory states are associated with loss of lean muscle mass (shrinking), low energy, decreased appetite, and the other symptoms of frailty. Newman and colleagues (2001) suggest that "the cost of surviving acute cardiovascular events may be that a chronic inflammatory state is maintained to continue to heal these extensive lesions, with resulting loss of strength, weight loss, inactivity, and poor appetite," (p. 165).

Frailty in the absence of chronic disease, then, may be a consequence of a disease process that has failed to cause frank disease, as in the end-organ damage hypothesis. Or frailty may be a consequence of the body's response to this disease process, as in the inflammatory hypothesis. More research is required to clarify which best characterizes its origins.

The significance of inflammatory processes for frailty and risk of disability has also been investigated in the Women's Health and Aging Study (WHAS) and Health, Aging, and Body Composition Study (Health ABC). High levels of interleukin-6 (IL-6) and C-reactive protein were shown to predict incident disability in the WHAS cohort, independently of other risk factors (Ferrucci et al., 1999). The mechanism for this effect is the catabolic effect of IL-6 on muscle, which leads to sarcopenia and hence loss of muscle strength in the lower extremities. This, in turn, leads to disability in both mobility and ultimately ADL. Examination of changes in knee extensor strength and walking speed suggests that IL-6 affects muscle mass, and that this effect is responsible for the increased risk of disability. That is, the effect of IL-6 on risk of disability was attenuated when changes in muscle mass were introduced into regression equations. This attenuation in risk suggests that "change in muscle strength is intrinsic to the causal pathway leading from high IL-6 to the development of new disability" (Ferrucci et al., 2002). This is an indirect demonstration of the causal mechanism, but it is consistent with other research showing an association between high levels of IL-6 and lower muscle mass and strength (Visser, Pahor, Taafe, Goodpaster, 2002), as well as lower muscle mass and poorer lower extremity function (Visser, Kritchevsky, Goodpaster, Newman, Nevitt, Stamm, Harris, 2002). A stronger demonstration would show an increased risk of disability among people whose IL-6 serum levels have increased (or a lower risk of disability in a group whose IL-6 levels have declined, perhaps as a result of a therapeutic intervention).

What do these findings on the biology of frailty imply for public health and the prevention of disability at older ages? We know that IL-6 increases with age (Hager et al., 1994); that a 1 sd increase in IL-6 level is associated with significantly lower strength (a 1.1.–2.4 kg difference in grip strength), a smaller muscle area, and greater fat infiltration (Visser, Pahor et al., 2002), raising the risk of disability; and that increases in IL-6 (as well as other proinflammatory cytokines) are a feature of both chronic medical conditions and a more general chronic inflammatory process.

These considerations suggest a number of intervention strategies. Certainly, reduction of the incidence of chronic disease, postponement of its onset, and attenuation of its effects would likely reduce inflammation from this source. This primary prevention approach might be supplemented with treatment strategies for elders who develop chronic conditions. Once elders have developed this inflammatory response, whether from disease or the more general process described earlier, pharmacologic agents might be used to prevent IL-6 and other cytokines from affecting muscle. Finally, exercise and strength training increases muscle mass in older people (Fiatarone et al., 1990). A carefully planned program of exercise and activity in frail elders may offer benefit, but to our knowledge no such trial has been conducted.

Preventing Falls

Falling is a common event among older people. About 30% of community-resident people aged 65+, and 40% of people aged 80+, fall each year (Tinetti et al., 1988). About 5% of these falls result in fractures and another 5% in serious soft-tissue injury requiring hospitalization or long-term immobilization and recovery. Falls occupy a prominent position in the case of deaths due to injury and also play a role in the institutionalization of older people.

In a study of non-nursing home elderly aged 75+, Tinetti and colleagues (1988) found that 32% fell during the course of a year; a quarter of the fallers had serious injuries and 6% fractures. Risk factors for falling in this cohort included sedative use, cognitive impairment, functional limitation in the lower extremities, poor reflexes, abnormalities of balance and gait, and foot problems. The many different risk factors for falling, representing disparate physiological systems, again suggest that falling is a geriatric syndrome (like urinary incontinence, slow gait speed, or lower extremity weakness), a syndrome of poor or inefficient function with many causes. People with none of the risk factors were very unlikely to fall; only 8% of this group reported a fall over 12 months. By contrast, people with all eight risk factors were extremely likely to fall: 78% of this group fell. Notably, only 10% of the falls occurred during acute illnesses and only 5% during hazardous activity.

An important finding from this study was the important role of environmental and ergonomic factors in falls. While 77% of the falls occurred at home, in a familiar environment, 44% involved modifiable home hazards. In these falls, people tripped over objects or slipped on stairs. Also, a majority of falls involved particular kinds of activities, mainly those that displaced a person's center of gravity. These activities included getting up or sitting down, bending over or reaching, or stepping up or down. These particular environmental and ergonomic factors, along with medical risk factors identified in this effort, suggest a number of interventions to reduce the risk of falling. In fact, a series of randomized clinical trials have shown that fall risk can be reduced. These trials were multifactoral: one addressed physical activity, hearing, vision, alcohol use, psychotropic drug use, and safety in the home (Wagner et al., 1994); a second examined psychotropic drug use, polypharmacy (see below), muscle weakness, problems with balance, gait, and transfers, and postural hypotension (Tinetti et al., 1994); and a third studied home modification, recommendations about physical activity, and health counseling (Hornbrook et al., 1994). All showed benefit.

One of the intervention studies is notable for explicitly linking reduction in the risk of falling to modification of particular fall risk factors. In the trial conducted by Tinetti and colleagues (1994), the Yale FICSIT trial (Frailty and Injuries Cooperative Studies of Intervention Techniques), 35% of the intervention group fell, compared to 47% of controls, over a 1-year period. In this trial, one inclusion criterion was use of four prescription medications, a risk factor for falling, and one target of this multifactorial intervention. As part of the intervention, medication use for people in the intervention group was evaluated and adjusted as needed. In this trial, 63% of the intervention group continued to take four or more medications, compared to 86% of controls. The trial also showed that many other risk factors for falling were modifiable, including balance impairment, difficulty with toilet transfer, and gait impairment. Each was modified through a combination of behavioral training, an exercise program, and-or environmental change. The prevalence of impairments in the intervention group declined relative to controls; this reduction appears to have been responsible for the reduction of falls.

One limitation in this trial was inability to establish that the lower incidence of falls was a direct consequence of reduction in risk factors. This issue was addressed in a follow-up analysis of this trial (Tinetti et al., 1996). Re-analyses showed that improvements in balance and reduction in blood pressure (to lower fall risk associated with orthostatic hypotension) were associated with lower rates of falling. Also, the reanalysis showed that fall risk declined in both treatment and control groups according to degree of reduction in a composite measure of fall risk. In the treatment group, the average number of risk factors declined by about one (of 7 different risks), but this degree of risk factor reduction was enough to reduce falls by about 35% (Buchner, 1999). Together, these findings suggest that altering or eliminating specific risk factors for falls can reduce fall risk.

This conclusion, straightforward and not surprising at first glance, is quite important. It is a clear demonstration that the pathway from impairment to disability, in this case fall risk, can be modified. Table 9.1 shows in detail the relevant risk factors, criteria for defining risk, and FICSIT interventions that successfully altered the risk factor. A meta-analysis of the FICSIT trials showed that exercise and balance interventions (which varied across studies in duration, intensity, and

TABLE 9.1 Risk Factors for Falls in Yale FICSIT Trial

Risk Factor	Criteria for Defining Risk	Intervention
Postural hypotension	≤20 mmHg drop or drop to ≤90 mmHg when moving from lying to standing position	Postural exercises; elevate head of bed; medication adjustment
Use of sedative-hypnotic agents	Use of benzodiazepines or other medications for sleeping	Taper off and discontinue; use of non-pharmacologic treatments
Use of 4 medications	Use of one centrally acting antihypertensive, nitrate diuretic, histamine blocker, or non-steroidal anti-inflammatory; report of fatigue, dizziness, or fall	Medication review and adjustment by physician
Unsafe tub or toilet transfer	Unsafe performance	Transfer training; environmental adjustments
Gait impairment	Defect in step length, height, symmetry, continuity, path deviation, trunk sway, turning	Gait training; use of assistive devices; exercise
Balance impairment	Defect in progressively hard static stances or retropulsion	Balance exercises
Strength or range-of-motion limitation, arms or legs	Less than full range against full resistance	Resistance exercises

Source: Tinetti, McAvay, Claus, 1996; Tinetti, Speechley, & Ginet, 1988.

type [including a tai chi dynamic balance component]) were associated with significant reductions in fall risk (Province et al., 1995).

An additional set of findings from the Seattle FICSIT study provides an important lesson in targeting fall prevention interventions (Buchner et al., 1997). HMO enrollees, all selected for lower extremity weakness or gait abnormalities and hence at risk for falling, were randomized to an exercise intervention or control group. The goal was to improve balance, gait, and self-reported physical health status to see if these improvements were associated with lower risk of falls over an 18-month follow-up period.

This trial was negative; gait, balance, and physical health did not significantly differ between intervention and control groups at the end of the trial, despite improvements in strength and aerobic capacity in the experimental group. However, fall risk was lower in the intervention group: 42% of intervention subjects reported a fall compared to 60% of controls. Buchner and colleagues (1997) note that the 42% rate is typical, as we have seen, of 1-year fall risk in community-resident elders; the exceptional finding, then, is the very high rate of falling (60%) in controls. They reason that the eligibility criteria for this study resulted in a sample on the verge of substantial decline. The exercise intervention prevented this decline. That is, without the intervention both groups would likely have shown fall rates of 60%. Selection criteria for this study identified a group with very little physical reserve and great risk of further decline. Thus, intervention outcomes must be interpreted in light of the position of elders on the curvilinear function that relates impairment to disability outcomes (see chapter 5) (Buchner et al., 1996). This intervention blunted the very high fall risk typical of older people with little physical reserve. Thus, while they did not lower fall risks typical of community elders in this study, fall interventions may offer benefit even to quite frail elderly.

Strengthening Independence

Can the skills required for independent living be taught or bolstered in such a way that the risk of disability is reduced? This is the premise of "pre-habilitation" (Gill et al., 2002) or "preventive occupational therapy" (Clark et al., 1997).

This preventive approach to disability has two targets. One involves factors extrinsic to aging that are nevertheless associated with disablement. These factors include safety awareness in the home and community (to prevent falls), efficient use of adaptive equipment or assistive technologies (to foster a sense of control and personal efficacy), exercise (to promote strength, balance, and stamina), energy conservation (to allow effective use of diminished capacities), and efficient use of public transportation. A second target, which sometimes overlaps with the first, includes the intrinsic features of aging that lead to disability. The primary target is functional limitation (see chapter 5), such as performance on tests of balance, strength, and mobility below norms expected for a given age group. Both sets of factors have served as targets for "prehabilitation" or remediation in randomized clinical trial settings.

Clark and colleagues (1997) compared an OT training group with two control groups, a social activity group and no treatment group, to assess remediation of extrinsic factors relevant to disablement. In this trial, the OT group received 2 hours of group training each week over 9 months, as well as 9 hours of individual OT training. "The key intent of the program was to help the participants better appreciate the importance of meaningful activity in their lives, as well as to impart specific knowledge about how to select or perform activities so as to achieve a healthy and satisfying lifestyle," (p. 1324). Participants received specific guidance in promoting safety, using transportation, making use of available adaptive equipment, exercise, and related areas. Use of the social-recreational control group allowed the researchers to separate the effect of OT-specific training from possible benefits of simple group participation.

Participants were residents of senior housing who volunteered in response to advertisements and posted announcements of the project. Outcomes in the research included a variety of health status measures: disability, life satisfaction, depressive symptoms, self-perceived health, and health-related quality of life. Attrition after randomization was about 15% in all three groups, and about 65% of participants randomized to the OT and social activity arms attended at least half the sessions, a measure of effective delivery of the behavioral intervention.

The social activity and non-intervention groups were equivalent in almost all outcomes, so the two groups were pooled and compared to the OT training intervention group. Participants in the OT program showed significant benefit in a variety of self-reported psychosocial outcomes, including quality of interaction, life satisfaction, health perception, pain, physical and role function, and mental health. Five of 15 outcomes (covering depression, IADL and ADL disability, social activity) did not show benefit, but may have been subject to ceiling effects (i.e., most people were already scoring low on measures of disability or depression). Clark and colleagues (1997) concluded that the program helped participants construct daily routines that were health promoting and meaningful given the context of their lives and in this way promoted well-being.

This is a provocative study, in that a relatively low-cost (and cost-effective [Hay et al., 2002]) intervention was associated with significant benefit, where the benefit also appears to be specific to OT training directed toward extrinsic sources of disability. However, the mechanism for this benefit is not completely clear. The authors suggest that health and subjective well-being improve when people are given greater opportunity to engage in health-promoting activities that are consistent with what they find important or meaningful. But no direct evidence is provided for this effect. Still, this is a first suggestive demonstration of the benefit of preventive occupational therapy training for healthy elderly.

The alternative approach, with remediation directed toward antecedent functional impairment before the onset of disability, was demonstrated in a randomized trial conducted by Gill and colleagues (2002). This controlled trial of prehabilitation recruited frail elderly, with a mean age of 83, from primary care practices. The intervention group received a physical therapy assessment and review of the home environment, with an average of 16 visits by the intervention team over 6 months. Particular regimens of exercise, home modification, and activity were designed according to results from individual evaluations. Disability outcomes in this group were compared to outcomes in a group receiving a health education program. The control group received monthly visits from a health educator over 6 months. Both groups received follow-up calls over an additional 6 months to maintain contact, answer questions, and provide encouragement.

In the intervention group, 65% completed the program. Withdrawal was due mainly to worsening health or other illness in families. Participants in the program, on the whole, followed through on exercise recommendations, with over 70% reporting completion of balance training, leg-conditioning, and arm-strengthening regimens. Of the control group, 78% completed the study.

Participants in the intervention reported less disability than the control group at 7 and 12 months. Benefit was more pronounced among participants who began the study with moderate, rather than severe, frailty. This is an important finding, as it suggests that prehabilitation can delay disablement, but also that different interventions may be required for the most frail elderly. The use of an active control here suggests that the mechanism for this reduction in disability risk was the linked physical therapy-exercise regimen rather than health education or attention from the study team.

Preventive Cognitive Remediation

If physical prehabilitation can retard disablement, could a program of preventive cognitive remediation have the same effect in the realm of cognitive decline? The Advanced Cognitive Training for Independent and Vital Elderly (ACTIVE) trial investigated this question in the setting of a randomized clinical trial (Ball et al., 2002). A volunteer sample of nearly 3,000 older adults without cognitive or physical impairment was randomized to one of three intervention groups or a no-contact control group. The three intervention arms involved 10 sessions devoted to training in memory skill (verbal episodic memory), reasoning (problem-solving strategies), or speed of processing (visual search and identification). The intervention program was delivered in small-group settings, with a focus on teaching strategies designed to improve memory, speed, or problem solving. Intervention groups were given exercises to practice and retain skills. In the memory training arm, for example, participants were instructed how to organize word lists into meaningful categories and to form visual images and mental associations to recall words and text. In this 2-year study, a subset of participants received booster training just before the 1-year evaluation.

Outcomes in the trial included ability on cognitive tests of these remediated skills, such as episodic memory, identification of patterns, and speed of processing. The trial also examined performance-based and self-reported everyday skills related to these cognitive domains. These included everyday problem-solving (e.g., the ability to handle medication information), everyday speed (e.g., the speed with which one looks up a telephone number), driving habits, and ADL and IADL disability.

The trial showed that these cognitive interventions helped normal elderly perform better on the specific cognitive skills for which they were trained. These benefits suggest that the slow cognitive declines reported for non-demented elders can be remediated. For example, ACTIVE participants receiving memory training improved about 0.25 sd over 2 years, while older adults without dementia typically decline at about this rate over a 7-year period. However, these proximal cognitive benefits did not translate into improvements in everyday performance. The authors suggest that the absence of transfer to real-world outcomes is best explained by a ceiling effect in the everyday performance measures. Most subjects were not impaired in driving, in looking up telephone numbers, or in reasoning about medications. The pronounced ceiling effect may have obscured true benefit in this area. In fact, the control group did not decline on many of the everyday performance measures. The authors conclude, "it is not yet clear whether differential functional decline across treatment groups will be observed in the future as this select cohort enters more fully into an age of functional loss" (Ball et al., 2002 p. 2280).

This important trial demonstrates that cognitive remediation in non-demented elders offers benefit that is sustained over 2 years. It does not follow from this finding that such training reduces the risk of impending dementia or disability, or that such remediation concurrently increases independence or activity in older people. The latter is an important limitation of the promise of cognitive remediation. It may be that ceiling effects prevented demonstration of benefit, but it may also be that these sorts of training are too limited to affect everyday function. For this translation to real-world outcomes we may be on safer grounds with the occupational and physical remediation efforts described earlier.

PROMOTING CHRONIC DISEASE MANAGEMENT

Five to 10% of older people incur 60–70% of the health care expenses of the older population (Boult & Pacala, 1999). An effective means of identifying this group at highest risk for medical care would be an important addition to the armamentarium of public health. As Boult and Pacala argue, "This dense concentration of morbidity and use of health-related services is unfortunate for those afflicted, but it offers hope for effectively focusing resources where they will do the most good," (p. 65).

Who is the high-risk senior? In ambulatory and hospitalized patients, one way to identify the high-risk elder is to identify factors associated with hospitalization (and repeated hospitalization). An effective tool for identifying the high-risk elder is the P_{ra}, the Probability of Repeated Admission (Pacala, Boult, Reed, & Aliberti, 1997). The 8 items of the P_{ra} reliably identify people with high likelihood of repeated hospital admissions. The items include self-rated health, hospital stays over the prior 12 months, number of physician visits in the prior 12 months, diabetes, heart disease (coronary heart disease, angina, myocardial infarction), gender, presence of a person "who would take care of you for a few days, if necessary," and age. Thus, a male with coronary artery disease, angina pectoris, diabetes in past year, and a self-rating of only "fair" health faces a high risk for hospitalization. He meets 5 of the 8 P_{ra} risk factors. Pacala and colleagues have developed regression equation weights for combining the factors into a single risk index. We could also add additional risk factors. If this person also has a medication regimen of 5 or more prescriptions and a medical condition that requires regular injections or catheter care, he would obviously be at even higher risk. The P_{ra} is useful for its identification of eight simple indicators that reliably identify high-risk elders.

Once the high-risk elder is identified, how should this person's medical care be managed to maximize effective treatment and minimize disability? Three areas of progress in this area, offering major benefit to older people, include geriatric evaluation and management, self-management of chronic disease, and reduction in polypharmacy.

Geriatric Evaluation and Management

The core of geriatric evaluation and management (GEM) is comprehensive geriatric assessment. This assessment includes a medical, psychological, and functional assessment that is integrated to develop an overall plan for treatment and follow-up (Boult & Pacala, 1999; Rubenstein,

Stuck, Siu, & Wieland, 1991). Interdisciplinary teams meet to establish a comprehensive care plan for each patient that takes into account the full picture of this person's medical risks, ongoing preserved abilities, personal resources, and preferences for care. GEM works best when the team making the care plan is also involved in its implementation; otherwise, recommendations from comprehensive geriatric assessment may go unfulfilled (Stuck, Siu, Wieland, & Rubenstein, 1993).

A meta-analysis of controlled clinical trials involving GEM showed that effects were stronger in inpatient than outpatient settings (Stuck et al., 1993). A number of randomized trials in inpatient settings have shown benefits for GEM in a variety of areas, such as improvement in diagnostic accuracy, reduction in disability risk, improvement in mental health, and reduction in nursing home admission and mortality. Elders in the treatment arms of these trials were more likely to report satisfaction with medical care, and their family caregivers also reported lower stress. Finally, some of the trials reported decreases in hospital and emergency department services. While the interventions usually involve greater use of home care and other long-term care services, these expenses are balanced and in some cases offset by lower hospitalization costs.

However, GEM results must be interpreted cautiously, that is, in light of the particular program elements involved and specific outcomes (and time frame) assessed. In a recent set of randomized clinical trials assessing GEM in inpatients, one showed no benefit in mortality risk, disability or health status over 12 months (Reuben et al., 1995). The 1-year mortality rate in the two arms of the study was about 25%, typical of mortality risk in older people discharged from hospitals. A second study showed no benefit in survival but significant reductions in disability risk and admission to long-term care facilities (Landefeld, Palmer, Kresevic, Fortinsky, & Kowal, 1995). However, the two studies are not truly comparable. The second only examined change from hospital admission to discharge, while the former involved a full year of follow-up.

Improvements in discharge status, as shown in this second GEM program, should translate into longer-term benefit. If they do not, as shown in the first trial, it may be because selection criteria in these trials do not always identify people likely to benefit (i.e., they may be too ill or, conversely, too healthy to show benefit), or because the trials take place in settings where control group participants already receive services and assessment protocols typical of GEM.

Table 9.2 shows key elements in the GEM program that successfully improved outcomes at hospital discharge. The program illustrates well how hospital care can be modified to promote appropriate discharge planning from the point of admission, using the many resources required for such a focus. The hospital environment was remodeled to

TABLE 9.2 Inpatient Geriatric Evaluation and Management Protocol

Key Element	Features
Prepared environment	Make hospital ward approximate adapted natural living conditions: carpeting, handrails, uncluttered hallways, large clocks, calendars; elevated toilet seats, door levers
Patient-centered care	Daily nursing assessment; nursing interventions to improve self-care, continence, nutrition, mobility, sleep, skin integrity, mood, cognition; daily multidisciplinary assessment
Planning for discharge	Emphasis on return to home; early involvement of case manager/social worker to develop appropriate discharge plan
Medical care review	Daily review of medications; protocols to minimize iatrogenesis

Source: Landefeld, et al., 1995.

concentrate on readying the patient for the return home, the patient-centered care protocol stressed skills and interventions that patients would need to bring with them when they returned home, and the barrier between the hospital and home care was broken down through active involvement of case management teams.

GEM has also been applied outside the inpatient and ambulatory care setting. In a randomized controlled trial of annual in-home GEM, Stuck and colleagues (1995) showed that a program of home visits by geriatric nurses, who consulted with geriatricians, reduced disability risk (12% vs. 22% in ADL) and nursing home admission (4% vs. 10%) over 3 years. These benefits came with the additional cost of significantly more visits to physicians, but the total incremental cost of the program was very favorable, about $6000 for each additional well (disability-free) year. Other in-home intervention studies have shown benefit with different program elements (i.e., preventive home visits without comprehensive geriatric assessment, one-shot comprehensive assessment with follow-up, telemedicine contact). Unfortunately it is not clear which element of the program was most responsible for the beneficial effect.

A less extensive application of GEM principles is visible in geriatric case management. In this approach, a specially trained case manager arranges social and health-related services and coordinates these services across long-term care settings. Results from this approach to GEM have been mixed. One randomized assessment of geriatric case management to increase access to primary care did not show a benefit in hospitalization or quality of life (Weinberger, Oddone, & Henderson, 1996). This was a study of veterans with a variety of conditions. Studies involving other elderly patient groups, such as patients with congestive heart failure, have shown benefit (Rich et al., 1995).

Making Patients and Families Partners in Medical Care

Chronic disease is highly prevalent among older people, as we have seen. People aged 60+ have a mean of over 2 chronic conditions, conditions that account for the vast majority of health care expenditures (Hoffman, Rice, & Sung, 1996; Rothenberg & Koplan, 1990). Clinical and personal experience suggests that people differ in their capacity to manage the disability and symptoms typical of chronic disease. Some adapt well and maintain relatively active lifestyles, while others are less able to do so. Given these differences, it would be valuable to know what is involved in successful management of chronic disease. Second, assuming these tasks can be identified, it would be valuable to know whether such skills can be taught. Finally, it would also be valuable to know if disease management in this sense is associated with important health outcomes, such as physician utilization or hospitalization.

Recent research has examined the elements of effective chronic disease self-management. Lorig and colleagues (1999) identified twelve common features of successful disease self-management. These allow people to adapt to states of limited health and minimize the effects of disease on function. They include "recognizing and acting on symptoms, using medication correctly, managing emergencies, maintaining nutrition and diet, maintaining adequate exercise, giving up smoking, using stress reduction techniques, interacting effectively with health providers, using community resources, adapting to work, managing relations with significant others, and managing psychological responses to illness" (p. 8). These elements have been incorporated into a program of patient education, the Chronic Disease Self-Management Program (CDSMP), which has been used to teach patients with a variety of chronic conditions to manage symptoms well, to communicate effectively with health professionals, and to develop realistic appraisals of the health risks they face. Principles of this program include use of peer patient educators, mobilization of small groups of patients who develop joint problem-solving strategies, and a stress on self-efficacy, that is, development of weekly action plans with realistic goals and expectations of success.

A randomized trial of this model involving different chronic disease groups showed encouraging results for a variety of outcomes. For the

664 participants in the self-management treatment arm, 108 CDSMP groups were convened. Outcomes for these patients were compared to the experience of a waiting-list control group (n = 476) over 6-months of follow-up. Participants were drawn from people with a diagnosis of chronic lung disease, heart disease, stroke, or arthritis. People in the treatment arm completed a mean of 5.5 of 7 program sessions, showing effective delivery of the intervention, an important consideration in behavioral interventions of this type.

The trial showed significant benefit for CDSMP on a variety of outcomes, including health behaviors (self-reports of exercise, symptom management, effective communication with physicians), health status (self-rated health, disability, fatigue, and distress over health), and health service use (physician visits, hospitalization). These benefits were maintained over two years (Lorig et al., 2001) and were replicated when the control was offered the intervention. Comparing the CDSMP group to other samples assessed with a common measure of disability (HAQ, the Health Assessment Questionnaire) showed that CDSMP participants were more or less stable in disability scores, where other samples, matched for age and health status, declined.

These are impressive findings, and as a result CDSMP has been embraced by large HMOs, such as Kaiser Permanente, and by the National Health Service's (UK) Expert Patient program (AHQR, 2002). Still, some caution is in order. Lorig and colleagues (1999) do not report participation rates in their initial randomization (i.e., how many patients randomized to the intervention declined to participate). They do report that only 72% of controls agreed to enter the intervention when offered the chance to do so after the end of the initial 6-month trial. This suggests that the intervention group may have been enriched with more highly motivated participants, that is, people able to benefit from the program or more motivated to self-manage their disease in any case. These selection effects are difficult to assess in behavioral trials.

CDSMP can also be faulted for ignoring a number of other factors that may be central to effective self-management. One is the availability of objective ways to monitor a chronic disease condition, such as urine or blood tests to identify hypoglycemia, as in the case of diabetics. Access to these indicators allows patients to monitor and adjust medications or behaviors (Tattersall, 2002). Another factor is fostering effective partnerships between patients and health professionals. The "copy letter," in which physicians send patients a copy of their recommendations and the results of jointly planned care plans, is one way to build such partnerships. Finally, more needs to be done from the physician side, especially giving patients approval, or permission, to take a more active role in their care. Tattersall (2002) suggests that many doctors and other healthcare professionals are uncomfortable with the idea of empowering their patients.

Apart from promotion of effective self-management of chronic disease, it is also worth asking how older people actually manage chronic conditions. In fact, for the most disabled and oldest patients, management usually involves a patient-physician-family triad, rather than the traditional patient-physician dyad. Little is known about self-management behaviors in the home, or outside of contact with physicians or other health professionals. Up to a third of older people are accompanied by other family in their physician consults (Silliman et al., 1996). Presumably, the patient's family plays an even larger role in management decisions beyond physician contact. This would be an important topic for future research on self-care.

Avoiding Inappropriate Medication Use and Managing Polypharmacy

Inappropriate medication use is a common problem in older people. One community-based study of people aged 75+ found that 14% were using at least one inappropriate drug (Stuck et al., 1994), and a second study found a higher prevalence of 23.5% over a 1-year period (Willcox, Himmselstein, & Woolhandler, 1994). Forty percent of nursing home residents have been reported to receive one or more inappropriate drugs (Beers et al., 1992). "Inappropriate medications" in these studies are defined as drugs that should generally be avoided by older people, as specified in expert consensus panels. The drugs have all been shown to be ineffective or have been replaced by safer alternatives. For example, long-acting benzodiazepines (sedative-hypnotic agents) have been replaced by short-acting benzodiazepines with better side effect profiles. The same is true for a number of antidepressant agents, antihypertensives, non-steroidal anti-inflammatory agents, oral hypoglycemic agents, analgesics, dementia therapies, platelet inhibitors, muscle relaxants, and gastrointestinal antispasmodic agents (Stuck et al., 1994).

In these efforts to identify inappropriate medication use, the authors obtained valuable information on the prevalence of medication use in older people generally. In the sample of community-resident people aged 75+, medication use was fairly high. People were taking an average of 2.4 prescription and 2.4 non-prescription medications. A very small proportion, less than 5%, managed to avoid all medications, and about a third were taking six or more. The 14% of the sample taking at least one inappropriate drug were more likely to be older, on an antidepressant, and taking many medications (Stuck et al., 1994).

A distinction should be drawn between inappropriate and excessive use of medications on the one hand, and polypharmacy on the other (Stuck, 2001). Inappropriate or excessive medication involves use of medications in which harm exceeds benefit, as described above. Polypharmacy, by contrast, is simply use of many medications, all potentially appropriate. It is a problem, however, because of the greater risk of adverse events associated with a greater number of medications, which is complicated further by interactions between medications (drug-drug interactions) and between medications and non-indicated medical conditions (drug-disease interactions). Also, the greater the number of medications, the less likely compliance, and hence the greater the risk that people will not take medications they should be taking.

One operational definition of polypharmacy is regular use of four or more prescription medications. By this definition, about 50% of the oldest old meet criteria for polypharmacy. A challenge to geriatric care is to determine which medications are inappropriate, because it is possible for diseases to be poorly managed and symptoms under-treated even with an excessive number of medications. The following tests can be used to determine the appropriateness of medications: Is there an indication for the drug and is the drug effective for the condition? Is the dosage correct (taking into account changes in renal clearance and other features of pharmacokinetics and pharmacodynamics associated with aging)? Are there drug-drug or drug-disease interactions? Are directions for administering the drug reasonable for the patients, that is, is the patient likely to be able to take the drug according to directions and for as long as indicated? Does the drug duplicate an existing drug? Can the drug be replaced with something less expensive? (Stuck, 2001).

In pursuit of proper polypharmacy, physicians may have to take patients off medications as part of a comprehensive examination of medication profiles. It is much easier to add a medication than to remove one, but good management of patients may also require taking patients off drugs. Evidence suggests that physicians, like patients themselves, are reluctant to remove medications that have been prescribed for a long time. For example, in-home evaluations of medicine cabinets show a great number of expired and obsolete medications, stored "just in case" (Rubenstein, 1999). Likewise, with passage of time patients are likely to accumulate medications, with a comprehensive assessment of medications undertaken by physicians only when adverse events or a medical event requires it.

The rational management of polypharmacy is a major challenge for public health and aging. Some success in this effort will likely come from new partnerships between physicians and pharmacists (Weinberger et al., 2002), as well as greater consumer awareness, and perhaps from increased regulatory pressure.

ENHANCING CUSTODIAL CARE

Kane (2003) has specified goals for the care of custodial populations, such as people with Alzheimer's disease or severe psychiatric illness, or people dependent on extensive medical technologies. For these populations, rehabilitation or cure is not a reasonable goal, nor, in some cases, is extended survival. That is, for the severely demented individual receiving formal home care services, or the older patient receiving ventilator care in a nursing home, excellent custodial care should be the goal but will most likely not extend survival or lead to regained function. What, then, are goals for enhanced custodial care? What outcomes would be reasonable targets for interventions in these populations? Table 9.3 shows supportive care goals for custodial populations.

These goals (for example, dignity, privacy, a sense of security, or the opportunity to participate in meaningful activity or reciprocal social relationships) are the essence of sensitive treatment of any person. The goals are no more difficult than ones we set for ourselves and expect in daily activity. Thus, an important conclusion from research with custodial populations is that the same goals apply. Privacy is as important in the nursing home as anywhere else. Allowing someone to maintain individuality, perhaps through the use of personal objects or "memory cases," is appropriate in institutions just as it is in homes. "Meaningful activity" is a goal even for someone with severe memory impairment, even if attempts at such activity strike the observer as terribly primitive or unsatisfying.

In fact, one additional conclusion from Kane's approach is that we cannot presume to know, without detailed investigation, the valence of behaviors for people with severe dementia. Agitation is almost always a negative behavior (patients appear distressed, risk injuring themselves,

TABLE 9.3 Goals for Enhanced Custodial Care

- Sense of security and order
- Enjoyment
- Meaningful activity (opportunity to accomplish goals)
- Social relationships (opportunity for reciprocity)
- Dignity
- Privacy
- Individuality (identity with past)
- Autonomy (opportunity to express preferences)
- Spiritual well-being
- Functional competence
- Physical comfort

After Kane, 2000.

and elicit negative responses both from caregivers and other patients). Likewise, a patient's demonstration of a preference, or assertion of continuity with the past, or clear pleasure in activity is easily recognized as positive behavior (as indicated by facial expressions of happiness, contentment, or interest) (Lawton, Van Haitsma, Perkinson, & Rutdeschel, 2001). But the valence of other behaviors is less clear (see Chapter 6). Wandering, perseveration, delusions, and vocalizations are disturbing to observers but may represent sources of pleasure or engagement to the person with severe dementia (Albert, 1997).

For custodial care populations, the following areas have recently become topics of research: recognition of older people's care preferences and designing care regimens that respect such preferences; upgrading home attendant and nursing assistant care; developing special care units for people with Alzheimer's disease; expanding options for supportive housing; supporting family caregivers; and upstreaming palliative care, that is, moving palliative care away from the point of death to allow the dying or chronically ill patient to benefit from the more intensive person-centered care typical of hospice. We examine each below.

Taking Older People's Care Preferences Seriously

Are family caregivers, even when they are in daily contact with dementia patients, good judges of patient preferences? Reason for doubt on the accuracy of caregiver perceptions is evident in Logsdon's finding of high correlations between caregiver mental health, particularly depression, and caregiver ratings of a patient's quality of life (Logsdon, Gibbons, McCurry, Teri, 2001). Depressive symptoms in caregivers were associated with lower ratings of patient quality of life, suggesting that caregivers are not accurate reporters, but rather transfer their own negative perceptions onto patients.

A related result is shown in Figure 9.1, which displays patient reports of enjoyment in activity, caregiver perceptions of patient enjoyment in activity, and the relationship between each of these reports and *patient* reports of depressive symptoms. The figure is based on reports from 161 patient-caregiver pairs in a clinical cohort of mildly demented Alzheimer's patients followed at Columbia University. Patient reports of enjoyment in activity were correlated with patient depressive symptoms. Caregiver reports of patient enjoyment were less clearly related to patient depressive symptoms. Thus, at least in the case of enjoyment of activity, patient reports may be more accurate than caregiver reports.

This situation contrasts with other domains of patient experience, in which caregiver reports may, in fact, be more accurate than patient

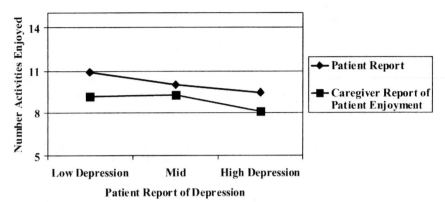

FIGURE 9.1 Mild Dementia: Patient Reports of Enjoyment in Activity Correlated with Patient-Reported Depressive Symptoms.
n = 161, ratings from patients with mild dementia and caregivers.

reports. In the same Columbia clinical cohort, for example, caregiver reports of the *frequency* of patient activity were significantly correlated with the patient's Mini-Mental Status score. By contrast, patient reports of activity frequency were not related to patient cognitive status. Thus, for these mildly demented elders reports of affective experience (enjoyment in activity) are likely to be more accurate than reports of the frequency of behaviors or symptoms.

A recent area of research has been the care and more general psychosocial preferences of community-dwelling elders. As Carpenter and colleagues point out, "Just as people have unique wishes about the medical care they receive [as in the case of advanced directives], they may have unique wishes about the personal care they receive as they become more dependent" (Carpenter, Van Haitsma, Ruckdeschel, & Lawton, 2000 p. 335). Documenting these preferences is useful for the concurrent delivery of care, but may also be useful for establishing an "advanced psychosocial directive," a statement about preferred care delivery and living situation that can be consulted when a person is no longer able to state these preferences. This approach would likely allow individualized care planning rather than current standard service plans.

In a pilot concept-mapping approach to psychosocial preferences, Carpenter and colleagues (2000) found that preferences for care and caregiving formed a well-defined cluster, distinct from other domains (such as "growth activities," "leisure," or "self-dominion"). On a scale of 1–5 to indicate importance, preferences in this domain ranged from 4.35 ("caregivers should know about my medical conditions and treatment") to 1.90 ("caregivers should address me by my first name"). Midrange preferences included "having friends involved in my care," "using alternative medicine providers," "having caregivers call me by a particular name," and "accepting restrictions for my safety." The investigators are conducting a larger study using a more extensive inventory to assess daily preferences, the Preferences for Everyday Living Inventory.

We used a modified version of this preference inventory to examine concordance between family and formal caregivers on the perceived preferences of people with dementia for particular activities. For this study, we enrolled patients with mild to moderate dementia who were attending an adult day care program at a senior center. We identified the primary family caregiver (the person making sure the needs of the patient were met, either directly or by arranging services). The formal caregiver in every case was a home attendant who provided care in the patient's home and also accompanied the elder to the adult day care program. The families and home attendants in this study were Spanish-speakers. We reasoned that concordance between the two different types of caregiver would indicate that mild to moderately demented patients are able to communicate preferences (even if they cannot state them in an interview or research questionnaire). Each type of caregiver was asked to rate how important particular behaviors or activities were to the patient on a 4-point Likert scale (very, some, little, or no importance).

Concordance between family and formal care providers was quite good. We examined the proportion of patients for whom family caregiver and home attendant maximally disagreed (i.e., where one said the activity was "very important" and the other said "no importance"). For activities with low frequency (< 25% of patients reported to consider it very important or of some importance), pairs were discordant less than 15% of the time. These preferences included the wish to be left alone, to have a challenging task, to talk about worries, and to keep to a particular routine. For more commonly preferred activities (reported to be preferred by > 40% of patients), such as choosing what clothes to wear, hearing the news, spending time outside, and having visitors, discordance was also relatively uncommon and was again about 15%. We conclude that mild to moderately demented patients can express preferences, as evident in joint recognition of such preferences by people who spend time with these elders.

Upgrading Home Attendant and Nursing Assistant Care

As we have seen, home care paraprofessionals are an important element in the long-term care spectrum. They provide support for elders with ADL needs severe enough to require nursing home levels of care.

These paraprofessionals do not have medical training and are barred from providing help with prescriptions or medical equipment. Low-income elders are eligible for Medicaid-waiver home attendant services, as in New York City's Home Care Services Program, which provides ADL support to 60,000 elders in the city. In fact, Health Care Financing Administration data show that New York City has the highest percentage of Medicaid recipients using home care services and the highest expenditures for such services (HCFA, 1997).

Nearly a third of the elders receiving home care through this program have moderate to severe dementia and half some degree of cognitive impairment (Hokenstad, Ramirez, Haslanger, & Finneran, 1997). In fact, in a study of elders with Alzheimer's disease living in the community, we noted that more than half the sample received ADL support from home care paraprofessionals. Moreover, a quarter of the sample received *all* ADL care from such paraprofessionals (Albert et al., 1998).

Home care paraprofessionals are typically referred to as "home attendants" (HA). A typical care arrangement might include a block of daily home attendant time (4, 8, 12, or 24 hours), with weekly visits from a visiting nurse service and quarterly re-evaluation of the elder by the home care-agency. Home care agency care coordinators supervise groups of attendants, and HA's are required to meet in-service requirements on a regular basis.

The difficulty of the HA–client relationship is apparent in a number of ways: HA's are family and not family; they perform roles typically assumed by family but are also performing a job. They may care for more than one client at a time, sometimes in "cluster care" arrangements. They are often asked to perform tasks outside the scope of their duties. They have to get along with other family members. They are isolated for a large part of the day with a person who has some authority over them but is also dependent on them.

We interviewed 70 home attendants, from two home health care agencies, in 1997–1998 to better understand their situation. These were seasoned paraprofessionals; inclusion criteria required that they had at least 1 year of experience. We found that HA's in New York City are almost exclusively female, members of minority groups, and largely immigrants. Their median age was 49 and the median length of time in the U.S. was 17 years, suggesting that these women were well-established breadwinners for their families. They had worked as HA's for a median of 9.5 years, and most were working full time (with overtime) in this capacity. The median number of clients they had been assigned over time was 12, with one of every four clients reported to be demented.

In their current situation, the median number of hours spent with the index client was 55.0/week over a median of 4 days per week. The high number reflects the large number of HA's spending 24 hours per day with clients for 3–4 days per week. It also reflects the low-wage nature of the work and the need for these women to work extremely long hours. In fact, 44% of the HA's had another client, and the median number of hours for such second clients was 12.0/week.

The median age of their clients was 82, of whom 86% were women. HA's reported that more than half the elders showed signs of depression and that about 40% had Alzheimer's disease or stroke. Symptoms of poor health were highly prevalent among clients. About a third were reported to suffer from dyspnea, difficulty swallowing, or severe pain. Cognitive symptoms were also highly prevalent: 62% were reported to have a memory problem, 32% were said to be disoriented, and 5% were said to be vegetative. HA's provided help with bathing, dressing, and outdoor mobility in almost every case, and the majority of clients were also receiving aid in toileting, indoor mobility, and bed/chair transfer. Half the client sample was incontinent, a third were limited to bed or chair, and 16% could not be taken outside. Thus, these elders were receiving support equivalent to nursing home care.

We asked home attendants to rate how difficult it was to provide care for their clients and examined correlates of these ratings. The strongest correlate of perceived "easiness" was client emotional status. "Easy" clients were reported to demonstrate positive affects more frequently than other clients ($r = 0.40$, $p < .01$). They were also seen as more satisfied with the care provided by the HA ($r = 0.30$, $p < .05$). The presence of daily medical symptoms was associated with greater difficulty in providing care ($r = -0.27$), but none of the other indicators of poor function or general medical status achieved statistical significance. Severity of functional deficit was not strongly associated with HA judgments of client difficulty, suggesting that HA's view this aspect of their work as a "job," without the emotional valence family caregivers attribute to such care.

We have found that almost all in-services for home attendants stress the physical demands of care, and not help with practical issues that might mitigate the more emotionally charged challenges of home care. We have developed a manual, based heavily on our interviews with home attendants, to remedy this gap (Albert, 2002). To give the flavor of this approach, Table 9.4, provides an excerpt from the manual.

Developing training in this practical approach to the dilemmas of home care would go a long way. A second approach would be to "credentialize" paraprofessional care, that is, make it more of a profession, with standardized training, licensure, and opportunity for continued training leading to nursing degrees. This would likely result in wage increases and improvement of work conditions.

Similar challenges appear to be at work among certified nursing assistants (CNA), who provide the bulk of care, as we have seen, in

TABLE 9.4 Excerpt: Home Attendants Speak About Home Care

What You Do . . . When You Feel You Can't Handle the Job but Feel You Can't Give the Job Up

Sometimes conditions in a home or with a particular client are just not acceptable. You can notify the agency and complain, or give up the job. But because of the wait to get a new long-term client assignment, you may be reluctant to complain or leave.

One home attendant reported that she did put up with a terrible home situation, where they would not even let her use the toilet, because she did not feel she could afford to give up the job. Another mentioned that she did not report neglect of the client to the agency for the same reason. She was afraid the agency would call the family, and that the family would dismiss her. As she put it, *"You cannot tell them. You have to walk into that house everyday. You don't know what they will do to you."*

But other home attendants disagreed. *"If you feel the family might threaten you or something, you don't want to be there. You don't go back there."* Or, as another said, *"I am not going to put myself in that kind of predicament. I will tell the agency that they better take me out of there."* Even home attendants who had put up with terrible conditions in the past because they felt they needed a job now agreed that it was not a good strategy. Better to quit the job than face abuse.

One complication, though, is concern for neglected or abused clients. *"If I see something like that, I don't stay on the job but you feel sorry for the client."* Still, no one benefits, neither you or the client, if you keep quiet about a situation of neglect or abuse. The welfare of clients requires that you report the problem to the agency. This allows the agency to arrange for the proper intervention.

How do you let the agency know about a problem with a client or home? Using the telephone in the home may be a problem because of privacy. Clients and families may listen in. One solution is to call while you are out doing errands: *"When I call the agency to speak to the coordinator, I always try to call when the client sends me to the store. So I call when I am out in the street."*

---

nursing homes. They provide almost all "bed and body work" for residents and, as a result, have the most daily contact with residents. As we have described in chapter 6, new efforts are underway to take advantage of CNA's greater contact with residents to improve resident care, especially in the setting of special care units for people with Alzheimer's disease (see below).

Do CNA's view residents the same way as nurses or nurse managers do? Or does their greater contact with residents lead them to rate residents differently? We examined this issue in a pilot study. Forty CNA's were asked to nominate a "difficult" and an "easy" resident under their care. They then completed eight questions regarding these residents' behaviors, which were drawn from the nursing home Minimum Data Set form. CNA ratings were compared to the nurse-rated MDS record within the same month.

On the whole, agreement between CNA ratings and MDS scores was low. For example, in the case of verbal abuse, 24 of 40 CNA's reported verbal abuse from the resident, which was recorded in only one MDS chart for this set of residents. On almost every indicator, CNA's reported more symptoms (depressive mood, memory problems, dependence in daily tasks, and physical abuse) than the MDS record. These findings need to be investigated further. It may be that CNA's use different criteria when completing MDS forms, or, more likely, daily contact with residents allows them to identify greater deficits. If CNA ratings were incorporated into MDS records, different resident assessment protocols would be triggered and perhaps more intensive care plans.

Special Care Units for People with Alzheimer's Disease

Freiman and Brown (2001) point out that today's nursing home population is more functionally and cognitively disabled and requires more skilled and/or specialized care than ever before. Special care units (SCU) for Alzheimer's disease have been developed to meet this need. The Medical Expenditures Panel Study (MEPS) found that over 10% of nursing homes in the United States, 2,130 homes, had an Alzheimer's unit, for a total of 73,400 SCU beds. These SCU's are relatively small, in keeping with the greater staff time and more specialized staff assignments typical of the units. The MEPS survey found that Alzheimer's units contained a mean of 34 beds (Freiman & Brown).

Despite the growth in specialized care for Alzheimer's disease, at this point there is still no standard definition of an SCU. Units called "SCU's" differ considerably in environmental design, physical separation from other units in nursing homes, specialized dementia care training for staff, staffing ratios, and activity programming (Morris, Emerson-Lombardo, 1994; Teresi, Holmes, Ramirez, & Kong, 1998). This variation has posed difficulties for the assessment of the SCU as a superior approach in Alzheimer's care.

Outcome studies have not found an SCU benefit in slowing the trajectory of functional or cognitive decline (McCann, Bienas, & Evans, 2000; Phillips et al., 1997). The SCU setting, however, may offer benefit in promoting participation in activity (as measured by behavior stream real-time observation) and resident well-being (as observed in ratings of resident affective expression) (Holmes, Teresi, & Ory, 2000).

While results to date have been mixed for SCU evaluations, the evaluation effort has been useful in drawing attention to features of environment and staffing that affect resident well-being. One finding of interest is that environmental simplification for residents with Alzheimer's in the absence of increased staffing may have negative effects (Van Haitsma, Lawton, & Kleban, 2000). On the other hand, changes in lighting may affect sleep patterns, which may in turn affect agitation behaviors (Kutner & Bliwise, 2000). Low levels of light, excess glare, noise, and other environmental sounds may be easily altered sources of excess morbidity for Alzheimer's patients (Sloan, Mitchell, Calkins, & Zimmerman, 2000). Changing staff assignments so that particular certified nursing aides (CNAs) are assigned to particular residents may promote resident participation in organized activity (Lindeman, Arnsberger, & Owens, 2000).

The role of nursing home staff, particularly the CNA, as an agent of resident well-being is only now being fully appreciated. Innovations in the delivery of nursing home care are now underway and undergoing evaluation to see if giving staff greater latitude to change the way they deliver care offers benefit to residents. For example, in one labor-management partnership in New York City, staff on certain demonstration units is free to assign more time to certain activities (such as bathing or feeding), based on their understanding of resident needs and unit dynamics. In another nursing home, CNAs are being encouraged to upgrade clinical skills, communicate information they have obtained about resident health, and participate in comprehensive care planning meetings for residents. The role of labor-management partnerships in this effort is critical.

Expansion of Options for Supportive Care and Housing

Kane (1995) has identified a series of policy challenges for home care that would give adequate scope to the preference of frail older people to live in homes, rather than institutions, and that would also give greater flexibility to service providers to cross current, fixed service categories. She urges policymakers to think beyond the rigid service categories that have been linked to particular living environments, such as home care, board and care or assisted living care, and nursing home care.

This change has already begun. "Home care" paraprofessionals now assist clients outside the home as they travel, shop, go to physician appointments, attend adult day care, or simply go outside for exercise or entertainment. "Home care" paraprofessionals also provide ADL care and housekeeping support to frail elderly who do not live in "homes" in the traditional sense, but who instead reside in group settings, such as board and care homes or single room occupancy hotels (that have become de facto sites for long-term care). This is a welcome development, for it suggests that people can hold on to "home" despite severe ADL needs, and that providing ADL support can be made flexible enough to accommodate different kinds of home settings and preferred personal lifestyles.

Implicit in this expansion of the home care concept is recognition that the nursing home is mostly a residence rather than a site for medical or nursing care. The 24–hour care designation of the nursing home is a fiction. Kane (1995) points out that these prescribed settings provide remarkably little nursing care. One study of nursing home care, reported by Kane, showed that 39% of residents received no care from a registered nurse in a 24–hour period. The mean duration of nursing care over this 24–hour period was quite small: for RN care, 7.9 minutes; for LPN care, 15.5 minutes; and for CNA care 76.9 minutes. Thus, the nursing home is mainly a residence, and care of this sort or degree could be brought into homes, though not necessarily in as cost-effective a manner. "This modest amount of care cannot be replicated at home for the same price because the nursing home efficiently provides stand-by assistance and can meet unscheduled, quickly arising needs" (Kane, 1995, p. 171). The program for All Inclusive Care of the Elderly (PACE) has developed models, however, that allow cost-effective home care service in lieu of nursing home care, provided that housing services are altered to create more easily serviced groups of elders.

While extending what we mean by "home care," it is also worth thinking about ways to extend the flexibility of "service provision." Two such efforts are underway. One is to allow greater delegation of nursing skills in home care settings. Traditionally, only nurses could administer medications, care for wounds, monitor vital signs, perform catheter or ostomy care, or suction patients who are on ventilators. Kane (1995) reminds us that families have always performed these tasks, and that family members learn these skills from nurses. There really is no reason less skilled formal caregivers, such as home care paraprofessionals, cannot take on these tasks. It would mean an upgrading of their skills, a boon to family members, and a significant cost savings.

A second development in the expansion of services is a shift in the balance of authority between home care providers and families. The "consumer-directed care" movement allows elders and their families to use funds assigned for a home care benefit (such as the Medicaid personal assistance home care benefit) to hire, train, and employ home care aides as they think best. In practice, families are helped by home care agencies in this process. The agencies suggest lists of potential workers, provide training and counseling on how to be an employer, and usually manage disbursement of funds. A major demonstration to assess consumer-directed care is underway for this program, which is likely to become more important.

Supporting Family Caregivers

Family caregiving, as we have mentioned earlier (chapters 5 and 6), is a major challenge in care of the frail or demented elder. Families overwhelmed by the stresses of caregiving may resort to nursing home placement even when this is not a preferred choice. They may simply feel they have no other option once the stresses of caregiving and lack of respite have undermined coping resources and family function. A program of psychosocial support might strengthen caregivers resources and help them manage the stresses of care better. Would such a program, if effectively delivered, also reduce rates of nursing home placement? This difference in outcome would be a powerful demonstration of the effects of psychosocial support to vulnerable families, and in the case of spouse caregivers, highly vulnerable elders.

Mittelman and colleagues designed such a program for caregiving spouses of people with Alzheimer's disease and tested it in a randomized controlled trial of nursing home placement. The intervention was designed to guide and support caregivers through the challenging period when spouses progressed to increasingly severe dementia. In the first 4 months of the study, spouses received two individual counseling sessions and four family sessions. "Counseling sessions were task oriented, promoting communication among family members, teaching techniques for problem solving and management of troublesome patient behavior, and improving both emotional and instrumental support for the primary caregiver." This phase was followed by participation in a support group and finally by continuing availability of contact with counselors. The control group received usual follow-up and information and referral. Thus, "if control subjects asked about obtaining paid help at home, they were given the names of service providers, whereas treatment subjects were given as much help as they needed to find and appropriately use such services" (Mittelman et al., 1996 p. 1729).

After 3.5 years, 58.7% of patients in this sample of 206 families had entered nursing homes and 26.2% had died at home. In addition, not all caregivers in the intervention group agreed to support group participation; only 72% joined support groups. However, 42% of controls joined such support groups. Despite this combined drop-out and "drop-in" dilution of the experiment, patients in the treatment group remained at home significantly longer than patients in the control group. Treatment group patients entered nursing homes about a year later than controls. This difference was obtained in survival models that controlled for age and gender of caregivers, socioeconomic resources, caregiver mental health, and severity of dementia.

Mittelman and colleagues (1996, p.1730) conclude that "continuously available support and information can enable spouse caregivers of AD patients to withstand the difficulties of caregiving and avoid or defer institutionalization of the patients." This conclusion is supported by the design of the experiment but also by absence of differences in patient care between intervention and control groups. For example, patients in the two groups were equally likely to receive psychotropic medications and medical care. Thus, the intervention appears to have affected caregivers rather than patients. Patients were equally likely to develop urinary incontinence and equally likely to receive medical care for the condition, but intervention group caregivers, through support from training and counseling, were better able to manage the demands of care related to incontinence.

This finding is reassuring, given the absence or unclear benefit for a variety of other interventions involving patient and caregiver outcomes, including respite programs (Lawton, Brody, & Pruchno, 1991) and home attendant care (Weissert, Chernow, & Hirth, 2003). On the other hand, benefit has been reported for caregiver mental health, as in the Medicare Alzheimer's Disease Demonstration (Newcomer, Spitalny, Fox, & Yordi, 1999). As the United States moves toward increasing incentives for family caregivers (mostly in the form of tax breaks) and a greater diversity of services that can be provided in homes, it will become increasingly important to figure out what kinds of resources families need to be effective caregiving units.

Upstreaming Palliative Care

In chapter 4 we already mentioned that most of the expense of medical care in late life is related to end-of-life care, and that the costs of dying decline with a greater age at death. We know also that the use of life-sustaining treatments at the end of life in older people is still quite high. For example, among people aged 80+ who died in the Hospitalized Elderly Longitudinal Project (HELP), 54% were admitted to an intensive care unit, 43% were put on ventilators, 18% received cardiopulmonary resuscitation, 18% had feeding tubes placed, 14% received blood transfusions, and 6% had hemodialysis—even though 70% stated they wanted comfort care only and 80% had completed do-not-resuscitate orders (Somogyi-Zalud, Zhong, Hamel, & Lynn, 2002).

Limiting aggressive care for people at the end of life should be complemented by greater use of palliative care principles when people are still outside the traditional window of eligibility for hospice services.

This window is currently 6 months, as established in the Medicare hospice benefit. Hospice benefits are available to Medicare beneficiaries if a physician certifies that the patient is terminally ill and has a life expectancy of less than 6 months (though the benefit can be extended if patients are recertified). Recipients must also sign a form that they accept the hospice benefit and are willing to forego curative treatment related to this terminal condition (but not necessarily curative treatment for other conditions). It is, of course, difficult to predict survival, as we have already shown (chapter 4). Currently, users of the Medicare benefit spend about 50 days on hospice (Gage, Miller, Mor, Jackson, & Harvell, 2000), suggesting underuse and missed opportunities for palliation even in the minority of dying elders who do make use of the benefit.

Moving palliative care back in time, that is, away from the point of death, is the premise of "upstreaming." It suggests a breaking down of the current mostly rigid boundary between curative and palliative care. What would happen if the hospice care benefit were offered to people with a life expectancy of 1 year, rather than 6 months? Or what outcomes would likely change if hospice services were made available earlier for people with specific progressive, terminal diseases? Would people accept the service? Would physicians suggest it? How might hospice service itself have to change to accommodate the needs of people 9 or 12 months from death? The current hospice benefit has saved the Medicare system significant expense. Would an expanded benefit result in further cost savings? These questions need to be investigated if the full benefits of the palliative orientation are to be realized.

SUMMARY

Preventing Frailty. Great progress has been made in understanding the origin of frailty in late life, which may suggest ways to reduce the risk of physical and cognitive disability in people who have already entered old age. Frailty in the absence of chronic disease may be a consequence of a disease process that has failed to cause frank disease, as in the end-organ damage hypothesis. Or it may be a consequence of the body's response to a disease process, as in the inflammatory hypothesis.

Reducing the Risk of Falling. Falls occupy a prominent position in the case of deaths due to injury and also play a role in the institutionalization of older people. The many different risk factors for falling, representing disparate physiological systems, suggest that falling is a geriatric syndrome (like urinary incontinence, slow gait speed, or lower extremity weakness), a syndrome of poor or inefficient function with many causes. Fall risk can be reduced if risk factors are addressed. In the FICSIT trials, improvements in balance and reduction in orthostatic hypotension were each associated with lower rates of falling.

Preserving Independence through Pre-habilitation. Can the skills or abilities required for independent living be taught or bolstered in such a way that the risk of disability is reduced? This is the premise of "pre-habilitation." Randomized clinical trials have addressed two targets for such pre-habilitation. One target includes factors extrinsic to aging that are nevertheless associated with disablement, such as safety awareness, efficient use of adaptive equipment, energy conservation, and efficient use of public transportation. The second target, which sometimes overlaps with the first, stresses functional limitation, an intrinsic feature of aging. Randomized clinical trials have shown benefit for both approaches.

Cognitive Remediation. A similar approach has been developed for cognitive disability. Cognitive interventions helped normal elderly perform better on the specific cognitive skills for which they were trained. These benefits suggest that the slow cognitive declines reported for nondemented elders can be remediated.

Identifying the At-Risk Elder and Effectively Managing Disease. The core of geriatric evaluation and management (GEM) is comprehensive geriatric assessment. This assessment includes medical, psychological, and functional assessment that is integrated to develop an overall plan for treatment and follow-up. GEM now includes a variety of program elements, which have been combined in many different ways, with mixed results. Still, the overall benefit of GEM is clear, provided that GEM units are able to see that recommendations are followed.

Promoting Self-Management and Family Involvement in Chronic Disease Care. People differ in their capacity to manage the disability and symptoms typical of chronic disease. It would be valuable to know what is involved in successful management of chronic disease. It would also be valuable to know whether such skills can be taught, and if disease management in this sense is associated with important health outcomes, such as physician utilization or hospitalization. The Chronic Disease Self-Management Program (CDSMP) has been used to teach patients to manage symptoms well, communicate effectively with health professionals, and develop realistic appraisals of the health risks they face. Randomized clinical trials of the program have shown the acceptability of the intervention and its ability to promote more effective use of health care services.

Managing Polypharmacy. Polypharmacy is not inappropriate medication use, but simply use of many medications, all potentially appropriate. It is a problem, however, because of the greater risk of adverse events associated with a greater number of medications. Also, the greater the number of medications, the less likely compliance, and hence the greater the risk that people will not take medications they should be taking. An important task for public health in aging is continual reassessment of medications and elimination of medications that have been supplanted or which can no longer be justified.

Enhancing Custodial Care. For the severely demented individual receiving formal home care services, or the older patient receiving ventilator care in a nursing home, excellent custodial care should be the goal but will most likely not extend survival or lead to regained function. What, then, are goals for enhanced custodial care? Dignity, privacy, a sense of security, and the opportunity to participate in meaningful activity or reciprocal social relationships are the essence of sensitive treatment of any person. Thus, goals for care in this case are no more difficult than ones we set for ourselves and expect in daily activity.

Taking the Care Preferences of Older People Seriously. It may be valuable to obtain the care preferences of people, just as we currently obtain advanced directives for hospital care. These preferences can be elicited and incorporated into care plans. Even mild to moderately demented patients express preferences, as evident in joint recognition of such preferences by people who spend time with these patients.

Upgrading Home Attendant and Certified Nursing Assistant Care. Training in the practical dilemmas of home care would go a long way in improving the position of home attendants, who provide an increasingly large amount of home care. A second approach would be to credentialize paraprofessional care, that is, make it more of a profession, with standardized training, licensure, and opportunity for continued training leading to nursing degrees. This would likely result in wage increases and improvement of work conditions.

Certified nursing assistants (CNA) in nursing homes face similar challenges. New efforts are underway to take advantage of CNA's greater contact with residents to improve resident care, especially in the setting of special care units for people with Alzheimer's disease.

Special Care Units for People with Alzheimer's Disease. Outcome studies have not found an SCU benefit in slowing the trajectory of functional or cognitive decline. The SCU setting, however, may offer benefit in promoting participation in activity and resident well-being. Because SCU's differ considerably in features, assessment of this benefit is difficult.

Expanding the Concept of "Home Care" and "Service Delivery." Home care now is delivered outside the home and to people who do not live in traditional homes. Likewise, people who traditionally did not deliver services now deliver services and consumers, rather than providers, now supervise the delivery of such services. This may be a positive development, as it allows greater autonomy for elders and greater flexibility for providers.

Supporting Family Caregivers. Providing support and information can enable caregivers of AD patients to cope with the challenges of home care and avoid or defer institutionalization of patients. These sorts of support are critical and are increasingly being recognized as important by providers and legislators.

Upstreaming Palliative Care. Hospice benefits are available to Medicare beneficiaries if a physician certifies that the patient is terminally ill and has a life expectancy of less than 6 months. Moving palliative care back in time, that is, away from the point of death ("upstreaming") would help break down the current mostly rigid boundary between curative and palliative care. It remains to be seen if early use of palliative care would be acceptable to patients and families, and how this change would affect outcomes in the last year of life.

References

Abrams, R. C., Lachs, M., McAvay, G., Keohane, D. J., & Bruce, M. L. (2002). Predictors of self-neglect in community-dwelling elders. *Am J Psychiatry, 159*(10), 1724–30.

Ahronheim, J. C., Morrison, R. S., Baskin, S. A., Morris, J., Meier, D. E. (1996). Treatment of the dying in the acute care hospital: Advanced dementia and metastatic cancer. *Arch Intern Med., 156*(18), 2094–2100.

Albert, S. M. Assessing health-related quality of life in elderly chronic care populations. In J. A. Teresi, M. P. Lawton, D. Holmes, & M. Ory (Eds.), *Measurement in elderly chronic care populations* (pp. 210–227). New York: Springer.

Albert, S. M. (1999). The caregiver as part of the dementia management team. *Disease Management and Health Outcomes, 5*(6), 329–337.

Albert, S. M. (2000). Time and function. In R. L. Rubinstein, M. Moss, & M. H. Kleban (Eds.), *The many dimensions of aging* (pp. 57–67). New York: Springer.

Albert, S. M. (2002). *Being There for Someone: Home Attendants Speak about Home Care.* Fan Fox & Leslie R. Samuels Foundation. New York.

Albert, S. M., & Brody, E. M. When elder care is viewed as child care: Significance of elders' cognitive impairment and caregiver burden. *Am J Geriatr Psychiat 4,* 121–130.

Albert, S. M., Castillo-Castaneda, C., Jacobs, D. M., Sano, M., Bell, K., Merchant, C., et al. (1999). Proxy-reported quality of life in Alzheimer's patients: Comparison of clinical and population-based samples. *J Mental Health and Aging, 5*(1), 49–58.

Albert, S. M., Cattell, M. G. (1994). *Old age in global perspective.* New York: G. K. Hall/McMillan.

Albert, S. M., Costa, R., Merchant, C., Small, S., Jenders, R. A., & Stern Y. (1999). Hospitalization and Alzheimer's disease: Results from a community-based study. *J Gerontology: Med Sci 54A,* M267–M271.

Albert, S. M., Del Castillo-Castaneda, C., Sano, M., Jacobs, D. M., Marder, K., Bell, K., Bylsma, F., Lafleche, G., Brandt, J., Albert, M., Stern Y. Quality of life in patients with Alzheimer's disease as reported by patient proxies. *J Am Geriatr Soc, 44*(11), 1342–1347.

249

Albert, S. M., Glied, S., Andrews, H., Stern, Y., & Mayeux, R. (2002). Primary care expenditures before the onset of Alzheimer's disease. *Neurology 59*(4), 573–578.

Albert, S. M., Im, A., & Raveis V. (2002). Public health and the second 50 years of life. *Am J Public Health 92,* 1214–1216.

Albert, S. M., Jacobs, D. M., Sano, M., Marder, K., Bell, K., Devanand, D., Brandt, J., Albert, M., & Stern, Y. (2001, Spring). Longitudinal study of quality of life in people with advanced Alzheimer's disease. *Am J Geriatr Psychiatry, 9*(2), 160–168.

Albert, S. M., Logsdon, R.G. (Eds.). (2001) *Assessing quality of life in alzheimer's disease.* New York: Springer.

Albert, S. M., Michaels, K., Padilla, M., Pelton, G., Bell, K., Marder, K., Stern, Y., & Devanand, D. P. (1999). Functional significance of mild cognitive impairment in elderly patients without a dementia diagnosis. *Am J Geriatric Psychiatry 7,* 213–220.

Albert, S. M., O'Neil, M., Muller, C., & Butler R. (2002). When does old age begin? Results from a national survey. New York: International Longevity Center.

Albert, S. M., Sano, M., Bell, K., Merchant, C., Small, S., & Stern, Y. (1998). Hourly care received by people with Alzheimer's disease: Results from an urban, community-based survey, *The Gerontologist, 38*(6), 704–714.

Albert, S. M., & Stern, Y. (2001). Cultural factors and risk of Alzheimer's disease. Gerontological Society of America, Chicago.

Albert, S. M., Tabert, M. H., Dienstag, A., Pelton, G., & Devanand D. (2002, February). The impact of mild cognitive impairment on functional abilities in the elderly. *Curr Psychiatry Rep, 4*(1), 64–68.

Albert, S. M., & Teresi, J. A. (2002) Quality of life, definition and measurement. In Eckert, DJ., ed. *Encyclopedia of Aging* (vol 4, pp. 1158–1161). New York: MacMillian.

Albert, S. M., & Teresi, J. A. (1999). Reading ability, education, and cognitive status assessment among older adults in Harlem, New York City. *Am J Public Health 89,* 95–97.

Albert, S. M. (1998). Defining and measuring quality of life in medicine. *JAMA, 279*(6), 429.

Alecxih, L. M. B., Zeruld, S., & Olearczyk, B. (2002). Characteristics of caregivers based on the survey of income and program participation. Internet Publication. Falls Church, VA: The Lewin Group.

Alexopoulos, G. S., Buckwalter, K., Olin, J., Martinez, R., Wainscott, C., & Krishnan, K. R. (2002, September 15). Comorbidity of late life depression: an opportunity for research on mechanisms and treatment. *Biol Psychiatry, 52*(6), 543–558.

Alzheimer's Association, Basic statistics on Alzheimer's Disease, 2000. *http://www.alz.org/AboutAD/Statistics.htm.*

Arias, E. (2002). United States life tables, 2000. (National Vital Statistics Reports, Vol. 51, No. 3). Hyattsville, MD: National Center for Health Statistics.

Ball, K., Berch, D. B., Helmers, K. F., Jobe, J. B., Leveck, M. D., Marsiske, M., Morris, J. N., Rebok, G. W., Smith, D. M., Tennstadt, S. L., Unverzagt, F. W., & Willis, S. L., for the ACTIVE Study Group. (2002). Effects of cognitive training interventions with older adults: A randomized controlled trial. *JAMA 288*, 2271–2281.

Baltes, P. B. (1993). The aging mind: potential and limits. *Gerontologist, 33*(5), 580–594.

Barrick, A. L., Rader, J., Hoeffer, B., & Sloane, P. (Eds.). (2002). *Bathing without a battle: Personal care of individuals with dementia.* New York: Springer.

Beekman, A. T., Geerlings, S. W., Deeg, D. J., Smit, J. H., Schoevers, R. S., de Beurs, E., Braam, A. W., Penninx, B. W., & van Tilburg, W. (2002). The natural history of late-life depression: A 6–year prospective study in the community. *Arch Gen Psychiatry 59*(7), 605–611.

Beers, M. H., Ouslander, J. G., Fingold, S. F., Morganstern, H., Reuben, D. B., & Rogeres, W. (1992). Inappropriate medication prescribing in skilled nursing facilities. *Ann Intern Med, 117,* 684–689.

Benton, A. L. (1955). *The Benton visual retention test.* New York: The Psychological Corporation.

Benton, A. L. (1967). *FAS test.* University of Victoria, Victoria, B.C.

Bergner, M., Bobbitt, R. A., Pollard, W. E., Martin, D. P., & Gilson, B. S. (1976, January). The sickness impact profile: validation of a health status measure. *Med Care, 14*(1), 57–67.

Berzon, R. A., Leplege, A. P., Lohr, K. N., Lenderking, W. R., & Wu, A. W. (1997, August). Summary and recommendations for future research. *Qual Life Res, 6*(6), 601–605.

Blackwell, D. L., Collins, J. G., Coles R. (2002). Summary health statistics for U.S. Adults: National Health Interview Survey, 1997. *Vital Health Stat 10*(205). National center for Health statistics.

Borson, S., Barnes, R. A., Kukull, W. A., Okimoto, J. T., Veith, R. C., Inui, T. S., et al.. (1986, May). Symptomatic depression in elderly medical outpatients. I. Prevalence, demography, and health service utilization. *J Am Geriatr Soc., 34*(5), 341–7.

Bortz, W. M. (1989). Redefining human aging. *J Am Geriatr Soc, 37*(11), 1092–1096.

Boult, C., Altmann, M., Gilbertson, D., Yu, C., & Kane, R. L. (1996). Decreasing disability in the 21ˢᵗ century: The future effects of controlling six fatal and nonfatal conditions. *Am J Public Health, 86*(10), 1388–1393.

Boult, C., Kane, R. L., Louis, T. A., Boult, L., & McCaffrey, D. (1994, January). Chronic conditions that lead to functional limitation in the elderly. *J Gerontol, 49*(1), M28–M36.

Boult, C., & Pacala, J. T. (1999). Care of older people at risk. In E. Calkins, C., Boult, E. H. Wagner, & J. T. Pacala (Ed.). *New ways to care for older people: Building systems based on evidence* (pp. 65–81). New York: Springer.

Brod, M., Stewart, A. L., & Sands, L. (2001). Conceptualization of quality of life in dementia. In S. M. Albert, R. G. Logsdon (Eds.). *Assessing quality of life in alzheimer's disease* (pp. 3–16). New York: Springer Publishing.

Brookmeyer, R., Corrada, N. M., Curriero, F. C., & Kawas, C. Survival following diagnosis of Alzheimer's disease. *Arch Neurol, 59*(11), 1764–1767.

Brookmeyer, R., Gray, S., & Kawas C. (1998, September). Projections of Alzheimer's disease in the United States and the public health impact of delaying disease onset. *Am J Public Health, 88*(9), 1337–1342.

Bruce, M. L., Seeman, T. E., Merrill, S. S., & Blazer, D. G. (1994). The impact of depressive symptomatology on physical disability: MacArthur Studies of Successful Aging. *Am J Public Health, 84*(11), 1796–1799.

Buchner, D. M., Cress, E., de LaTour, B. J., Essleman, P. C., Margherita, A. J., Price, R., et al. (1997). The effect of strength and endurance training on gait, balance, fall risk, and health services use in community-living older adults. *J Gerontol: Med Sci, 52A*, M218–M224.

Buchner, D. M., Larson, E. B., Wagner, E. H., Koepsell, T. D., & de Lateur, B. J. (1996). Evidence for a non-linear relatationship between leg strength and gait speed. *Age and Aging, 25*, 386–391.

Buchner, D. M. (1999). Prevention of frailty. In E. Calkins, E., C. Boult, E. H. Wagner, & J. T. Pacala (Eds.). *New ways to care for older people: Building systems based on evidence* (pp. 3–19). New York: Springer Press.

Bushke, H., & Fuld, P. A. (1974). Evaluating storage, retention, and retrieval in disordered memory and learning. *Neurology, 24*(11), 1019–1025.

Butler, R. N. (1969). Age-ism: Another form of bigotry. *Gerontologist, 9*(4), 243–6.

Callahan, D. (1987). Setting the limits: Medical goals in an aging society. Washington, D.C.: Georgetown University Press.

Carey, J. R., Liedo, P., Orozco, D., & Vaupel, J.W. (1992). Slowing of mortality rates at older ages in large medfly cohorts. *Science, 258*, 457–461.

CDC. (2000, July 24). Deaths, United States, 2000. *National Vital Statistics Reports, Vol 48, No 11.* Hyattsville, MD: National Center for Health Statistics.

Cummings, J. L. (1997, May). The Neuropsychiatric Inventory: assessing psychopathology in dementia patients. *Neurology, 48*(5 Suppl 6), S10–S16.

Carey, J. R., Liedo, P., Muller, H. G., Wang, J. L., Vaupel, J. W. (1998). Dual modes of aging in Mediterranean fruit fly females. *Science, 281*(5379), 996–998.

Carpenter, B. D., Van Haitsma, K., Ruckdeschel, K., & Lawton, M. P. (2000, June). The psychosocial preferences of older adults: a pilot examination of content and structure. *Gerontologist, 40*(3), 335–348.

Health Care Financing Administration. (1997). *Office of the Actuary: Data from the Office of National Health Statistics.* Baltimore, MD: Office of the Actuary.

Carstensen, L. L. (1992). Social and emotional patterns in adulthood: Support for socioemotional selectivity theory. *Psychol Aging, 7*(3), 331–338.

Cella, D. F., & Bonomi, A. E. (1996). The Functional Assessment of Cancer Therapy (FACT) and Functional Assessment of HIV Infection (FAHI) quality of life measurement system. In B. Spilker (Ed.), *Quality of life and pharmacoeconomics in clinical trials* (pp. 203–225). Philadelphia: Lippincott-Raven.

Centers for Disease Control and Prevention. (2003). Trends in aging—United States and worldwide. *MMWR, 53*, 102–106.

Clark, F., Azen, S. P., Zemke, R., Jackson, J., Carlson, M., Mandel, D., et al. (1997). Occupational therapy for independent-living older adults. *JAMA, 278*(16), 1321–1325.

Coon, D. W., Ory, M. G., & Schulz, R. (2002). Family caregiving: Enduring and emergent themes. In D. W. Coon, D. Gallagher-Thompson, & L. W. Thompson (Eds.), *Innovative interventions to reduce dementia caregiver distress* (pp. 3–27). New York; Springer.

Corder, E. H., Saunders, A. M., Risch, N. J., Strittmatter, W. J., Schmechel, D. E., Gaskell, P. C. Jr., et al. (1994). Protective effect of apolipoprotein E type 2 allele for late onset Alzheimer disease. *Nat Genet, 7,* 180–184.

Costa, D. (2000). Understanding the twentieth century decline in chronic conditions among older men." *Demography 37*(1), 53–72.

Crews, D. E. (1990). Anthropological issues in biological anthropology. In R. Rubenstein (Ed.), *Anthropology and aging: Comprehensive reviews* (pp. 11–39). Dordrecht: Kluwer Academic Publishers.

Crews, J. E., & Smith, S. M. (2003). Public health and the second 50 years of life: Response to Albert, Im, & Raveis. *Am J Public Health, 93*(5), 700–701.

Crimmins, E. M., Hayward, M. D., & Saito Y. (1996). Differentials in active life expectancy in the older population of the United States. *The Journals of Gerontology, Psychological Science and Social Sciences, 51*(Bn3), S111–S120.

Crimmins, E. M., Saito, Y., & Reynolds, S. L. (1997). Further evidence on recent trends in the prevalence and incidence of disability among older Americans from two sources: The LSOA and the NHIS. *The Journal of Gerontology, Psychological science and social sciences, 52*B(2), S59–S71.

Crook, T., Bartus, R. T., Ferrish, S. H. (1986). Age-associated memory impairment: Proposed diagnostic criteria and measures of clinical change. Report of a National Institute of Mental Health Work Group. *Dev Neuropsychol, 2,* 261–276.

Crum, R. M., Anthony, J. C., Bassett, S. S., Folstein, M. F. (1993, May 12). Population-based norms for the Mini-Mental State Examination by age and educational level. *JAMA, 269*(18), 2386–2391.

Day, J. C. (1996). *Population projections of the United States by age, sex, race, and Hispanic origin: 1990–2050. (Current Population Reports,* Publication 25–1130). Washington, DC: US Government Printing Office.

Derogatis, L. R., Lipman, R. S., Rickels, K., Uhlenhuth, E. H., & Covi, L. (1974, January). The Hopkins Symptom Checklist (HSCL): A self-report symptom inventory. *Behav Sci, 19*(1), 1–15.

Devanand, D. P., Sano, M., Tang, M. X., Taylor, S., Gurland, B. J., Wilder, D., Stern, Y., & Mayeux, R. (1996, February). Depressed mood and the incidence of Alzheimer's disease in the elderly living in the community. *Arch Gen Psychiatry, 53*(2), 175–182.

Dolan, P., Gudex, C., Kind, P., & Williams A. (1996, April). Valuing health states: a comparison of methods. *J Health Econ, 15*(2), 209–231.

Dooneief, G., Marder, K., Tang, M. X., & Stern, Y. (1996, June). The Clinical Dementia Rating scale: community-based validation of "profound' and "terminal' stages. *Neurology, 46*(6), 1746–1749.

DSM-IV. Diagnostic and Statistical Manual of Mental Disorders, Fourth Edition. (2000). Washington, DC: American Psychiatric Association.

Elo, I. T., & Preston, S. H. (1996). Educational differentials in mortality: United States, 1979–85. *Social Science and Medicine 42*(1), 47–57.

Erickson, P., Wilson, R., & Shannon, I. (1995). *Years of healthy life. Healthy People 2000, Statistical Notes, No. 7.* Atlanta, GA: Centers for Disease Control.

Evans, J. E. (2002). What does the epidemiology of aging tell us now? Valencia Forum (Mardid-UN). http://www.valenciaforum.com/Keynotes/ge.html

Evers, M. M., Purohit, D., Perl, D., Khan, K., & Marin D. B. (2002, May). Palliative and aggressive end-of-life care for patients with dementia. *Psychiatr Serv, 53*(5), 609–613.

Fabiszewski, K. J., Volicer, B., & Volicer, L. (1990, June 20). Effect of antibiotic treatment on outcome of fevers in institutionalized Alzheimer patients. *JAMA, 263*(23), 3168–3172.

Farrer, L., & American College of Medical Genetics/American Society of Human Genetics Working Group on ApoE and Alzheimer Disease. (1995). Statement on Use of Apolipoprotein E Testing for Alzheimer Disease. *JAMA, 274*, 1627–1629.

Feder, J., Komisar, H. L., & Niefeld, M. (2001). Long-term care in the United States: An overview. *Health Affairs 19*(3), 40–56.

Federal Interagency Forum on Aging-Related Statistics. (2000). Older Americans 2000: Key indicators of well-being. http://www.agingstats.gov/chartbook2000/default.htm

Feeny, D., Furlong, W., Boyle, M., & Torrance, G. W. (1995, June). Multiattribute health status classification systems. Health Utilities Index. *Pharmacoeconomics, 7*(6), 490–502.

Feher, E. P., Larrabee, G. J., Sudilovsky, A., Crook, T. H. (1994). Memory self-report in Alzheimer's disease and in age-associated memory impairment. *J Geriatric Psychiatry Neurology, 6*, 58–65.

Feinstein, A. R., Josephy, B. R., & Wells, C. K. (1986, September). Scientific and clinical problems in indexes of functional disability. *Ann Intern Med, 105*(3), 413–420.

Ferrucci, L., Guralnik, J. M., Buchner, D., Kasper, J., Lamb, S. E., Simonsick, E. M., & Corti, M. C., Bandeen-Roche, K., Fried, L. P. (1997, September). Departures from linearity in the relationship between measures of muscular strength and physical performance of the lower extremities: the Women's Health and Aging Study. *J Gerontol A Biol Sci Med Sci, 52*(5), M275–M285.

Ferrucci, L., Guralnik, J. M., Simonsick, E., Salive, M. E., Corti, C., & Langlois J. (1996). Progressive versus catastrophic disability: A longitudinal view of the disablement process. *J Gerontol A Biol Sci Med Sci, 51*(3), M123–30.

Ferrucci, L., Harris, T. B., Guralnik, J. M., Tracy, R. P., Corti, M. C., Cohen, H. (1999). Serum IL-6 level and the development of disability in older persons. *J Am Geriatr Soc, 47*, 639–646.

Ferrucci, L., Penninx, B. W., Volpato, S., Harris, T. B., Bendeen-Roche, K., Balfour, J., Leveille, S. G., Fried, L. P., & Guralnik, J. M. (2002). Change in muscle strength explains accelerated decline of physical function in older women with high interleukin-6 serum levels. *J Am Geriatr Soc, 50,* 1947–1954.

Fiatarone, M. A., Marks, E. C., Ryan, N. D., Meredith, C. N., Lipsitz, L. A., & Evans, W. J. (1990). High-intensity strength training in nonagenerians: Effects on skeletal muscle. *JAMA, 263,* 3029–3034.

Fillenbaum, G., Heyman, A., Peterson, B., Pieper, C., Weiman, A. L. (2000). Frequency and duration of hospitalization of patients with AD based on Medicare data: CERAD XX. *Neurology, 54*(8), 740–743.

Fisher, A. G. (1997). *Assessment of motor and process skills* (2nd ed.). Fort Collins, CO: Three Star Press.

Ford, A. B. (1999). "Overview of community-based long-term care," In E. Calkins, C. Boult, E. H. Wagner, J. T. Pacala (Eds.), *New ways to care for older people: Building systems based on evidence.* New York: Springer, pp. 135–142.

Forette, F., Seux, M. L., Staessen, J. A., Thijs, L., Babarskiene, M. R., Babeanu, S., Bossini, A., Fagard, R., Gil-Extremera, B., Laks, T., Kobalava, Z., Sarti, C., Tuomilehto, J., Vanhanen, H., Webster, J., Yodfat, Y., & Birkenhager, W. H. (2002). Systolic Hypertension in Europe Investigators. The prevention of dementia with antihypertensive treatment: New evidence from the Systolic Hypertension in Europe (Syst-Eur) study. *Arch Intern Med, 162*(18), 2046–52.

Freedman, V. A., Hakan, A., Martin, L. G. (2001). Aggregate changes in severe cognitive impairment among older Americans: 1993 and 1998. *The Journals of Gerontology, Psychological sciences and social sciences, 56*B(2), S100–S111.

Freedman, V. A., Hakan, A., & Martin, L. G. (2002). Another look at aggregate changes in severe cognitive impairment: Further investigation into the cumulative effects of three survey design issues. *The Journals of Gerontology, Psychological sciences and social sciences, 57*B(2), S126–S131.

Freedman, V. A., & Martin, L. G. (1998, October). Understanding trends in functional limitations among older Americans. *Am J Public Health, 88*(10), 1457–1462.

Freedman, V. A., & Martin, L. G. (1999, November). The role of education in explaining and forecasting trends in functional limitations among older Americans. *Demography, 36*(4), 461–473.

Freedman, V. A., Martin, L. G., & Schoeni, R. F. (2002). Recent trends in disability and functioning among older adults in the United States: A systematic review. *JAMA, 288*(24), 3137–3146.

Freiman, M., & Brown, E. (2001). Research Findings No. 6: Special Care Units in Nursing Homes—Selected Characteristics, 1996. Medical Expenditures Panel Study. AHQR. http://www.meps.ahrq.gov/Papers/RF6_99–0017/RF6.htm

Freund, A. M., & Baltes, P. B. (1998, December). Selection, optimization, and compensation as strategies of life management: Correlations with subjective indicators of successful aging. *Psychol Aging, 13*(4), 531–543.

Fried, L. P., Bandeen-Roche, K., Kasper, J. D., & Guralnik, J. M. (1999, January). Association of comorbidity with disability in older women: The Women's Health and Aging Study. *J Clin Epidemiol, 52*(1), 27–37.

Fried, L. P., Bandeen-Roche, K., Williamson, J. D., Prasada-Rao, P., Chee, E., Tepper, S., & Rubin, G. S. (1996, September). Functional decline in older adults: Expanding methods of ascertainment. *J Gerontol A Biol Sci Med Sci 51*(5), M206–M214.

Fried, L. P., Herdman, S. J., Kuhn, K. E., et al. (2001). Preclinical disability: Hypotheses about the bottom of the iceberg. *J Aging Health, 47,* 747–760.

Fried, L. P., Tangen, C. T., Walston, J., Newman, A. B., Hirsch, C., Gottdiener, J., Seeman, T., Tracy, R., Kop, W. J., Burke, G., & McBurnie, M. A. (2001). Frailty in older adults: Evdience for a phenotype. *J Gerontol: Med Sci, 56A,* M146–M156.

Friedland, R. P., Fritsch, T., Smyth, K. A., Koss, E., Lerner, A. J., Chen, A. H., Petot, G. J., & Debanne, S. M. (2001). Patients with Alzheimer's disease have reduced activities in midlife compared with healthy control-group members. *Proceedings of the National Academy of Sciences, 98,* 3440–3445.

Fries, J. F. (1983). The compression of morbidity. *Milbank Mem Fund Q Health Soc 61*(3), 397–419.

Fries, J. F. (2002). Reducing disability in older age. *JAMA, 288*(24), 3164–3165.

Fry, C. L. (1980). Cultural dimensions of age: A multidimensional scaling analysis. In C. L. Fry (Ed.), *Aging in culture and society: Comparative viewpoints and strategies* (pp. 42–64). Brooklyn: JF Bergin.

Gage, B., Miller, S. C., Mor, V., Jackson, B., & Harvell J. (2000). Synthesis and analysis of medicare's hospice benefit: Executive summary and recommendations. MEDSTAT. http://aspe.hhs.giv/daltcp/reports/samhbes.htm

Gallo, J. J., Rabins, P. V., & Anthony, J. C. (1999, March). Sadness in older persons: 13–year follow-up of a community sample in Baltimore, Maryland. *Psychol Med, 29*(2), 341–350.

Gallo, J. J., Rabins, P. V., Lyketsos, C. G., Tien, A. Y., Anthony, J. C. (1997, May). Depression without sadness: Functional outcomes of nondysphoric depression in later life. *J Am Geriatr Soc, 45*(5), 570–578.

Ganguli, M., Seaberg, E., Belle, S., Fischer, L., Kuller, L. H. (1993, October). Cognitive impairment and the use of health services in an elderly rural population: The MoVIES project. Monongahela Valley Independent Elders Survey. *J Am Geriatr Soc, 41*(10), 1065–1070.

Gill, T. M., Baker, D. I., Gottschalk, M., Peduzzi, P. N., Allore, H., Byers A. (2002). A program to prevent functional decline in physically frail, elderly persons who live at home. *NEJM, 347*(14), 1068–1074.

Gill, T. M., Feinstein, A. R. (1994, August 24–31). A critical appraisal of the quality of quality-of-life measurements. *JAMA, 272*(8), 619–626.

Gill, T. M., Kurland B. (2003). The burden and patterns of disability in activities of daily living among community-living older persons. *J Gerontol A Biol Sci Med, 58*(1), M70–M75.

Gill, T. M., Robison, J. T., Tinetti, M. E. (1997, December). Predictors of recovery in activities of daily living among disabled older persons living in the community. *J Gen Intern Med 12*(12), 757–762.

Gill, T. M. , Williams, C. S., Richardson, E. D., & Tinetti, M. E. (1996). Impairments in physical performance and cognitive status as predisposing factors for functional dependence among nondisabled older persons. *J Gerontol A Biol Sci Med Sci, 51*(6), M283–M288.

Gill, T. M., Williams, C. S., Robison, J. T., & Tinetti, M. E. (1999, April). A population-based study of environmental hazards in the homes of older persons. *Am J Public Health, 89*(4), 553–556.

Gillick, M. R. (1994). *Choosing medical care in old age: What kind, how much, when to stop.* Cambridge, MA: Harvard University Press.

Ginzburg-Walter, A., Blumstein, T., Chetrit, A., & Modan B. (2002). Social factors and mortality in the old-old in Israel: The CALAS study. *J Gerontol: Soc Sci, 57*B, S308–S318.

Goldberg, T. H., & Chavin, S. I. (1997, March). Preventive medicine and screening in older adults. *J Am Geriatr Soc, 45*(3), 344–354.

Grady, D., Yaffe, K., Kristof, M., Lin, F., Richards, C., & Barrett-Connor, E. (2002). Effect of postmenopausal hormone therapy on cognitive function: The Heart and Estrogen/Progestin Replacement Study. *Am J Med, 113*(7), 543–548.

Green, C. R., Mohs, R. C., Schmeidler, J., Aryan, M., & Davis, K. L. (1993). Functional decline in Alzheimer's disease: A longitudinal study. *J Am Geriatr Soc, 41,* 654–661.

Green, R. C., Cupples, L. A., Go, R., Benke, K. S., Edeki, T., Griffith, P. A., Williams, M., Hipps, Y., Graff-Radford, N., Bachman, D., Farrer, L. A.; MIRAGE Study Group. (2002, January 16). Risk of dementia among white and African American relatives of patients with Alzheimer disease. *JAMA, 287*(3), 329–36.

Gregg, E. W., Yaffe, K., Cauley, J. A., Rolka, D. B., Blackwell, T. L., Narayan, K. M., Cummings, S. R. (2000, January 24). Is diabetes associated with cognitive impairment and cognitive decline among older women? Study of Osteoporotic Fractures Research Group. *Arch Intern Med, 160*(2), 174–180.

Greiner, P. A., Snowdon, D. A., Schmitt, F. A. (1996, January). The loss of independence in activities of daily living: The role of low normal cognitive function in elderly nuns. *Am J Public Health, 86*(1), 62–66.

Guralnik, J. M., Land, K. C., Blazer, D., Fillenbaum, G. G., & Branch, L. G. (1993, July 8). Educational status and active life expectancy among older blacks and whites. *N Engl J Med, 329*(2), 110–116.

Guralnik, J. M., Ferrucci, L., Simonsick, E. M., Salive, M. E., & Wallace, R. B. (1995, March 2). Lower-extremity function in persons over the age of 70 years as a predictor of subsequent disability. *N Engl J Med, 332*(9), 556–561.

Guralnik, J. M., Fried, L. P., Simonsick, E. M., Kasper, J. D., & Lafferty, M. E. (Eds.). (1995b). *The Women's Health and Aging Study* (NIH 95–4009). National Institutes of Health.

Guralnik, J. M., Land, K. C., Blazer, D., Fillenbaum, G. G., & Branch, L. G. (1993, July 8). Educational status and active life expectancy among older blacks and whites. *N Engl J Med, 329*(2), 110–116.

Guralnik, J. M., Simonsick, E. M., Ferrucci, L., Glynn, R. J., Berkman, L. F., Blazer, D. G., Scherr, P. A., & Wallace, R. B. (1994, March). A short physical performance battery assessing lower extremity function: Association with self-reported disability and prediction of mortality and nursing home admission. *J Gerontol, 49*(2), M85–M94.

Gurland, B. J., Wilder, D. E., Chen, J., Lantigua, R., Mayeux, R., & Van Nostrand J. (1995). A flexible system of detection for Alzheimer's disease and related dementias. *Aging, (Milano) 7*(3), 165–72.

Hadley, E. (1992). Cause of death among the oldest old. In R. M. Suzman, D. P. Willis, K G. Manton (Eds.), *The oldest old* (pp. 183–198). New York: Oxford University Press.

Hager, K., Machein, U., Krieger, S., Platt, D., Seefried, G., & Bauer, J. (1994). Interleukin-6 and selected plasma proteins in healthy persons of different ages. *Neurobiol Aging, 15*, 771–772.

Hay, J., Labree, L., Luo, R., Clark, F., Carlson, M., Mandel, D., Zemke, R., Jackson, J., & Azen S. (2002). Cost-effectiveness of preventive occupational therapy for independent living adults. *J Am Geriatrics Society, 50*, 1381–1388.

Hayward, M. D., & Heron, M. (2001). Racial inequality in active life among adult Americans. *Demography, 36*(1), 77–91.

Helmes, E., Csapo, K. G., Short, J-A. (1987). Standardization and validation of the Multidimensional observation scale for elderly subjects (MOSES). *J Gerontol, 42*, 395–405.

Hennessey, C. H., Moriarty, D. G., Scherr, P. A., & Brackbill R. (1994). Measuring health-related quality of life for public health surveillance. *Public Health Reports, 109*(5), 665–672.

Hochschild, R. (1989). Improving the precision of biological age determinations. Part 2: Automatic human tests, age norms and variability. *Exp Gerontol, 24*, 301–316.

Hogan, C., Junney, J., Gabel, J., & Lynn J. (2001). Medicare beneficiaries' costs of care in the last year of life. *Health Affairs, 20*(4), 188–195.

Hogervorst, E., Yaffe, K., Richards, M., & Huppert, F. (2003). Hormone replacement therapy to maintain cognitive function in women with dementia (Cochrane Review). *The Cochrane Library, Issue 2.* Oxford: Update Software Ltd. http://www.cochrane.org/cochrane/revabstr/ab003799.htm

Hokenstad, A., Ramirez, M., Haslanger, K., & Finneran K. (1997). *Medicaid home care services in New York City: Demographics, health conditions, and impairment levels of New York City's Medicaid home care population.* New York: United Hospital Fund.

Holmes, D., Teresi, J. A., & Ory, M. G. (2000). Overview of the volume. In D. Holmes, J. A. Teresi, M. G. Ory (Eds.), *Special care units* (pp. 7–18). Paris: Serdi; New York: Springer.

Hooyman, N., Gonyea, J., & Montgomery, R. (1985, April). The impact of in-home services termination on family caregivers. *Gerontologist, 25*(2), 141–145.

Horiuchi, S. (in press). Age patterns of mortality. In P. Demeny & G. McNicoll (Eds.), *The encyclopedia of population.* Farmington Hills, MI: Macmillan Reference.

Hornbrook, M. C., Stevens, V. J., Wingfield, D. J., Hollis, J. F., Greenlick, M. R., & Ory, M. G. (1994). Preventing falls among community-dwelling older persons: Results from a randomized trial. *The Gerontologist, 34,* 16–23.

Hughes, C. P., Berg, L., Danziger, W. L., Cohen, L. A., Martin, R. L. (1982). A new clinical scale for the staging of dementia. *Br J Psychol, 140,* 566–572.

Hurley, A. C., Volicer, B. J., Hanrahan, P. A., Houde, S., Volicer, L. (1992). Assessment of discomfort in advanced Alzheimer patients. *Res Nursing Health, 15,* 369–377.

Inouye, S. K., Bogardus, S. T. Jr., Charpentier, P. A., Leo-Summers, L., Acampora, D., Holford, T. R., & Cooney, L. M. Jr. (1999, March 4). A multicomponent intervention to prevent delirium in hospitalized older patients. *N Engl J Med, 340*(9), 669–676.

Jaeschke, R., Singer, J., & Guyatt, G. H. (1989, December). Measurement of health status: Ascertaining the minimal clinically important difference. *Control Clin Trials, 10*(4), 407–415.

Jarvik, G. P., Wijsman, E. M., Kukull, W. A., Schellenberg, G. D., Yu, C., & Larson, E. B. (1995). Interaction of apolipoprotein E genotype, total cholesterol level, and sex in prediction of Alzheimer disease in a case-control study. *Neurology, 45,* 1092–1096.

Jette, A. M., Assmann, S. F., Rooks, D., Harris, B. A., & Crawford, S. (1998, September). Interrelationships among disablement concepts. *J Gerontol A Biol Sci Med Sci, 53*(5), M395–M404.

Jorm, A. F., Christensen, H., Korten, A. E., Jacomb, P. A., Henderson, A. S. (2000, July). Informant ratings of cognitive decline in old age: Validation against change on cognitive tests over 7 to 8 years. *Psychol Med, 30*(4), 981–985.

Judge, J. O., Schechtman, K., & Cress, E. (1996, November). The relationship between physical performance measures and independence in instrumental activities of daily living. The FICSIT Group (Frailty and Injury: Cooperative Studies of Intervention Trials). *J Am Geriatr Soc, 44*(11), 1332–1341.

Kane, R. A. (1995). Expanding the home care concept: blurring distinctions among home care, institutional care, and other long-term-care services. *The Milbank Quarterly, 73*(2), 161–186.

Kane, R. A. (2003, April). Definition, measurement, and correlates of quality of life in nursing homes: Toward a reasonable practice, research, and policy agenda. *Gerontologist, 43 Spec No 2,* 28–36.

Kaplan, E., Goodglass, H., & Weintaub, S. (1983). *Boston naming test.* Phila., PA: Lea & Febiger.

Kaplan, R. M., Anderson, J. P. (1996). The General Health Policy Model: An integrated approach. In B. Spilker (Ed.), *Quality of life and pharmacoeconomics in clinical trials* (pp. 203–225). Philadelphia: Lippincott-Raven.

Karagiozis, H., Gray, S., Sacco, J., Shapiro, M., & Kawas C. (1998, February). The Direct Assessment of Functional Abilities (DAFA): A comparison to an indirect measure of instrumental activities of daily living. *Gerontologist, 38*(1), 113–121.

Katz, S., Ford, A. B., Moscowitz, A. W., et al. (1963). Studies of illness in the aged: The index of ADL: A standardized measure of biological and psychosocial function. *JAMA, 185,* 914–919.

Katz, S., Branch, L. G., Branson, M. H., Papsidero, J. A., Beck, J. C., & Greer, D. S. (1983). Active life expectancy. *New Engl J Med, 309,* 1218–1224.

Kemper, P., & Murtaugh, C. M. (1991, February 28). Lifetime use of nursing home care. *N Engl J Med, 324*(9), 595–600.

Kirkwood, T. B. L. (1985). Comparative and evolutionary aspects of longevity. In E. L. Schneider, J. W. Rowe (Eds.), *Handbook of the biology of aging* (pp. 27–44). New York; van Nostrand.

Kleemeier, R. W. (1962). *Intellectual change in the senium* (pp. 290–295). In proceedings of the Social Statistics Section of the American Statistical Association. Washington, D.C.: American Statistical Association.

Kluger, A., Gianutos, J. G., Golumb, J., Ferris, S. H., George, A. E., Franssen, E., & Reisberg, B. (1997). Patterns of motor impairment in normal aging, mild cognitive decline, and early Alzheimer's disease. *J Gerontology: Psychol and Social Sci, 52,* P28–P39.

Knopman, D. S., Berg, J. D., Thomas, R., Grundman, M., Thal, L. J., & Sano M. (1999). Nursing home placement is related to dementia progression: Experience from a clinical trial. Alzheimer's Disease Cooperative Trial. *Neurology, 52,* 714–718.

Knopman, D. S., Rocca, W. A., Cha, R. H., Edland, S. D., Kokmen, E. (2003, January). Survival study of vascular dementia in Rochester, Minnesota. *Arch Neurol, 60*(1), 85–90.

Kochanek, K. D., Smith, B. L., Anderson, R. N. (2001). Deaths: Preliminary Data for 1999. *National Vital Statistics Reports, 49*(3). Hyattsville, MD: National Center for Health Statistics.

Kovar, M. G., (1986). Aging in the eighties: Preliminary data for the Supplement on Aging to the National Health Interview Survey, US, Jan-June, 1984. Advance Data from Vital and Health Statistics, No. 115 DHHS 86–1250. Hyattsville, MD: National Center for Health Statistics. http://www.cdc.gov/nchs/data/ad/ad115acc.pdf

Kovar, M. G., & Lawton, M. P. (1994). Functional disability: Activities and instrumental activities of daily living. *Ann Rev Geriatr Gerontol, 14,* pp. ??–??. New York: Springer.

Kramer, B. J., Thompson, E. H. (Eds.). (2002). *Men as caregivers: Theory, research, and service implications.* New York: Springer.

Kuh, D., Bassey, J., Hardy, R., Sayer, A. A., Wadsworth, M., & Cooper C. (2002). Birth weight, childhood size, and muscle strength in adult life: Evidence from a birth cohort study. *Am J Epidemiol, 156,* 627–633.

Kutner, N. G., & Bliwise, D. L. (2000). Observed agitation and the phenomenon of "sundowning" among SCU residents. In D. Holmes, J. A. Teresi, M. G. Ory (Eds.), *Special care units* (pp. 151–162). Paris: Serdi; New York: Springer.

Lachs, M. S., Williams, C. S., O'Brien, S., & Pillemer, K. A. (2002, August). Adult protective service use and nursing home placement. *Gerontologist, 42*(6), 734–739.

References 261

Lachs, M. S., Williams, C. S., O'Brien, S., Pillemer, K. A., & Charlson, M. E. (1998). The mortality of elder mistreatment. *JAMA, 280*(5), 428–432.
LaCroix, A. Z., Leveille, S. G., Hecht, J. A., Grothaus, L. C., & Wagner, E. H. (1996). Does walking decrease the risk of cardiovascular disease hospitalizations and death in older adults? *J Am Geriatr Soc, 44*(2), 113–20.
Landefeld, C. S., Palmer, R. M., Kresevic, D. M., Fortinsky, R. H., & Kowal J. A randomized trial of care in a hospital medical unit especially designed to improve functional outcomes of acutely ill older patients. *New Engl J Med, 332,* 1338–1344.
Larson, R., Zuzanek, J., & Mannell, R. (1985, May). Being alone versus being with people: Disengagement in the daily experience of older adults. *J Gerontol, 40*(3), 375–381.
Launer, L. J., Anderson, K., Dewey, M. E., Lentenneur, L., Ott, A., Amaduci, L. A., Brayne, C., Copeland, J. R. M., Dartigues, J.-F. Kragh-Sorensen, P., Lobo, A., Martinez-Lage, J. M., Stijnen, T., & Hofman, A. (1999). Rates and risk factors for dementia and Alzheimer's disease: Results from EURODEM pooled analyses. *Neurology, 52,* 78–84.
Lawton, M. P. (1972). *Environment and aging.* Monterey, CA: Brooks/Cole.
Lawton, M. P. (1980). *Environment and aging.* Monterey, CA: Brooks/Cole Series in Social Gerontology.
Lawton, M. P. (1991). A multidimensional view of quality of life in frail elders. In J. E. Birren (Ed.), *The concept and measurement of quality of life in the frail elderly.* San Diego, CA: Academic Press.
Lawton, M. P., & Brody, E. M. (1969). Assessment of older people: Self-maintaining and instrumental activities of daily living. *Gerontologist, 9*(3), 179–86.
Lawton, M. P., Brody, E., & Pruchno, R. (1991). *Respite for Caregivers of Alzheimer Patients: Research and Practice.* New York: Springer.
Lawton, M. P., Moss, M., & Glicksman, A. (1993). The quality of the last year of life of older pertsons. *Milbank Quarterly, 68,* 1–28.
Lawton, M. P., Parmelee, P. A., Katz, I. R., & Nesselroade, J. (1996, November). Affective states in normal and depressed older people. *J Gerontol B Psychol Sci Soc Sci, 51*(6), P309–P316.
Lawton, M. P., Van Haitsma, K., Perkinson, M., & Ruckdeschel K. (2001). Observed affect and quality of life in dementia. In S. M. Albert & R. G. Logsdon (Eds.), *Assessing quality of life in Alzheimer's disease* (pp. 3–16). New York: Springer.
Lazaridis, E. N., Rudberg, M. A., Furner, S. E., & Cassel, C. K. (1994). Do activities of daily living have a hierarchical structure? An analysis using the longitudinal study of aging. *Journal of Gerontology, 49*(2), M47–M51.
Leplege, A., & Hunt, S. (1997, July 2). The problem of quality of life in medicine. *JAMA, 278*(1), 47–50.
Levy, G., Tang, M. X., Louis, E. D., Cote, L. J., Alfaro, B., Mejia, H., Stern, Y., & Marder K. (2002, December 10). The association of incident dementia with mortality in PD. *Neurology, 59*(11), 1708–1713.
Levy, R. (1994). Aging-associated cognitive decline. *International Psychogeriatrics, 6,* 63–68.

Liao, Y., McGee, D. L., Cao, G., & Cooper, R. S. (2000). Quality of life in the last year of life of older adults: 1986 vs. 1993. *JAMA, 283*(4), 512–518.

Lieberman, A. (2002). Dementia in Parkinson's Disease. National Parkinson's Disease Foundation. http://www.parkinson.org/pddement.htm

Liebson, C., Owens, T., O'Brien, P., WAring, S., Tangalos, E., Hanson, V. (1999). Use of physician and acute care services by persons with and without Alzheimer's disease: A population-based comparison. *J Am Geriatrics Soc, 47,* 864–869.

Lindeman, D. A., Arnsberger, P., & Owens D. (2000). Staffing and specialized dementia care units: Impact of resident outcomes. In D. Holmes, J. A. Teresi, M. G. Ory (Eds.), *Special care units* (pp. 217–228). Paris: Serdi; New York: Springer.

Lindenberger, U., & Baltes, P. B. (1997). Intellectual functioning in old and very old: Cross-sectional results from the Berlin Aging Study. *Psychology and aging, 12,* 410–432.

Lindenberger, U., Singer, T., & Baltes, P. B. (2002, November). Longitudinal selectivity in aging populations: Separating mortality-associated versus experimental components in the Berlin Aging Study (BASE). *J Gerontol B Psychol Sci Soc Sci, 57*(6), P474–P482.

Logsdon, R. G., Gibbons, L. E., McCurry, S. M., & Teri L. (2001). Quality of life in Alzheimer's disease: Patient and caregiver reports. In S. M. Albert, R. G. Logsdon (Eds.), *Assessing quality of life in Alzheimer's disease* (pp. 17–30). New York: Springer.

Lopez, O. L., Kuller, L. H., Fitzpatrick, A., Ives, D., Becker, J. T., & Beauchamp, N. (2003). Evaluation of dementia in the cardiovascular health cognition study. *Neuroepidemiology, 22*(1), 1–12.

Lorig, K., Ritter, P., Stewart, A. L., Sobel, D., Brown, B. W., Bandura, A., Gonzalez, V. M., Laurent, D., Holman, H. R. Chronic disease self-management program: Two-year health status and health care utilization outcomes. *Med Care* 39(11), 1217–1223, 2001.

Lorig, K., Sobel, D., Stewart, A. L., Brown, B. W., Bandura, A., Ritter, P., Gonzalez, V. M., Laurent, D., Holman, H. R. (1999). Evidence suggesting that a chronic disease self-management program can improve health status while reducing hospitalization: A randomized trial. *Med Care, 37*(1), 5–14.

Loewenstein, D. A., Arguelles, S., Bravo, M., Freeman, R. Q., Arguelles, T., Acevedo, A., et al. (2001). Caregivers' judgments of the functional abilities of the Alzheimer's disease patient: A comparison of proxy reports and objective measures. *Journal Gerontology B Psychology Science Social Science, 56*(2), P78–P84.

Lubitz, J. D., & Riley, G. R. (1993). Trends in Medicare payments in the last year of life. *New England J Med, 328*(15), 1092–1096, 1993.

Luchsinger, J. A., Tang, M. X., Stern, Y., Shea, S., Mayeux R. Diabetes mellitus and risk of Alzheimer's disease and dementia with stroke in a multiethnic cohort. *Am J Epidemiol* 154(7), 635–641.

Lunney, J. R., Lynn, J., & Hogan C. (2002). Profiles of older Medicare decdents. *J Amer Geriatrics Society 50,* 1108–1112.

Lydick, E., & Epstein, R. S. (2001). Interpretation of quality of life changes. *Quality of Life Research, 2,* 221–226.

Lynn, J. (2001). Serving patients who may die soon and their families: The role of hospice and other services. *JAMA, 285,* 925–932.

Maestre, G., Ottman, R., Stern, Y., Gurland, B., Chun, M., Tang, M. X., Shelanski, M., Tycko, B., & Mayeux, R. (1995, February). Apolipoprotein, E. and Alzheimer's disease: ethnic variation in genotypic risks. *Ann Neurol, 37*(2), 254–259.

Magaziner, J., Simonsick, E. M., Kashner, T. M., Hebel, J. R. (1988). Patient-proxy response comparability on measures of patient health and functional status. *J Clin Epidemiol, 41*(11), 1065–1074.

Manly, J. J., Jacobs, D. M., Touradji, P., Small, S. A., Stern, Y. (2002, March). Reading level attenuates differences in neuropsychological test performance between African American and White elders. *J Int Neuropsychol Soc, 8*(3), 341–348.

Manton, K. G. (1992). Mortality and life expectancy changes among the oldest old. In R. M. Suzman, D. P. Willis, K. G. Manton (Eds.), *The oldest old* (pp. 157–182). New York: Oxford University Press.

Manton, K. G., Corder, L. S., & Stallard E. (1993). Estimates of change in chronic disability and institutional incidence and prevalence rates in the U.S. elderly population from the 1982, 1984, and 1989 National Long Term Care Survey. *J Gerontol, 48*(4), S153–S166.

Manton, K. G., Corder, L., & Stallard E. (1997, March 18). Chronic disability trends in elderly United States populations: 1982–1994. *Proc Natl Acad Sci U S A, 94*(6), 2593–2598.

Manton, K. G., & Gu, X. (2001). Changes in the prevalence of chronic disability in the United States black and nonblack population above age 65 from 1982 to 1999. *Proc Natl Acad Sci USA 98*(11), 6354–6359.

Manton, K. G., Stallard, E., & Corder L. (1995). Changes in morbidity and chronic disability in the U.S. elderly population: Evidence from the 1982, 1984, and 1989 National Long Term Care Surveys. *The Journal of Gerontolgy, Psychological science and social sciences, 50*(Bn4), S194–S204.

Manton, K. G., Suzman, R., & Willis, D. (Eds.). (1992). *The oldest old.* New York: Oxford University Press.

Manton, K. G., & Vaupel, J. W. (1995). Survival after the age of 80 in the United States, Sweden, France, England, and Japan. *New Engl J Med, 333,* 1232–1235.

Mattis, S. (1976). Mental status examination for organic mental health syndrome in the elderly patient. In L. Bellek, T. B. Karasu (Eds.), *Geriatric psychiatry* (pp. 77–121). New York: Grune & Stratton.

Mausner, J. S., & Kramer, S. (1985). *Epidemiology: An introductory text.* Philadephia: Saunders.

Mayeux, R., Small, S. A., Tang, M., Tycko, B., & Stern Y. (2001). Memory performance in healthy elderly without Alzheimer's disease: effects of time and apolipoprotein-E. *Neurobiol Aging, 22*(4), 683–689.

McCann, J. J., Bienas, J. L., Evans, D. A. (2000). Change in performance tests of activities of daily living among residents of dementia special care and traditional nursing home units. In D. Holmes, J. A. Teresi, M. G. Ory (Eds.), *Special care units* (pp. 141–150). Paris: Serdi; New York: Springer.

McCluskey, A. (2000, November). Paid attendant carers hold important and unexpected roles which contribute to the lives of people with brain injury. *Brain Inj, 14*(11), 943–957.

McKhann, G., Drachman, D., Folstein, M., Katzman, R., Price, D., & Stadlan, E. M. (1984, July). Clinical diagnosis of Alzheimer's disease: Report of the NINCDS-ADRDA Work Group under the auspices of Department of Health and Human Services Task Force on Alzheimer's Disease. *Neurology, 34*(7), 939–944.

Meier, D. (1999). Impact of palliative interventions and mortality rate in hospitalized patients with advanced dementia. In van der Heiude, A., ed. *Clinical and epidemiological aspects of end of life decision-making* (pp. 217–227). Akad. Van Wetensch Verhandl. Natuur. Reeks 2, 102 Netherlands: Amsterdam.

Miller, T. (2001). Increasing longevity and Medicare expenditures. *Demography, 38,* 215–226.

Minino, A. M., & Smith, B. L. (2001). *Deaths: Preliminary data for 2000.* (National Vital Statistics Reports, Vol. 49, No. 12). Hyattsville, MD: National Center for Health Statistics.

Mittelman, M. S., Ferris, S. H., Shulman, E., Steinberg, G., & Levin, B. (1996). A family intervention to delay nursing home placement of patients with Alzheimer's disease. *JAMA 276*(21), 1725–1731.

Mohs, R. C., Doody, R. S., Morris, J. C., Ieni, J. R., Rogers, S. L., Perdomo, C. A., Pratt, R. D. (2001). A 1–year, placebo controlled preservation of functional survival study of donepezil in AD patients. *Neurology, 57,* 481–488.

Moritz, D. J., Kasl, S. V., & Berkman, L. F. (1995). Cognitive functioning and the incidence of limitations in activities of dailyliving in an elderly community sample. *Am J Epidemiol, 141,* 41–49.

Morris, J. C., Storandt, M., Miller, J. P., McKeel, D. W., Price, J. L., Rubin, E. H., & Berg, L. (2001). Mild cognitive impairment represents early-stage Alzheimer's disease. *Arch Neurol, 58,* 397–405.

Morris, J. N., & Emerson-Lombardo, N. (1994). A national perspective on SCU service richness: Finings from the AARP survey. *Alzheimer Dis Assoc Disorders 8*(suppl), S87–S96.

Morrison, R. S., & Siu, A. L. (2000, July 5). Survival in end-stage dementia following acute illness. *JAMA, 284*(1), 47–52.

Moss, M., & Lawton, M. P. (1982). Time budgets of older people: A window on four lifestyles. *J Gerontol, 37,* 115–123, 1982.

Mossey, J., & Moss M. (2002). Subthreshold depression in elders living at home: A public health problem. *Am Public Health Association,* Phila., PA. Abstract #51804.

Muharin, R. K., DeBettignies, B. H., & Pirozzolo, F. J. (1991). Structured assessment of independent living skills: Preliminary analysis of functional abilities in dementia. *J Gerontol: Psychol Sci, 46,* P58–P66.

Murray, C. J., & Lopez, A. D. (1996, November 1). Evidence-based health policy—lessons from the Global Burden of Disease Study. *Science,* *274*(5288), 740–743.

Myers, R. H., Schaefer, E. J., Wilson, P. W. F., D'Agostino, R., Ordovas, J. M., Espino, A., et al. (1993). Apolipoprotein E allele 4 is associated with dementia in a population based study: the Framingham Study. *Neurology,* *46*(3), 673–677.

National Center for Health Statistics. (2001). *Health, United States.* http://www.cdc.gov/nchs/products/pubs/pubd/hus/hus.htm

National Center for Health Statistics. (2002). National Health Interview Survey, 2000. *Early Release of Selected Estimates Based on Data From the January-June 2002 NHIS.* http://www.cdc.gov/nchs/about/major/nhis/released200212.htm

National Council on Aging. (2001). Myths and Realities of Aging, 2000. New York: Harris Interactive.

Nelson, H. D., Humphrey, L. L., Nygren, P., Teutsch, S. M., & Allan, J. D. (2002, August 21). Postmenopausal hormone replacement therapy: Scientific review. *JAMA, 288*(7), 872–881.

Newcomer, R., Clay, T., Luxenberg, J. S., & Miller, R. H. (1999). Misclassification and selection bias when identifying Alzheimer's disease solely from Medicare claims records. *J AM Geriatr Soc, 47,* 215–219.

Newcomer, R., Spitalny, M., Fox, P., & Yordi C. (1999, August). Effects of the Medicare Alzheimer's Disease Demonstration on the use of community-based services. *Health Serv Res, 34*(3), 645–667.

Newman, A. B., Gottdiener, J. S., McBurnie, M. A., Hirsch, H. H., Kop, W. J., Tracy, R., Walston, J. D., Fried, L. P; Cardiovascular Health Study Research Group. (2001). Associations of subclinical disease with frailty. *J Gerontol: Med Sci, 56A,* M158–M166.

Olshansky, S. J., Carnes, B. A., & Cassel C. (1990). In search of Methuselah: Estimating the upper limits to human longevity. *Science, 250*(4981), 634–640.

Østbye, T., & Crosse, E. (1994). Net economic costs of dementia in Canada. *Canadian Med Assoc J, 151*(10), 1457–64.

Pacala, J. T., Boult, C., Reed, R. L., & Aliberti, E. (1997). Predictive validity of the P_{ra} instrument among older recipients of managed care. *J Am Geriatrics Soc, 45,* 614–617.

Palmore, E. B. (1999). *Ageism.* New York: Springer.

Patrick, D. L., & Erikson P. (1993). *Health status and health policy.* Oxford: Oxford University Press.

Patrick, D. L., & Peach, H. (1989). *Disablement in the community.* Oxford; Oxford University Press.

Patrick, D. L., Danis, M. L., Southerland, L. I., & Hong, G. (1988). Quality of life following intensive care. *J Gen Intern Med, 3,* 218–223.

Patrick, D. L., Sittampalam, Y., Somerville, S. M., Carter, W. B., & Bergner M. (1985, December). A cross-cultural comparison of health status values. *Am J Public Health, 75*(12), 1402–1407.

Pearlin, L. I., & Schooler, C. (1978). The structure of coping. *J Health Soc Behav, 19*(1), 2–21.

Penninx, B. W., Ferrucci, L., Leveille, S. G., Rantanen, T., Pahor, M., & Guralnik, J. M. (2000). Lower extremity performance in nondisabled older persons as a predictor of subsequent hospitalization. *J Gerontol: Med Sci, 55A,* M691–M697.

Penninx, B. W., Guralnik, J. M., Ferrucci, L., Simonsick, E. M., Deeg, D. J., & Wallace, R. B. (1998, June 3). Depressive symptoms and physical decline in community-dwelling older persons. *JAMA, 279*(21), 1720–1726.

Penninx, B. W., Leveille, S., Ferrucci, L., van Eijk, J. T., & Guralnik, J. M. (1999, September). Exploring the effect of depression on physical disability: longitudinal evidence from the established populations for epidemiologic studies of the elderly. *Am J Public Health, 89*(9), 1346–1352.

Perls, T. T., Wilmoth, J., Levenson, R., Drinkwater, M., Cohen, M., Bogan, H., Joyce, E., Brewsters, Kunkel, L., & Puca A. (2002). Life-long sustained mortality advantage of siblings of centenarians. *Proc Nat Acad Sci 99,* 8442–8447.

Peterson, R. C. (2000). Mild cognitive impairment: Transition between aging and Alzheimer's disease. *Neurologia, 15,* 93–101.

Peterson, R. C., Smith, G. E., Waring, S. C., Ivnik, R. J., Kokmen, E., & Tangelos, E. G. (1997). Aging, memory, and mild cognitive impairment. *International Psychogeriatrics, 9,* 65–69.

Peterson, R. C., Stevens, J. C., Ganguli, M., Tangalos, E. G., Cummings, J. L., DeKosky, S. T. (2001). Practice parameter: Early detection of dementia: Mild cognitive impairment (an evidence-based review). *Neurology, 56,* 1133–1142.

Pfeffer, R. I., Kurosaki, C. H., Chance, J. M., & Filos, S. (1982). Measurement of functional activities in older adults in the community. *J Gerontology, 37,* 323–329.

Phillips, C. D., Sloan, P. D., Hawes, C., Koch, G., Han, J., Spry, K., Dunteman, G., & Williams, R. L. (1997). Effects of residence in Alzheimer disease special care units on functional outcomes. *JAMA, 276,* 1341–1343.

Pickle, L. W., Mungiole, M., Jones, G. K., & White, A. A. (1996). *Atlas of United States Mortality.* Hyattsville, MD: National Center for Health Statistics.

Pillemer, K., & Finkelhor, D. (1988, February). The prevalence of elder abuse: a random sample survey. *Gerontologist 28*(1), 51–57.

Pollard, A. H., Yusuf, F., & Pollard, G. N. (1974). *Demographic techniques,* 2nd Edition. Sydney: Pergamon Press.

Posner, H. B., Tang, M. X., Luchsinger, J., Lantigua, R., Stern, Y., & Mayeux, R. (2002, April 23). The relationship of hypertension in the elderly to AD, vascular dementia, and cognitive function. *Neurology, 58*(8), 1175–1181.

Poulshock, S. W., Deimling, G. T. Families caring for elders in residence: Issues in the measurement of burden. *Journal of Gerontology, 39*(2), 230–239.

Province, M. A., Hadley, E. C., Hornbrook, M. C., Lipsitz, L. A., Miller, J. P., Mulrow, C. D., Ory, M. G., Sattin, R. W., Tinetti, M. E., Wolf, S. L. (1995). The effects of exercise on falls in elderly patients. A preplanned meta-analysis of the FICSIT Trials. Frailty and Injuries: Cooperative Studies of Intervention Techniques. *JAMA, 273*(17), 1341–1347.

Rabins, P. V., Black, B. S., Roca, R., German, P., McGuire, M., Robbins, B., Rye, R., & Brant, L. (2000, June 7). Effectiveness of a nurse-based outreach program for identifying and treating psychiatric illness in the elderly. *JAMA, 283*(21), 2802–2809.

Rabins, P., Jasper, J., Kleinman, L., Black, B. S., Patrick, D. L. (2001). Concepts and methods in the development of the ADQOL: An instrument for assessing health-related quality of lfie in persons with alzheimer's disease. In S. M. Albert, & E. R. Logsdon (Eds.), *Assessing Quality of life in Alzheimer's disease* (pp. 51–68). New York: Springer.

Rabkin, J. G., Wagner G. J., & Del Bene, M. (2000, March–April). Resilience and distress among amyotrophic lateral sclerosis patients and caregivers. *Psychosom Med, 62*(2), 271–279.

Rantanen, T., Guralnik, J. M., Ferrucci, L., Leveille, S., & Fried, L. P. (1999). Coimpairments: strength and balance as predictors of severe walking disability. *J Gerontol: Med Sci, 54*(4), M172–M176.

Rantanen, T., Guralnik, J. M., Foley, D., Masaki, Leveilk, S., Curb, J. D., et al. (1999). Midlife hand grip strength as a predictor of old age disability. *JAMA, 281,* 558–560.

Rantanen, T., Guralnik, J. M., Sakari-Rantala, R., Leveille, S., Simonsick, E. M., Ling, S., & Fried, L. P. (1999, February). Disability, physical activity, and muscle strength in older women: the Women's Health and Aging Study. *Arch Phys Med Rehabil, 80*(2), 130–135.

Rantanen, T., Masaki, K., Foley, D., Izmirlian, G., Whitle, L., & Guralnik, J. M. (1998). Grip strength changes over 27 years in Japanese Americans. *J Appl Physiol, 85,* 2047–2053.

Reuben, D. B., Borok, G. M., Wolde-Tsadik, G., Ershoff, D. H., Fishman, L. K., Ambrosini, V. L., Liu, Y., Rubenstein, L. Z., & Beck, J. C. (1995). A randomized trial of comprehensive geriatric assessment in the care of hospitalized patients. *New Engl J Med, 332,* 1345–1350.

REVES, Reseau Esperance de Vie en Sante. (1995). Contribution of the Network on Health Expectancy and the Disability Process to the World Health Report. J. M. Robine, I. Romieu, E. Cambois, H. P. A. van de Water, H. C. Boshuizen (Eds.). Geneva: WHO.

Rice, D. P., & LaPlante, M. P. (1992). Medical expenditures for disability and disabling comorbidity. *Am J Public Health, 82*(5), 739–41.

Rich, M. W., Beckkam, V., Wittenberg, C., Leven, C. V., Freedland, K. E., & Carney, R. M. (1995). A multidisciplinary intervention to prevent the readmission of elderly patients with congestive heart failure. *New Engl J Med, 333,* 1190–1195.

Richards, M., Touchon, J., Ledesert, B., Ritchie, K. (1999). Cognitive decline in ageing: Are AAMI and AACD distinct entities? *International J Geriatric Psychiatry, 14,* 534–540.

Ritchie, K., Artero, S., & Touchon, J. (2001, January 9). Classification criteria for mild cognitive impairment: a population-based validation study. *Neurology, 56*(1), 37–42.

Ritchie, K., Robine, J. M., Letenneur, L., & Dartigues, J. F. (1994, February). Dementia-free life expectancy in France. *Am J Public Health, 84*(2), 232–236.

Roberts, R. E., Kaplan, G. A., Shema, S. J., & Strawbridge, W. J. (1997, September). Prevalence and correlates of depression in an aging cohort: the Alameda County Study. *J Gerontol B Psychol Sci Soc Sci, 52*(5), S252–S258.

Robine, J.-M. (1992). Disability-free life expectancy. In J.-M. Robine, M. Blanchet, J. E. Dowd (Eds.), *Health expectancy.* First Workshop of the International Healthy Life Expectancy Network (REVES). London: HMSO, Studies on Medical and Population subjects, No. 54. (pp. 1–22).

Robine, J.-M., & Allard M. (1998). The oldest human. *Science, 279*(5358), 1834–1835.

Robine, J. M., Blanchet, M., Dowd, J. E. (Eds.). (1992). Health expectancy: First workshop of the International Healthy Life Expectancy Network (REVES). *Studies on Medical and Population Subjects, 54,* 1–22.

Robine, J. M., & Ritchie, K. (1991, February 23). Healthy life expectancy: evaluation of global indicator of change in population health. *BMJ, 302*(6774), 457–460.

Robine, J. M., Romieu, I., Cambois, E., van de Water, H. P. A., & Boshuizen, H. C. (1995). *Contribution of the Network on Health Expectancy and the Disability Process. World Health Report* WHR95. World Health Organization.

Rodgers, W., & Miller B. (1997, May). A comparative analysis of ADL questions in surveys of older people. *J Gerontol B Psychol Sci Soc Sci, 52*(Spec No.), 21–36.

Rosen, W. (1981). *The Rosen drawing test.* Veteran's Administration Medical Center, Bronx, NY.

Roses, A. D. (1994). Apolipoprotein E affects the rate of Alzheimer disease expression: beta-amyloid burden is a secondary consequence dependent on APOE genotype and duration of disease. *J. Neuropathol Exp Neurol, 53,* 429–437.

Roses, A. D., Strittmatter, W. J., Pericak-Vance, M. A., Corder, E. H., Saunders, A. M., & Schmechel, D. E. (1994, June 18). Clinical application of apolipoprotein E genotyping to Alzheimer's disease. *Lancet, 343*(8912), 1564–1565.

Ross, G. W., Abbott, R. D., Petrovitch, H., Masaki, K. H., Murdaugh, C., Trockman, C., Curb, J. D., & White, L. R. (1997, March 12). Frequency and characteristics of silent dementia among elderly Japanese-American men. The Honolulu-Asia Aging Study. *JAMA, 277*(10), 800–805.

Rothenberg, R. B., & Koplan, J. P. (1990). Chronic disease in the 1990's. *Annual Rev Public Health, 11,* 267–296.

Roubenoff, R., & Castaneda C. (2001). Sarcopenia—Understanding the dynamics of aging muscle. *JAMA, 286*(10), 1230–1231.

Rowe, J. W. (2002, February). Address to Harvard University commencement.

Rowe, J. W., & Kahn, R. L. (1987). Human Aging: usual and successful. *Science, 237,* 143–149.

Rozzini, R., Frisoni, G. B., Sabatini, T., & Trabucchi M. (2002, February). The association of depression and mortality in elderly persons. *J Gerontol A Biol Sci Med Sci, 57*(2), M144–M145.

Rubenstein, L. Z. (1999, January). The importance of including the home environment in assessment of frail older persons. *J Am Geriatr Soc.* 47(1), 111–112.

Rubenstein, L. Z., Schairer, C., Wieland, G. D., & Kane R. (1984, November). Systematic biases in functional status assessment of elderly adults: effects of different data sources. *J Gerontol, 39*(6), 686–691.

Rubenstein, L. Z., Stuck, A. E., Siu, A. L., Wieland, G. D. (1991). Impacts of geriatric evaluation and management programs on defined outcomes: Overview of evidence. *J Am Geriatrics Soc, 38S,* 8S–16S.

Russell, D. W., Cutrona, C. E., de la Mora, A., & Wallace, R. B. (1997). Loneliness and nursing home admission among rural older adults. *Psychology & Aging 12*(4), 574–589.

Ryan, E. B., Bourhis, R. Y., Knops, U. (1991). Evaluative perceptions of patronizing speech addressed to elders. *Psychol Aging, 6*(3), 442–450.

Sanders, B. S. (1964). Measuring community health levels. *Am J Public Health 54*(7), 1063–1070.

Saunders, A. M., Strittmatter, W. J., Schmechel, D., George-Hyslop, P. H., PEricak-Vance, M. A., Joo, S. H., et al. (1993). Association of apolipoprotein E allele epsilon-4 with late-onset familial and sporadic Alzheimer's disease. *Neurology, 43,* 1467–1472.

Schoeni, R. F., Freedman, V. A., & Wallace, R. B. (2001). Persistent, consistent, widespread, and robust? Another look at recent trends in old-age disability. *J of Gerontology 56B*(4), S206+.

Schulz, R., & Beach, S. R. (1999, December 15). Caregiving as a risk factor for mortality: the Caregiver Health Effects Study. *JAMA, 282*(23), 2215–2219.

Schulz, R., Beach, S. R., Lind, B., Martire, L. M., Zdaniuk, B., Hirsch, C., Jackson, S., & Burton L. (2001, June 27). Involvement in caregiving and adjustment to death of a spouse: findings from the caregiver health effects study. *JAMA, 285*(24), 3123–3129.

Scitovsky, A. (1994). The high costs of dying revisited. *Milbank Quarterly, 72,* 561–591.

Sehl, M. E., & Yates, F. E. (2001). Kinetics of human aging: I. Rates of senescence between ages 30 and 70 years in healthy people. *J Gerontol: Biol Sci, 56A,* B198–B208.

Silliman, R. A., Bhatti, S., Khan, A., et al. (1996). The care of older persons with diabetes mellitus: Families and primary care physicians. *J Am Geriatrics Soc, 44*(11), 1314–1321.

Sloan, P. D., Mitchell, C. M., Calkins, M., & Zimmerman, S. I. (2000). Light and noise levels in Alzheimer's disease special care units. In D. Holmes, J. A. Teresi, M. G. Ory (Eds.), *Special care units.* Paris: Serdi; New York: Springer.

Small, S. A., Tsai, W. Y., DeLaPaz, R., Mayeux, R., & Stern, Y. (2002, March). Imaging hippocampal function across the human life span: is memory decline normal or not? *Ann Neurol, 51*(3), 290–295.

Snowdon, D. A., Kemper, S. J., Mortimer, J. A., Greiner, L. H., Wekstein, D. R., & Markesbery, W. R. (1996, February 21). Linguistic ability in early life and cognitive function and Alzheimer's disease in late life. Findings from the Nun Study. *JAMA, 275*(7), 528–532.

Somogyi-Zalud, E., Zhong, Z., Hamel, M. B., Lynn, J. (2002). The use of life-sustaining treatments in hospitalized persons aged 80 and older. *J Am Geriatr Soc, 50*(5), 930–934.

Sonn, U., Frandin, K., & Grimby G. (1995). Instrumental activities of daily living related to impairments and functional limitation in 70 year olds. *Scand J Rehab Med, 27,* 119–128.

Spain, Daphne and Suzanne M. Bianchi. (1996). *Balancing act.* New York: Russell Sage Foundation.

Special Committee on Aging, United States Senate. (1991). *Lifelong learning for an aging society—An information paper.* (Serial No. 102). Washington, DC: U.S. Government Printing Office.

Spilker, B., Revicki, D. A. (1999). Taxonomy of quality of life. In B. Spilker (Ed.), *Quality of life and pharmacoeconomics in clinical trials.* Philadelphia: Lippincott-Raven.

Stern, Y., Albert, S. M., Sano, M., Richards, M., Miller, L., Folstein, M., Albert, M., Bylsma, F., & Lafleche G. (1994). Assessing dependency in Alzheimer's disease. *J Gerontol: Med Sci, 49,* M216–M221.

Stern, Y., Gurland, B., Tatemichi, T. K., Tang, M. X., Wilder, D., & Mayeux R. (1994). Influence of education and occupation on the incidence of Alzheimer's disease. *JAMA, 271*(13), 1004–1010.

Stern, Y., Tang, M. X., Albert, M. S., Brandt, J., Jacobs, D. M., Bell, K., Marder, K., Sano, M., Devanand, D., Albert, S. M., Bylsma, F., & Tsai, W. Y. (1997, March 22). Predicting time to nursing home care and death in individuals with Alzheimer disease. *JAMA, 277*(10), 806–812.

Strawbridge, W. J., Wallhagan, M. I., & Cohen, R. D. (2002). Successful aging and well-being: self-rated compared with Rowe and Kahn. *The Gerontologist, 42*(6), 727–733.

Stewart, A. L., Greenfield, S., Hays, R. D., Wells, K., Rogers, W. H., & Berry, S. D., McGlynn, E. A., Ware, & J. E., Jr. (1989, August 18). Functional status and well-being of patients with chronic conditions. Results from the Medical Outcomes Study. *JAMA, 262*(7), 907–913.

Stuck, A. E. (2001). Management of polypharmacy in community-dwelling older persons. Very Old Patient Centered Medicine: Assessment and management of geriatric syndromes. http://www.healthandage.com/html/min/eama/eama4/publi/

Stuck, A. E., Aronow, H. U., Steiner, A., Alessi, C. A., Bula, C. J., Gold, M. N., Yuhas, K. E., Nisenbaum, R., Rubenstein, L. Z., & Beck, J. C. (1995). A trial of annual in-home comprehensive geriatric assessments for elderly people living in the community. *New Engl J Med, 333,* 1184–1189.

Stuck, A. E., Beers, M. H., Steine, A., Aronow, H. U., Rubenstein, L. Z., & Beck, J. C. (1994). Inappropriate medication use in community-resident older persons. *Arch Intern Med, 154,* 2195–2200.

Stuck, A. E., Siu, A. L., Wieland, G. D., & Rubenstein, L. Z. (1993). Comprehensive geriatric assessment: A meta-analysis of controlled trials. *Lancet, 342,* 1032–1036, 1993.

Stuck, A. E., Walthert, J. M., Nikolaus, T., Bula, C. J., Hohmann, C., & Beck, J. C. (1999). Risk factors for functional status decline in community-living elderly people: a systematic literature review. *Social Science and Medicine, 48,* 445–469.

Sullivan, D. F. (1966). Conceptual Problem in Developing an Index of Health. Vital and Health Statistics, Data Evaluation and Methods Research. *National Center for Health Statistics, 2*(16), 1–18.

Sullivan, D. F. (1971). A single index of mortality and morbidity. *HSMHA Health Reports, 86*(4), 347–354.

Surgeon General's Report on Mental Health. (1999). http://www.surgeongeneral.gov/library/mentalhealth/home.html

Susser, M. (1997). Steps toward discovering causes: Divergence and convergence of epidemiology and clinical medicine. *Epidemiol Prev, 21*(3), 160–168.

Symonds, T., Berzon, R., Marquis, P., Rummans TA; Clinical Significance Consensus Meeting Group. (2002). The clinical significance of quality-of-life results: practical considerations for specific audiences. *Mayo Clin Proc, 77*(6), 572–583.

Tabert, M. H., Albert, S. M., Borukhova-Milov, L., Camacho, Y., Pelton, G., Liu, X., Stern, Y., & Devanand, D. P. (2002). Informant-versus self-reported functional deficits in patients with mild cognitive impairment predict Alzheimer's disease at follow-up. *Neurology, 58*(5): 758–764.

Talbot, C., Lendon, C., Craddock, N., Shears, S., Morris, J. C., & Goate, A. (1994). Protection against Alzheimer's disease with apoe e2. *Lancet, 343,* 1432–1433.

Tang, M.-X., Cross, P., Andrews, H., Jacobs, D., Small, S., Bell, K., Merchant, C., Lantigua, R., Costa, R., Stern, Y., & Mayeux, R. (2001). Incidence of AD in African-Americans, Carribean Hispanics, and Caucasians in northern Manhattan. *Neurology, 56,* 49–56.

Tang, M.-X., Jacobs, D., Stern, Y., Marder, K., Schofield, P., Gurland, B., Andrews, H., & Mayeux R. (1996). Effect of oestrogen during menopause on risk and age at onset of Alzheimer's disease. *Lancet, 348*(9025), 429–432.

Tang, M.-X., Stern, Y., Marder, K., Bell, K., Gurland, B., Lantigua, R., Andrews, H., Feng, L., Tycko, B., & Mayeux R. (????). The APOE-ε4 allele and the risk of Alzheimer disease among African-Americans, whites, and Hispanics. *JAMA, 279,* 751–755.

Tattersall, R. (2002). The expert patient: A new approach to chronic disease management for the twenty-first century. *Clinical Med, 2*(3), 227–229.

Teresi, J. A., Holmes, D., Ramirez, M., & Kong J. (1998). Staffing patterns, staff support, and training in special care and nonspecial care units. *J Mental Health Aging, 4*(4), 443–458.

Testa, M. A., & Simonson, D. C. (1996). Assessment of Quality-of-Life Outcomes. *New Engl J Med, 334*(13), 835–840.

Tierney, M. C., Szalai, J. P., Snow, W. G., Fisher, R. H., Nores, A., Nadon, G., et al. (1996). Prediction of probable Alzheimer's disease in memory-impaired patients: A prospective longitudinal study. *Neurology, 46,* 661–665.

Tinetti, M. E., Baker, D. I., McAvay, G., Claus, E. B., Garrett, P., Gottschalk, M., Koch, M. L., Trainor, K., & Horwitz, R. I. (1994). A multifactorial intervention to reduce the risk of falling among elderly people living in the community. *New Engl J Med, 331,* 821–827.

Tinetti, M. E., Inouye, S. K., Gill, T. M., et al. (1995). Shared risk factors for falls, incontinence, and functional dependence—Unifying the approach to geriatric syndromes. *JAMA, 273,* 1348–1353.

Tinetti, M. E., McAvay, G., & Claus E. (1996). Does multiple risk factor reduction explain the reduction in fall rate in the Yale FICSIT trial? *Am J Epidemiol, 144,* 389–399.

Tinetti, M. E., Speechley, M., Ginter, S. F. (1988). Risk factors for falls among elderly persons living in the community. *New Engl J Med, 319,* 1701–1707.

Torrance, G. W. (1987). Utility approach to measuring health-related quality of life. *J Chronic Dis, 40*(6), 593–603.

Touchon, J., & Ritchie, K. (1999). Prodromal cognitive disorder in Alzheimer's disease. *International J Geriatric Psychiatry, 14,* 556–563.

Trinh, N.-H., Hoblyn, J., Mohanty, S., & Yaffe K. (2003). Efficacy of cholinesterase inhibitors in the treatment of neuropsychiatric symptoms and functional impairment in Alzheimer's disease. *JAMA, 289,* 210–216.

United States General Accounting Office. (1998, January). *Report to the Secretary of Health and Human Services: Alzheimer's Disease, Estimates of Prevalence in the United States.*

Unutzer, J., Patrick, D. L., Marmon, T., Simon, G. E., Katon, W. J. (2002). Depressive symptoms and mortality in a prospective study of 2,558 older adults. *Am J Geriatr Psychiatry, 10*(5), 521–530.

U.S. Census Bureau, International Data Base. (2002). http://www.census.gov/ipc/www/idbnew.html

U.S. Task Force Preventive Health Services. (2002). *Guide to clinical preventative services.* http://odphp.osophs.dhhs.gov/pubs/guidecps/

van der Steen, J. T., Ooms, M. E., van der Wal, G., Ribbe, M. W. (2002, October). Pneumonia: the demented patient's best friend? Discomfort after starting or withholding antibiotic treatment. *J Am Geriatr Soc, 50*(10), 1681–1688.

van Duijn, C. M., de Knijff, P., Wehnert, A., De Voecht, J., Bronzova, J. B., Havekes, L. M., et al. (1995). The apolipoprotein E epsilon-2 allele is associated with an increased risk of early-onset Alzheimer's disease and a reduced survival. *Ann. Neurol, 37,* 605–610.

Van Haitsma, K., Lawton, M. P., & Kleban, M. H. (2000). Does segregation help or hinder? Examining the role of homogeneity in behavioral and emotional aspects of quality of life in persons with cognitive impairment in the nursing home. In D. Holmes, J. A. Teresi, M. G. Ory (Eds.), *Special care units* (pp. 163–178). Paris: Serdi; New York: Springer.

Vaupel, J. W. (1997, December 29). The remarkable improvements in survival at older ages. *Philos Trans R Soc Lond B Biol Sci, 352*(1363), 1799–1804.

Verbrugge, L. M., & Jette, A. M. The disablement process. *Soc Sci Med. 38,* 1–14.

Verbrugge, L. M., & Patrick, D. L. (1995). Seven chronic conditions: Their impact on US adults' activity levels and use of medical services. *Am J Public Health, 85,* 173–182.

Verbrugge, L. M., & Sevak, P. (2002, November). Use, type, and efficacy of assistance for disability. *J Gerontol B Psychol Sci Soc Sci, 57*(6), S366–S379.

Visser, M., Kritchevsky, S. B., Goodpaster, B. H., Newman, A. B., Nevitt, M., Stamm, E., & Harris, T. B. (2002). Leg muscle mass and composition in relation to lower extremity performance in men and women aged 70 to 79: The Health, Aging, and Body Composition Study. *J Am Geriatr Soc 50,* 897–904.

Visser, M., Pahor, M., Taafe, D. R., Goodpaster, B. H., Stimonsick, E. M., Newman, A. B., et al. (2002). Relationship of interleukin-6 and tumor necrosis factor-(alpha) with muscle mass and muscle strength in elderly men and women: The Health ABC Study. *J Gerontol, 57A,* M326–M332.

Wagner, E. H., LaCroix, A. Z., Grothaus, L., Leveille, S. G., Hecht, J. A., Artz, K., Odle, K., & Buchner, D. M. (1994). Preventing disability and falls in older adults: A randomized trial. *Am J Public Health, 84,* 1800–1806.

Waidmann, T. A., & Liu, K. (2000, September). Disability trends among elderly persons and implications for the future. *J Gerontol B Psychol Sci Soc Sci, 55*(5), S298–S307.

Wallace, R. B. (1997). Variability in disease manifestations in older adults: Implications for public and community health programs. In T. Hickey, M. A. Spears, T. R. Prahaska (Eds.), *Public health and aging* (pp. 75–86). Baltimore: Johns Hopkins University Press.

Ware, J. E., & Stewart, A. L. (1992). *Measuring Function and Well-Being.* Cambridge, MA: Harvard University Press.

Wechsler, D. (1981). *Wechsler adult intelligence scale-revised.* New York: The Psychological Corporation.

Weinberger, M., Murray, M. D., Marrero, D. G., Brewer, N., Lykens, M., Harris, L. E., Seshadri, R., Caffrey, H., Roesner, J. F., Smith, F., Newell, A. J., Collins, J. C., McDonald, C. J., & Tierney, W. M. (2002). Effectiveness of pharmacist care for patients with reactive airways disease: a randomized controlled trial. *JAMA, 288*(13), 1594–1602.

Weinberger, M., Oddone, E. Z., & Henderson, W. G. (1996, May 30). Does increased access to primary care reduce hospital readmissions? Veterans Affairs Cooperative Study Group on Primary Care and Hospital Readmission. *N Engl J Med, 334*(22), 1441–1447.

Weiner, J. M., Hanley, R. J., Clark, R., & Van Nostrand, J. F. (1990). Measuring the activities of daily living: Comparisons across national surveys. *J Geront 45*(6), S229–S237.

Weissert, W., Chernew, M., & Hirth R. (2003, February). Titrating versus targeting home care services to frail elderly clients: An application of agency theory and cost-benefit analysis to home care policy. *J Aging Health, 15*(1), 99–123.

Wells, K. B., Stewart, A., Hays, R. D., Burnam, M. A., Rogers, W., Daniels, M., Berry, S., Greenfield, S., & Ware J. (1989, August 18). The functioning and well-being of depressed patients. Results from the Medical Outcomes Study. *JAMA, 262*(7), 914–919.

West, C. G., Reed, D. M., & Gildengorin, G. L. (1998). Can money buy happiness? Depressive symptoms in an affluent older population. *Journal of the American Geriatrics Society 46*(1), 49–57.

Whalley, L. J., Starr, J. M., Athawes, R., Hunter, D., Pattie, A., & Deary, I. J. (2000). Childhood mental ability and dementia. *Neurology 55,* 1455–1459.

Willcox, S. M., Himmelstein, D. U., & Woolhandler, S. (1994). Inappropriate drug prescribing in the community-dwelling elderly. *JAMA, 272,* 292–296.

Wilmoth, J. R., & Horiuchi, S. (1999). Rectangularization revisited: Variability of age at death within human populations. *Demography 36*(4), 475–495.

Wilson, R. S., Beckett, L. A., Bienas, J. L., Evans, D. A., & Bennet, D. A. (2003, in press). Terminal drop in cognitive function. *Neurology, ??.*

Wolfson, C., Wolfson, D. B., Asgharian, M., M'Lan, C. E., Ostbye, T., Rockwood, K., and Hogan, D. B. (2001, April 12). Clinical Progression of Dementia Study Group. A reevaluation of the duration of survival after the onset of dementia. *N Engl J Med, 344*(15), 1111–1116.

World Bank. (1995). The disability-adjusted life year (DALY) definition, measurement, and potential use. Human Capital Development and Operations Policy, HCO Working Papers. www.worldbank.org/html.

World Health Organization. (1981). Development of Indicators for monitoring progress towards health for all by the year 2000. (Health for All, Series 4). Geneva, WHO.

World Health Organization. (1981). *International classification of impairment, disability, and handicap.* Geneva: WHO.

World Health Organization. (2001). *International Classification of Functioning, Disability and Health.* Geneva: WHO.

Yaffe, K., Blackwell, T., Gore, R., Sands, L., Reus, V., & Browner, W. S. (1999). Depressive symptoms and cognitive decline in nondemented elderly women: a prospective study. *Arch Gen Psychiatry, 56*(5), 425–430.

Yaffe, K., Browner, W., Cauley, J., Launer, L., & Harris, T. (1999, October). Association between bone mineral density and cognitive decline in older women. *J Am Geriatr Soc, 47*(10), 1176–1182.

Yesavage, J. A., Brink, T. L., Rose, T. L., Lum, O., Huang, V., Adey, M. B., & Leirer, V. O. (1983). Development and validation of a geriatric depression screening scale: A preliminary report. *Journal of Psychiatric Research 17,* 37–49.

Index

275